What Animals Want

LARRY CARBONE

What Animals Want

Expertise and advocacy in
laboratory animal welfare policy

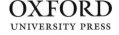

OXFORD
UNIVERSITY PRESS

2004

OXFORD
UNIVERSITY PRESS

Oxford   New York
Auckland   Bangkok   Buenos Aires   Cape Town   Chennai
Dar es Salaam   Delhi   Hong Kong   Istanbul   Karachi   Kolkata
Kuala Lumpur   Madrid   Melbourne   Mexico City   Mumbai   Nairobi
São Paulo   Shanghai   Taipei   Tokyo   Toronto

Library of Congress Cataloging-in-Publication Data
Carbone, Larry.
What animals want : expertise and advocacy in laboratory
animal welfare policy / Larry Carbone.
p.   cm.
Includes bibliographical references and index.
ISBN 0-19-516196-3
1. Animal experimentation. 2. Laboratory animals.
3. Animal welfare.   I. Title.
HV4915.C37 2004
179'4 —dc22   2003058032

9 8 7 6 5 4 3 2 1

Printed in the United States of America
on acid-free paper

For David

Acknowledgments

I COULD NEVER GET ENOUGH OF ANIMALS AS A CHILD; MY CAREER IN VETERINARY medicine was inevitable. But neither my love for animals nor my veterinary training prepared me for the conflicting feelings that life in an animal laboratory would bring; those conflicts led me to write this book.

A first book is a time to thank everyone who has brought the author to the point of publication. Older first-time authors and those who have needed the most help are challenged to highlight a few dozen from the cast of thousands.

My parents encouraged my animal mania, despite the parade of strange animals that it brought into their house. Mentors and coworkers over the years helped me develop my knowledge and skills. Five stand out for pushing me to put that fascination with animals into a moral context of human responsibility. For this, I thank Fred Quimby, Richard Farinato, Katherine O'Rourke, Jerry Shing, and, especially, Barbara Lok. They lectured me more than I was comfortable with when I slacked, but mostly, they stand out more for the roles they modeled than for the words they spoke.

Two people's illness and death brought pain and sadness to my years of writing. My father, John Carbone, died of Alzheimer's disease at the start of this project, while my friend Joe DelPonte passed away midway through. They gave me love through the years, while their illnesses taught me that, no, I cannot call for an abolition to animal research, no matter my oath as a veterinarian to relieve animal suffering.

Several people read drafts of various chapters or provided historical and photographic resources, trusting me to do right by what they offered. For their assistance, some of it stretching out a decade or more, I thank Douglas Allchin, Tim Allen, Donna Artuso, Marc Bekoff, Gary Block, Nathan Brewer, Clive Coward, Mary Dallman, Jerry Depoyster, Katie Eckert, John Gluck, Steve Hilgartner, Katherine Houpt, Sheila Jasanoff, Mike Kreger, Hugh LaFollette, Hal Herzog, Christina Johnson, Susi D. Jones, Erin Kalagassy, Ron Kline, Monica Lawlor, Cathy Liss, Joy Mench, Adrian Morrison, David Morton, Anne Neill, Barbara Orlans, Trevor Pinch, Will Provine, Fred Quimby, Christopher Read, Viktor Reinhardt, and Martin Stephens, as well as the staffs of the Animal Welfare Information Center, the Animal Welfare Institute, the Institute for Laboratory Animal Resources, the Foundation for Biomedical Research, and the Animal and Plant Health Inspection Service. I especially thank my quartet of unofficial academic advisers—Arnie Arluke, Bernie Rollin, Jerry Tannenbaum, and Andrew Rowan—and my Oxford University Press editors, Kirk Jensen, Anne Rockwood, Heather Hartman, and Karla Pace.

My hosts in disparate places allowed me to stretch limited research dollars through their hospitality. Thus I thank Eva, Ned, and Emily Butler, Richard and Ari Entlich, Ilene Gaffin, Susi D. Jones, the late Richard LaFarge, the Mogan/King family, Anita Piccolie, Pat Roos, and Jae Wise. Robert Nagell took me in on several occasions during my travels, while Rod Hudson gave me free rein in his home during my several months of work in our nation's capital: may anyone who reads this open their homes generously to them on my behalf. Those research dollars, by the way, came from a National Science Foundation Ethics and Values Studies dissertation improvement grant (SBR-9411547), from an NSF Research and Training Grant through Cornell's Science and Technology Studies program, and from my Fellowship in Animal Welfare from the William and Charlotte Parks Foundation.

I thank the dozens of people who consented to grant me interviews, though they remain anonymous in this work. My interviews were invaluable sources of information, and they gave me a chance to meet the leaders in the fields of animal research and animal protection, as well as confirmation that good people can disagree profoundly on matters of moral import.

For the early years of this project I shared my life and home with Jerry Shing, Freddie, Vito, and Nicholas. Jerry is a gentle, intelligent man and an awesome veterinarian. Freddie and Nicholas gave me perspective whenever I read scientists' studies of what dogs want; both always seemed to know what two dogs in particular wanted, and never skimped on their efforts to enlighten. Vito was my poster boy for life after the laboratory, a laboratory-cat adoption success story.

I could not have written this book without the *constant* assistance, vision, and love of my partner, editor, teacher, traveling companion, fan, muse, font of knowledge, adviser, running coach, and best friend, David Takacs. David has kept me on task and kept me laughing, and he has read far more drafts of my work than anyone should ever have to. I really do not know how to thank him enough for what he has brought into my life.

Contents

What Animals Want

Introduction: What animals want

I TELL PEOPLE I MEET THAT I AM A VETERINARIAN AND THEIR FACES LIGHT UP. PEOPLE feel good about veterinarians and so I listen to stories about their pets' ailments or antics, or about how they, too, always wanted to be a veterinarian. It's a nice feeling; in a 1999 Gallup survey, veterinarians were rated the third most trusted profession, right behind nurses and pharmacists, just ahead of physicians (Gallup Poll 1999).

Folks who know a bit about veterinary practice invariably ask, "Small or large animal?" The fact is that I work with animals great and small—some very small, actually—but not with anybody's pets. I work with scientists' laboratory animals— their mice and frogs and monkeys and dogs and sheep. Smiles of recognition of who vets are and what vets do invariably give way to something more serious when I explain my field of practice. People feel discomfort at having to think beyond the happy stereotype. They must stop and think seriously, for however briefly, about how we use animals and how we treat animals in our society. The responses I elicit to my unusual line of work are what brought me to this write this book.

People with no connection to animal research must somehow reconcile the person before them—nice guy, doesn't eat meat, smiles at stories about their pets— with whatever images the mention of animal research conjures. "Is it painful for the animals?" "Is it really necessary?" "Are the scientists cruel to them?" Some people want to know more, to get some actual feel for how good people can do bad things to animals in the pursuit of medical progress. Others prefer to have their heroes and villains neatly delineated. "Good thing you're in there on the animals' side," they'll say to me as they look me in the eye with understanding and encouragement, though they barely have a clue of who I am or what I do, or that I think of myself as also being on the scientists' side. They might say, "So you keep them healthy until the scientists can make them sick." And yes, that's part of it.

Animal activists protest outside our doors. They may never have visited a laboratory, but they are sure that what happens inside must be stopped (figure 1.1). In the coming chapters I present something of a behind-the-scenes look at animal research. I am not writing about whether animals should be in laboratories or whether people have a right to use them in experiments. Rather, I start with the reality that I experience on the job: animals *are* in laboratories, and they are going to be there for many years to come. My goal here is to understand efforts over the past

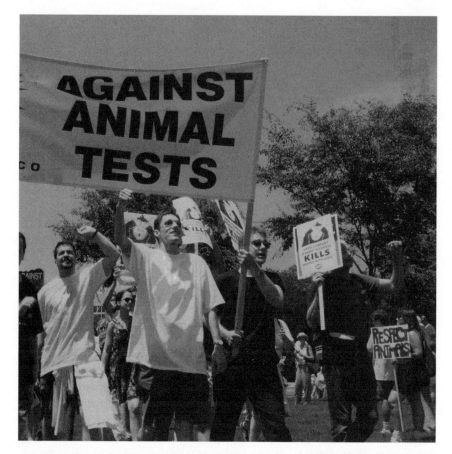

Fig. 1.1 Animal rights protesters. PHOTO COURTESY OF HAL HERZOG.

few decades to establish and maintain standards of animal welfare for those animals, in pursuit of improved lives for future animals.

This book is about the people who would speak for animals in laboratories, by which I mean two things. On the one hand, people vie to speak on animals' behalf in the policy arena, to advocate for them in a forum in which they have no direct voice. Animal protectionists are immediately obvious in this role, but so are veterinarians, other animal care professionals, and many scientists. On the other hand, speaking for animals means interpreting them, translating their animal minds into human language; it's a claim of expertise and knowledge rather than commitment and advocacy. But the two are intimately intertwined, and many of the policy debates that I examine are about these two ways of speaking for animals. Appointing themselves to speak as animals' champions, animal protectionists base their case for larger cages, oversight committees, and exercise programs on their ability to speak for animals, to know what matters to them. Similarly claiming a deep commitment to animal welfare, research advocates could call for very different policies, though based again on their own claims to be able to speak, expertly and authoritatively, for animals.

This book is written for people who want to know more about animal research. Some may grant its validity, want science and medicine to progress, but also want to be sure that animal suffering is minimal. I offer this book to those people like myself, who are hoping for some sort of balance that promotes animal welfare *and* biomedical progress, not platitudes or irrelevant rules with no real impact in the animals' lives.

I am writing as well for the people at the two poles in the animal research debates. To those who think that laboratory animals live a life of constant pain in meaningless experiments, and those who counter that all is well with the animals and any regulation unreasonable, I offer some history that should make them think differently. The debates over the past two decades have been simultaneously too personal and too impersonal. Caricatures of animal rights activists as violent, deluded misanthropes, or of scientists as cruel-hearted technocrats, distort the picture. Us-versus-them rhetorics serve only to inflame the issue and thwart the potential for incremental improvements in animal welfare.[1] On the other hand, philosophical writers similarly have focused on sharp dichotomies between liberationist philosophies that would ban animal research entirely and human-centered approaches that could leave animals without protections. Both miss the texture of daily life in the laboratory, the competing urges at both the individual and institutional levels to take responsible care of animals without paralyzing scientific progress.

I came to my work on this book much as I started my clinical work in laboratory animal medicine, convinced that though most of the scientists I know are decent, bright, caring people, they can lose their focus on animal welfare as they perform their experiments, or sometimes just don't know enough about animals to assure their welfare. I have had high expectations of the potential of laboratory animal veterinarians, more than anyone else, to blend expertise and advocacy on animals' behalf. At times, I have been frustrated and disillusioned at my own and other veterinarians' limitations—of commitment, of information, of authority—to be strong and effective advocates for animals. This book is my attempt to find the reasons for those limitations and to offer some ways to transcend them.

The book is rooted in a period from the late 1960s to the present during which a great deal of writing, talking, protest, study, and legislation was devoted to animals in general and to laboratory animals in particular. My concerns are not restricted just to animals in laboratories, but to animals in zoos, on the farm, in shelters, and in homes as well. Convinced that what we do about animals—the policies we adopt, the ways we treat them—has everything to do with what we think we know about them, my goal in this book is to examine closely some of those varied things that people claim to know about animals and how they claim to know them. Two features set this book apart from other books on animal welfare. One is the sociological approach I bring to examining these knowledge claims. The other is the inclusion of my own experiences and observations as a veterinarian in animal research. My hope is to change the ways that people who vie to shape animal use policies—whether animal protectionists, research advocates, veterinarians, or others—talk about animal welfare. I want to bring a more nuanced and balanced view than I have generally encountered of the animals whose pain and suffering we exploit in the quest to alleviate our own. I call for a multiplicity of voices—impassioned, empathetic, scientific, experiential—that will more fully capture the complex reality of animals' lives. I do this because I hope to change our practices and encourage efforts to give the animals in our laboratories the richest lives they can possibly have.

These are the major points that I hope to argue convincingly: that science is but one of several legitimate ways of knowing about animals; that veterinarians can and should be advocates for animals; that political, social, professional, and philosophical factors shape this advocacy potential and must be reckoned with; that these same human factors profoundly shape what we think we know about animals and what matters to them; and that animal welfare is bigger and more complicated than simply keeping animals fed, free of infections, free of pain, and free of pathology—something best described with words like "fun," "happy," "fulfilled," and "thriving."

Social theory and animal welfare science

What sets animal welfare policy studies apart from most other policy studies is that animals have no direct voice.[2] They enter policy dialogues only through those people who would speak for them. Though my initial training is in veterinary medicine, I have found it vitally important to study people as well as animals, particularly those people who would speak for animals.

Recent years have seen several sociological studies of animal rights activists and of the animal research controversy (Birke and Michael 1995; Groves 1997; Herzog 1993; Jamison and Lunch 1992; Jasper and Nelkin 1992; Matfield 1995; Michael and Birke 1994; Sperling 1988). Sociologists have ventured into animal laboratories to study the people who study the animals. Mary Phillips (1993) observed how laboratory workers deal with animal pain; she found them defining it so narrowly as to convince themselves and others that it is a rarity in research, thus making use of painkilling analgesics equally rare. Arnold Arluke (1994) studied the ethical socialization of animal researchers and has been struck by how new workers in animal laboratories quickly learn to stop asking questions about the justification of the work and adapt to the prevailing ethos. Julian McAllister Groves (1997) attended antivivisectionists' meetings and laboratory animal veterinarian's staff meetings to compare activists' and workers' perceptions of laboratory animal welfare. Michael Lynch (1988) observed animal use in neuroscience laboratories and described the scientist's transformation of the "naturalistic" animal in the cage into the "analytic" animal of data and electron micrographs, through the metaphor of sacrifice. Beyond this, ethnographic studies and participant observations of people in animal laboratories have been rare.

To this body of work I contribute a new dimension: my focus on the knowledge claims that people bring to the animal welfare policy arena. What are the facts about animals that should influence policy? Let's start by asking what count as scientific facts in the first place. I view knowledge, expertise, and even facts as rhetorical tools that must be carefully constructed if they are to be wielded by opposing parties in political settings. In this close examination of knowledge and expertise in the policy setting, I align my work with Steven Epstein's (1996) study of AIDS activism, David Takacs's (1996) examination of conservation biologists, Steven Yearley's (1991) look at environmental movements, and Sheila Jasanoff's (1990) analysis of environmental regulation, all four of which have influenced my thinking. By the company it keeps and the questions it asks, my work is situated in the academic discipline of science studies, also known by its practitioners as science and technology studies.

Science studies is an interdisciplinary blend of sociology, philosophy, history, and policy analysis. It is characterized by its focus on science and scientific ways of knowing as aspects of human culture, rather than as something separate and transcendent. Much of science studies has a constructivist approach to knowledge, whereas most current work in animal welfare studies takes a more realist approach.[3] Animal welfare studies could benefit from some of the constructivist's insights, much as those insights challenge a scientist's usual beliefs about science.

I summarize the difference between constructivists and realists in quantitative terms: the relative weight each gives the "real world" versus social factors in deciding what to accept as fact. A realist position is that if you can minimize social and personal values and biases to their absolute minimum, what will emerge as scientific facts are those things that really are more true than available alternatives. That is, nature determines which theories, interpretations, or fact claims will survive, while scientists' human sides (biases, theoretical commitments, funding issues, subjective opinions, personal rivalries, rhetorical practices) are the noise in the system that can be tamed through careful technique, anonymous peer review, replications of crucial experiments, and objective methodologies.

Constructivists and relativists, in contrast, assign nature a smaller role in all of this (with the more radical theorists allowing nature virtually no role) and focus instead on the active construction of facts as an intensely human activity.[4] What we know we know only through a human lens that is inescapably dependent on context, ideology, politics, theory, and social interactions. It's not that nature's reality has no role in this (no one, for instance, would posit a theory of gravity that had objects flinging away from the earth instead of toward it) but that there is typically enough room for flexible interpretations consistent with the available data to allow all sorts of social, rhetorical, and political factors to decide which theory or facts will persist.

I focus heavily in my case studies on scientific facts, not as neutral, objective statements about animals or the world, but as social constructions. It's the subtle difference between a fact being a bit of nature's reality versus being a statement about natural reality, the difference from being in nature versus being about nature. From this perspective, facts exist on a continuum with opinions and hunches and proposals and hypotheses, and they ascend to the status of fact only when the relevant stakeholders are convinced and agree. Truth is "whatever we all agree on, or whatever becomes too difficult or too expensive to contravene" (Takacs 1996, p. 117). I follow Takacs (1996) and Rudwick (1985) in believing that scientific knowledge is not entirely about either the construction or the discovery of truth, but that it is shaped by the interaction of the observer and the observed. Takacs writes:

> Constructivist sociologists of science have convincingly shown that theory shapes even apparently neutral observation, that culture constrains framing of questions, appropriate attitudes, likelihood of accepting or rejecting facts, what counts as reasonable evidence. . . . Yet, at the same time, nature intransigently insists on challenging our portraits of it. . . . Using a core of natural reality, scientists mold verifiable knowledge. (Takacs 1996, p. 117)

From this perspective, objectivity is both a myth and an ideal, but it is also a political tool, usually used by power holders within the scientific establishment to bolster their own interpretations and silence dissenters (Martin and Richards 1995). Thus, it is important to look not just at how claims are worked into facts, but at which parties in controversies are advancing which facts. How might veterinarians' facts differ from those of animal protectionists, from scientists, from your own?

My suspicion that much could be learned from examining the pivotal role of laboratory animal veterinarians in animal welfare debates led me to the work of the social historian Andrew Abbott. Abbott (1988) theorizes that understanding a professional group's history and development requires looking contextually at competition among professionals for jurisdiction over particular tasks.[5] Laboratory animal veterinarians have actively shaped their professional identity (with all the standard trappings of a full-fledged profession, including training and certification programs, their own journals, and codes of conduct) from the post–World War II era on, securing jurisdictional control over the tasks, initially, of laboratory animal care, and later on, of laboratory animal use. One part of this professionalization has involved issues of advocacy, as veterinarians have chosen whether to identify themselves as champions of animal welfare, as defenders of unrestricted freedom of scientific inquiry, or, most often, as standard bearers for an ideology that there is no conflict between animal welfare and scientific progress. The other aspect of the professionalization of laboratory animal veterinarians has required constructing an expertise that was uniquely their own, at once more generalized and applied than that of the specialized scientists whose animals they cared for, yet more technical and scientific than that of the animal protectionists.

Throughout the 1980s, many research advocates and laboratory animal veterinarians called for regulations that were "science-based" and "objective," distancing themselves and their expertise from what they saw as anthropomorphism by animal protectionists. Thus they used their expert scientific knowledge as a way to draw the boundaries of their profession. But drawing science-based boundaries around a profession requires some attention to the boundaries of what counts as science.[6]

How do you define science? By its content, the subject of its examinations? By its methods? By its underlying epistemological assumptions? By who does it? Among all the calls for science-based regulations, in all the disputes over who had the better animal welfare science with which to build a better Animal Welfare Act, I find nothing in the record to indicate that anyone has ever seen a need to clarify what they mean by "science." Thomas Gieryn (1995) has argued that the borders of science are imprecise and open to social and political negotiation, and I would add that they are particularly imprecise in dealing with questions of consciousness, experience, feelings, ethics, and animal minds—all the subjects most central to animal welfare policy. The use of science to close the decades-old controversy over what exercise provisions to mandate for caged dogs illustrates this point about science and its boundaries and underscores its importance.

Claims about canine needs and preferences were prevalent in discussions of dog exercise regulations in the 1980s. Reports of dog behavior abound. Suppose we want to restrict ourselves to the scientific ones—which ones are they? Elizabeth Marshall Thomas (1993) took to her bicycle and closely observed a few dogs roaming the streets of Cambridge, Massachusetts. Her observations of these individuals, and the implications she drew for dogs in general, were published in her bestseller *The Hidden Life of Dogs*. Around the same time, Howard Hughes, Sarah Campbell, and Cheryl Kenney (1989) set video cameras on six laboratory beagles who "traveled" more in small cages than in larger ones. Their observations of these individuals, and the implications they drew for dogs in general, were published in the journal *Laboratory Animal Science* and became one of the few articles that the U.S. Department of Agriculture (USDA) directly cited in writing its Animal Welfare Act regulations.

Now, what makes Thomas's work anecdote and Hughes's science? The subject of investigation, what dogs choose to do when left to their own devices, is precisely the same in both studies. The tools are different—bicycle and the naked eye versus computer-based videography—but the basic methodology (observation of dog behavior) seems about the same. What would it mean to label, and dismiss, Thomas's work as nonscience: does it mean that she didn't really follow the dogs she claims to have followed, or see the behaviors that she describes? Is it something to do with how reliably we can generalize from her observations to dogs as a whole? If science tells us things about dogs that her observations of this dog do not match, are her observations invalid (too particular, individual, unscientific, or just plain wrong)? Or is it simply that she is an author writing in a popular medium while Hughes is a scientist (if we veterinarians count as scientists) writing in an academic peer-reviewed journal?

The point is not trivial. For the USDA to privilege Hughes's study of caged dogs over Thomas's study of roaming dogs as the scientific basis for dog exercise laws, someone must place the former comfortably within the boundaries of science and exclude the latter.

Scientists evaluate not just the quality of scientific work, but the boundaries of what shall count as scientific work. Philosophers also engage in boundary work even when they tacitly leave scientists' information about animals unchallenged and focus instead on ethical issues as a separate entity. Many of the scientist/veterinarians whose work I examine are trying to do the same thing for themselves, presenting their findings as objective so that no one will challenge the inherent values and biases that they bring to their work, so that their assessments of animal welfare issues will carry more weight than those of people whom they exclude as unscientific or nonobjective. This is not some Machiavellian plot hatched in secret collusion between philosophers and scientists. Those of us in the animal welfare business desperately want the guidance that philosophy might hold and the information that science could yield. How much cleaner it all might be if philosophers could rely on scientists' data as the simple uncomplicated truth upon which to build their ethical pronouncements. Keeping the boundaries clear allows both scientists and philosophers to proceed with their contributions to animal welfare policy.

Still, people keep tinkering with the science/ethics boundary. The philosopher Bernard Rollin challenges it, though at heart he too, like most scientists, is a realist. Rollin believes that if we can tame the noise in the system, the biases and ideologies that distort scientists' view of the world, then the right studies will allow nature to tell us what is really true about animals. His spin is that although he is just a philosopher, as an intelligent and informed outsider, he can give scientists guidance to making better science that tells us more real things about animal welfare. In *The Unheeded Cry,* Rollin (1989) describes the ideological biases that led behaviorists to discount animals' feelings and the motives in their explanations of animal behavior, and the implications this view could have for animal welfare practices. He does not note, however, how the ethology with which he would replace behaviorism also carries its own biases and limitations. Ethology is not just different science, as Rollin promotes it; it is better science.[7]

Like Rollin, I want to challenge the sanctity of claims about animals and their subjective feelings, and I do not believe that the label "scientific" legitimates that sanctity. Where Rollin looks at behaviorists' discussions of animal mind, I examine some other animal studies, such as inquiries into dog exercise, rodent caging, methods of killing animals. In the process, Rollin and I are doing what the sociologist of science Bruno Latour calls "opening the black box" (Latour and Woolgar 1979). Latour argues that scientists create black boxes around bodies of knowledge, separating the information therein from the social and historical circumstances of its creation (Latour and Woolgar 1979). Epstein (1996) describes the progression, from a scientists' observation, as it is labeled "discovery," advanced as a "claim," then accepted by others as "fact," and finally, as "common knowledge" (too obvious to even merit a footnote) (p. 28). Information that has been securely established as fact or common knowledge appears divorced from the human hands that shaped it; it is black-boxed and need not be reexamined in the process of building on it. Epstein writes:

> Fact-making—the process of closing a black box—is successful when contingency is forgotten, controversy is smoothed over, and uncertainty is bracketed. Before a black box has been closed, it remains possible to glimpse human actors performing various kinds of work—examining and interpreting, inventing and guessing, persuading and debating. . . . Those who want to challenge a claim that has been accepted as fact must effectively "re-open" the black box. (Epstein 1996, pp. 28–29)

Much in veterinary medicine is already securely black-boxed. No one feels a need these days, for instance, to discuss the germ theory of disease in presenting their findings on the efficacy of a new antibiotic, even though that theory was once highly controversial among medical experts. In many of the behavior and welfare cases I examine, that process of black-boxing is not so far along, and some heavy-handed practices to speed the process are evident. The most obvious of these are the attempts to scientize claims about animal welfare by incorporating various technologies (computer-based video cameras, brain-wave recorders, measurement of various stress hormones) and to bundle an amalgam of published data, ethical norms, and on-the-job experience into expert documents (such as the *Guide for the Care and Use of Laboratory Animals*; ILAR 1965–1996) written in the depersonalized voice of academic prose.

My claim is not that I have the better interpretation of whether the rodent guillotine hurts rats or how guinea pigs and dogs use cage space, but that the data support several interpretations depending on your theoretical starting point. The final policy settlements will depend on all sorts of human factors and on multiple, valid ways of knowing about animals. I offer some of my own interpretations (that the conclusions of Hughes's dog study, for example, are implausible to at least one person, myself, who has worked for many years with caged dogs) that have some value and should be considered, but which are hardly the final word on animal welfare.

If I can successfully engage you to think about facts and objectivity and value and bias in this way and to think about expertise as a social issue, rather than some objective assessment of who has the most and best knowledge, then I can create space to theorize about the political landscape of how animal welfare policy is shaped. I can discuss why some issues capture attention and others are downplayed, why some people take the stances they do, how different sorts of arguments or information are brought to bear in favor of one policy or another. My task here is to present one plausible narrative of the historical developments in animal welfare policy and a credible interpretation of why things have developed as they have, to explain why I think the way I do, and to explain why I think you should agree with my interpretation. Ultimately, I hope to broaden the range of voices and knowledges that will influence animal welfare policy, not just scientific studies (which have their utility) but also the impassioned voices of animal protectionists, the clinical perspective of veterinarians, the emotional bond between animal care-givers and the animals, the thoughtful critiques of philosophers, and scientists' own creative searches for alternatives to harmful animal experiments.

Research methodology

In this book, I describe some current trends in laboratory animal welfare policy and how they developed. To tell this multifaceted story, I weave four basic sources of information together: (1) my twenty years of training and work experience as a veterinarian; (2) a review of published literature in a variety of forums; (3) correspondence the USDA received in the late 1980s (Regulatory Analysis and Development 1986, 1987, 1989, 1990); and (4) my conversations and interviews with several dozen people involved in various ways with animal welfare policy. Let's look at each in turn.

(1) My identity and experience as a laboratory animal veterinarian are crucial to this work. They have shaped what I see as the big issues, given me some behind-the-scenes look of how policy translates into action, and convinced me that the actions of laboratory animal veterinarians are worthy of examination to explain why policy has developed as it has. To this task, I bring Abbott's (1988) theories on the sociology of professions as one lens through which to interpret the history of welfare policy and the role of veterinarians. That perspective has some obvious limitations, of course. The campuses on which I have worked may or may not be typical of other labs, and I am certainly only representative of laboratory animal veterinarians in some respects.

One strength of my perspective as a laboratory animal veterinarian relates to so-called controversy studies—situations in which scientists are still in disagreement about a particular issue—which are a frequent focus of science studies research. Controversy studies can be useful for sociologists to examine because, as Dorothy Nelkin writes, "in the course of disputes, the special interests, vital concerns, and hidden assumptions of various actors are revealed" (Nelkin 1992, p. vii). Given my scientific and technical training, I have been able to articulate some of these critiques of animal welfare studies, even for issues that have failed to bring all the contending interpretations out of the woodwork. So, for example, I am not just reporting on what others have said when I draw distinctions between thinking about the average decapitated rat's time to flat-line EEG rather than the longest individual's time to flat-line; that is a lesson I have learned through years of relating population data to my animal patients at hand (Carbone 1997c).

(2) Reviews of published literature and media make up the most publicly accessible of my four sources of data. The published materials I use are varied. I have paid very close attention to historical developments in a few key texts of animal welfare policy in America: the Animal Welfare Act and its associated regulations and the seven editions of the National Academy of Science's and the National Institutes of Health's (NIH's) *Guide for the Care and Use of Laboratory Animals* (Animal Care Panel 1963; ILAR 1965–1996). These documents provide an interesting

contrast to each other. The Animal Welfare Act is imposed upon scientific research from the outside, a congressional law heavily influenced by lobbying of animal protectionists (and by resistance of research advocates, to be sure). The *Guide*, in contrast, is almost exclusively the creation of scientists and laboratory animal veterinarians (more of the latter than the former), though clearly cognizant of the concerns of animal protectionists.[8] In addition, I bring in philosophical works in animal ethics, which have mushroomed in number over the last few decades, veterinary texts and journals, conference proceedings, and primary scientific literature.

(3) My third source of data is the rich collection of letters that the USDA received in the late 1980s during its update of Animal Welfare Act regulations. Congress had amended the 1966 act in 1985, adding provisions for animal care and use committees and requirements to consider alternatives to painful animal studies, and it authorized the USDA to set standards for exercise for caged laboratory dogs and caging environments that would promote the psychological well-being of captive monkeys and apes. It took the USDA five years and several drafts of proposed regulations before it finalized its updated rules in 1991. During that period, it counted and responded to some 36,000 comments from scientists, animal protectionists, patient and research advocacy groups, veterinarians, and others. Quotes from these letters are cited collectively by the docket under which they are filed in the USDA's Office of Regulatory Analysis and Development, where they are held for twenty years (Regulatory Analysis and Development 1986, 1987, 1989, 1990).

The first methodological decision was whether to use these data qualitatively or quantitatively, or rather, what balance of qualitative versus quantitative to strike. The large number of correspondents should have been a statistician's dream, until you look at it more closely. Too much reliance on counting would overlook the fact that this was very much a mixed bag of apples, oranges, and other fruits. Official, multi-issue letters written on university letterhead by high-level administrators in consultation with several faculty and veterinarians are counted by the USDA (once) alongside the signatures on an opinion poll circulated in Philadelphia's Rittenhouse Square on whether monkey cages should be taller than currently mandated (each signature counted as one, for a total of 7275). In between these extremes are the numerous submissions of form letters written at the behest of the Animal Welfare Institute (AWI), the National Association for Biomedical Research (NABR), and the Humane Society of the United States.

The USDA's boxes of correspondence took up approximately 30 feet of shelf space, and that bulk had to be tamed somehow. My approach was to read through everything once, taking notes as I went along, as new issues showed up and as multiple copies of form letters became apparent. I then photocopied several hundred pieces of correspondence for closer analysis, including everything written by or about veterinarians; everything written by someone I expected to interview; everything submitted by the large research advocacy and animal protection organizations; and everything else I thought was unique or illuminating.

Other reasons to favor qualitative over quantitative analysis were my interest in the range of responses more than their statistical distribution and my desire to carefully examine the subtleties of argument and rhetoric in a manageable number of representative pieces. Who decided what to consider representative? I did. Both of those considerations met my interests far more than trying to count how many people were pro or con a particular initiative, how strongly they were pro or con, and so on. What would those numbers mean? How effectively the AWI or NABR could mobilize their memberships? How strongly those issues resonate with various people? What the "typical" or the majority of laboratory animal veterinarians or antivivisectionists really believes, or believes to be persuasive? I do make roughly quantitative statements about this USDA correspondence, even as I resist getting too precise in my counting. I use words like "many" and "a few" and "rarely" in my analysis of this correspondence with no direct correlation to numbers. A few times I mention how many comments the USDA reported on a particular issue. I report the USDA's count as an indicator of what that agency perceived public opinion to be; that is, I am talking about the USDA's perceptions, not making a claim about what the public really thinks.

(4) I spent much of 1995 on the road, talking to people who had been influential in shaping animal welfare policy or the profession of laboratory animal medicine, or who for other reasons might have interesting viewpoints to share. These people were generous and open about meeting with me, with rare exceptions. Despite the polarity on animal research issues, most animal protectionists gave me the benefit of the doubt as a research insider seriously concerned with animal welfare. Establishing a rapport with a few influential leaders in the movement enabled me greater access to some of the other animal protectionists I interviewed; most seemed eager to share their side of the story. On the other hand, being a laboratory animal veterinarian at a prestigious veterinary college gave me easy access to scientists and other laboratory animal veterinarians. Even those I expected to find me a little too sympathetic to animal activists or a little too harsh on the veterinary profession spoke freely to me, often confiding their admission that much of the progress in laboratory animal care was owed to the political pressures of animal protectionists.

I chose my interviewees for the breadth of information they could provide, focusing more on meeting a select group of highly influential people than a representative cross-section of protectionists, research advocates, or veterinarians. The two questions I asked almost all the people I interviewed were: "How did you get involved in this issue?" and "Is it your belief that things have gotten better for lab animals over the years?" Beyond that, the interview was uniquely determined by the people involved, reflecting the unique reasons for which I sought the interview. The list of potential questions that would pertain to the full range of people I met with— congressional aides and laboratory animal veterinarians and animal rights-oriented veterinarians and lobbyists and behaviorists and philosophers and activists—is rather short and sparse.

I tape-recorded and transcribed more than fifty interviews (as approved by the Cornell University Human Subjects Committee) and took only written notes on about twenty-five others. Many of my conversations at work and at conferences verged on data-gathering interviews, in which case I usually informed people of the nature of my study before the conversation proceeded. Though many gave me permission to quote and identify them, others withheld permission to identify pending what I wrote. On an issue as polarized as this, it would be impossible to write something that all of them would agree with, of course. When possible, I have chosen published material over interview excerpts for inclusion here. This allows critical readers to see quoted comments in their fuller cited context and ensures that people are not quoted for words they did not deliberately write for general consumption. My interviews challenged, changed, or confirmed my thinking, and many led me to other resources to look at. However, none of my claims or conclusions in this work are based solely on interview material.

Positionality and bias

This book is about the stories people tell about animals. Every story has a narrator, whether the narration takes the form of autobiographical narrative or the formalized language of a scientific report. And every storyteller has biases of what information to look for and report, how to analyze it, how to relate it to other stories, and how to convince audiences of its truth.

In this book, I closely examine several of the scientific studies that various narrators have put forth to speak for animals and to uncover what they want in their lives. I aim to show how, though written in the objective and impersonal language of a scientific report, these narratives nevertheless are deeply imbued with their narrators' personal beliefs, theories, and ideologies. They tell us as much about the human narrator as they do the animal subjects. I look closely at the studies of dogs and exercise in which computerized video cameras are used to eliminate the bias of the human element of interpretation. The authors report that dogs in small cages "travel" more than dogs in larger enclosures, with the clear policy message that regulations to give caged dogs more exercise are not needed (Hughes et al. 1989).The authors tell their story in the language of a scientific journal article. In that tradition, they cite the work of five other authors, and use the depersonalized passive voice throughout. They work to convince us of their story's truth, but it remains very much their personal story, with their own biases of what information counts and why it is compelling. Why, for instance, is dog behavior in front of a camera more important to report than behavior with people? Is that how the dogs would see it, did the authors' computer system tell them that, or is this just the authors' assumption? The supposed objectivity of a human-programmed computer-video system begins to lose some of its rhetorical punch in the face of these questions, long before we get to asking about motives, about why a medical school or a drug company would perform such a study just as regulations are being promulgated that would get these dogs out of those little cages.

As I critique the claims to objectivity of those who would use their scientific studies and credentials to speak for animals, the light immediately shines back on me—who am I to make the claims that I do? How can I objectively assess these people's work?

My first response to concerns about objectivity and bias-free writing is to question them as ideals in the first place, as either achievable or universally desirable. What's so bad about bias, or, conversely, what's so good about objectivity? Most academic writers, whether in the sciences or the humanities, are striving to make believable claims about what they have learned about the world and to convince their reader that the conclusions they have drawn have validity. A founder of the sociology of science, Robert Merton, worried about the conspicuously biased science of Nazi Germany, in which ideology so transparently shaped the information scientists published as fact. As a guard against this, he postulated the norms of disinterestedness and communalism—the less personal or political stake a scientist has in the outcome of any given experiment, the more credible his published findings (Merton 1942). Scientists (and scholars in many fields) use the impersonal passive voice in their writing as a sign of their attempts to remove their particular interests and biases from their project at hand.[9] They pose as mere bystanders, objectively reporting nothing but the facts, dispassionately explaining what those facts mean. Nature speaks through them.

But scientists can remove themselves from their science only so much. The projects they choose, the data they collect or leave uncollected, the decision to keep or reject some outlying data point, the imaginative leap from theory to prediction to data to interpretation and back again to theory—these are the very personal, even passionate, acts in the art of doing science. They are what separates the brilliant scientists from the drones. Each passively worded scientific publication is a rhetorical appeal to other scientists, saying: "Believe me. Believe my observations and the meaning I find in them. These are the steps I took and the instruments I used to get my data; this is how I worked to remove all taint of bias (all laid out as materials and methods and statistical analyses). These are the elders (works cited) on whom my work builds; see how we stand together. See how elegantly I have reasoned to harmonize data and theory, each supporting the other."

Historical writing is not so very different from scientific writing. I, too, want my readers to find my work credible. I describe my sources: archives, interviews, published work, direct observation. I explain the theories that guide my interpretation of those materials. I cite the community of scholars whose company enhances my credibility. But really, the work I report here is no more or less objective than the scientific writing I encounter every day as a veterinarian on an academic campus. The difference is ideological: most scientists want their work to be objective and hope to approach that ideal by removing themselves from the picture; I have no faith that they or I can become so transparent.

In truth, I do not claim objectivity because subjectivity is such a strong part of the expertise and authority I claim. Our subjective, personal intimate experiences of animals are just as important as the scientific studies and, indeed, can never be wholly separated from them. Certainly I must outline as clearly as I can the biases and commitments I bring to this work and share the evidence that I believe makes my observations valid. My story is not the only explanation of how policy has developed and how it translates into practice in the animal laboratories, but I hope to convince my readers that it is nonetheless a plausible and heartfelt examination to which they should assent.

The first bias to own up to is that I am writing a practitioner's account of the field in which I have worked. What I have seen is a reflection of the places and the time in which I have worked. For eighteen years, I worked in the laboratory animal program of Cornell University, a large research campus with strong emphases in the life sciences, agriculture, and veterinary medicine. More recently, I joined the veterinary staff at University of California-San Francisco, a major medical college focused on human health and disease. I came to this laboratory animal work with a background in zoo keeping, a college degree in evolutionary biology, and a deep suspicion about anyone who would experiment on animals. By the time I entered the field, first as an animal caretaker, and eventually as a laboratory animal veterinarian, the profession of laboratory animal medicine was well established as a veterinary specialty, as were certification programs for paraprofessional laboratory animal technicians and technologists. The Animal Welfare Act was then about fifteen years old and the NIH's *Guide for the Care and Use of Laboratory Animals,* first published in 1963, was in its fifth edition. The histories I describe of the early days of professionalization and standardization therefore predate my employment in this field, and I see myself as part of a third generation of laboratory animal veterinarians in America.

My instinct as a veterinary clinician has been to keep my explorations of policy, ethics, and politics rooted in the pragmatic. I want a "rat-side" view of animal welfare policy that closely attends to what the animals in my charge are experiencing. Frequently, it has been my professional responsibility as their veterinarian to make pronouncements on their behalf. The Institutional Animal Care and Use Committee will expect me to tell them how painful a particular experimental procedure is, or what drugs will ease that pain. Animal care staff will want my decision on whether a particular animal is in ill health and must be removed from the experiment in which she is being used. It is this challenge of making daily animal welfare decisions based on my all-too-human reading of these animals that informs the story I am telling.

Work as a laboratory animal veterinarian has convinced me of the enormous potential of that profession to be the strongest possible in-house advocate for research animals, and I will not drop my conviction that this is what laboratory animal veterinarians should strive to be. They should have the best combination of institutional authority, daily contact with animals, high-level professional knowledge, clinical focus on the experiences of individual patients, and personal commitment for that role, and they should do everything in their power to minimize any conflicts with that role.

Rather than a fatal source of bias, my standpoint as a practicing laboratory animal veterinarian is my strength. My veterinary identity grounds this book's forays into philosophy, history, and sociology. It is my touchstone. So, when I hear animal protectionists' claims that research animals are routinely tortured without anesthesia, or researchers' counterclaims that animal pain is rare in the laboratory, I retain my skepticism: I have seen plenty of animal pain *and* plenty of anesthetics in use, and know, if nothing else, that these claims about animal pain and painlessness are very complicated to evaluate and substantiate. When I hear either group claim that animals want, need, choose, or act in a particular way, I check back to the animals I have known in my professional life and ask, "Is this what I have seen? Does this respect the animals and experiences of my personal and professional life?"

If the things people tell me about animals do not reflect the things I have known, then those people have some explaining to do. I am full of skepticism when I hear that dogs do not profit from having a chance to run and play, that cutting rats' heads off with no anesthesia is a harmless procedure, that an animal who struggles or screams at the surgeon's knife is only resisting restraint, is uncomfortable but not painful, is displaying a mindless reflex. That is what my lifelong work as an "animal person" brings to this project. The challenge I faced in writing every page of this book was to bring a symmetrical skepticism to claims that *do* ring true to my experience, for every feint at impartial observation is colored by my training, experiences, assumptions, values, emotions, theories, and perspectives. In short, my experiences of animals are important, but they are not the final word, and they must be read in the context of my choices to work in animal research, to enjoy the fruits of that research (whether as patient or clinician), and to claim a deep commitment to animal well-being.

No one in my profession can talk about animal research without at least some nod to what I call the "big question": Do we have a right to use animals in research at all? That basic question lurks every time we evaluate a proposal to conduct a new animal experiment, and yet laboratory animal veterinarians have a surprising ability to sidestep it. Animals *are* being used in research, right now, every day, in thousands of laboratories around the country and the world. Regardless of whether you approve or not, millions of animals are undergoing experimentation, living in laboratory cages, and a laboratory animal veterinarian has all he can do in a day to keep up with their care. Some days are fueled by the excitement of discovery, the satisfaction of contributing to science and to animal welfare; some are fueled by anger, frustration, self-righteousness, and caffeine. Most days though, the big question seems pretty irrelevant, academic, in the face of the job at hand.

But let me not be coy: I wish there were no animal research. Animals have been my professional life, and almost every day, I have seen their welfare (as I interpret it) compromised, not in the grand torture that the animal rights activists describe, but in a thousand and one smaller ways: students awkwardly handle struggling mice and rats, dogs and cats sit alone day after day in small cages, technicians kill animals by the dozens or hundreds when they have outlived their usefulness. So much of animal research is a balance of the needs of science against the costs to the animals. Laboratory animal professionals (not just veterinarians, but the unsung animal caregivers and veterinary technicians) are uniquely poised to see nothing but the animal costs (the costs to the animals, that is), there in front of our eyes, rather than the medical advances that may eventually result, many years and many, many animal experiments later.

And yet, I am not ready to bite the bullet and call for an end to animal experimentation. I think of my mother's angioplasty and cardiac bypass, miraculous procedures, really, in whose development animal studies played a crucial role. I think of the animal patients for whom I have prescribed vaccines and antibiotics developed in animal research laboratories. Like chimpanzee veterinarian James Mahoney (1998), I conclude that we may not have a right to experiment on animals, only a very pressing need.

Of course, if animal experimentation is useless or misleading, then all the animal welfare guidelines in the world cannot justify it. Science advocates are so overwhelmingly convinced of its utility that they frequently resort to nothing more than a laundry list of medical advances to argue their case. What animal suffering could possibly weigh against it (Foundation for Biomedical Research 1990; Leader and Stark 1987)? Others (e.g., philosophers Hugh LaFollette and Niall Shanks [1996]) raise serious challenges to their reasoning or question the whole scientific, reductionistic Western approach to medicine that encourages vivisection in the first place.

I offer neither defense nor indictment of the utility of animal research here. I restrict myself to what I know best, the costs to animals, and leave the assessment of the benefits of research for others to argue. Could human ingenuity have come up with the medical advances we have were we committed from the start to avoiding animal harm? Might we now have different scientific tools, cures for some diseases that currently thwart us but not for some we currently seem to have conquered? These are not questions I am able to answer, important as they are.

The plan of the book

Who says what animals really want, and by what right? Those questions lie at the root of most current controversies in laboratory animal welfare policy. And those policies determine how millions of animals live and die every year in American laboratories.

In chapter 2, I offer a behind-the-scenes tour of an animal laboratory. To understand the issues that have dominated policy debates, you need to understand what an animal experiment actually is, who performs what roles in the laboratory, and what the rules and regulations have been.

Philosophers speak for animals, claiming rights for them, or denying them rights altogether. In chapter 3, I guide a brief tour of some of the major philosophical treatments of animal ethics, but with a twist: My focus is less on the philosophical reasoning per se than on the facts about animals, the knowledge claims, that philosophers bring to their argument. Are animals sentient? Can they feel pain? Can they respect human rights if humans decide to respect theirs? All these questions have implications for how we ought to treat animals, but how good is the philosophers' handling of these questions?

Rats and mice were shut out of Animal Welfare Act coverage for years, their welfare issues not deemed worthy of the cost of including them. Controversy over this exclusion heated up in the 1980s and remains hot today. In chapter 4, I discuss the significance of animal species in laboratory animal policy debates. The various species have one or more different identities in our society—the faithful dog, the intelligent but untamed monkeys, the small defenseless mouse cum vermin—that have played into anti- and pro-vivisection propaganda. I argue that different species identities, a blend of real facts about the animals as well as our cultural constructs, fit better or worse with shifting moral philosophies of rights, contractarian reciprocity, or feminist ethics of care.

Laboratory life means caged life for most animals, and so rules about housing animals have been part of public policy for decades. Animal protectionists have always pushed for larger cages no matter the cost. In chapter 5, I show how research advocates responded by promoting the regulatory innovation of "performance standards" as a more affordable approach to cage-size (and other) regulations. This plea for flexibility could only work if researchers could convincingly speak for what animals want and need.

Veterinarians in animal laboratories have long walked a delicate line between promoting animals and promoting animal research. Andrew Abbott's sociological analysis of professional competition is the theoretical core of chapter 6, in which I show how veterinarians carved out a limited niche for themselves without impinging on the liberty of researchers to use animals as they saw fit. Veterinarians had consolidated their domain of animal care (as opposed to animal use) through their focus on controlling animal infections and disease, but their medicalized conception of animal welfare left them ill prepared for the conceptual shift in animal welfare policy in the 1980s, with its new focus on animal behavior, subjectivity, emotion, and psychological well-being.

Veterinarians' promotion on health and hygiene could not allay animal protectionists' presumptions that the life of the laboratory animal is a life of pain. Pain management might be seen as the expertise of veterinarians, but within the laboratories it was part of research methodology—the scientists' autonomous domain of animal use. In chapter 7, I describe how pain became the driving wedge that eroded the care/use jurisdictional divide between veterinarians and scientists and opened the door to greatly expanded regulation in the 1980s.

While veterinarians and scientists tussled on the basis of their expertise in the 1980s, animal protectionists sought again to shift the discourse. Who really cares about the animals, protectionists wanted to know, and they trusted neither the scientists nor the veterinarians. At stake was the "nonaffiliated member's" seat on the newly mandated Institutional Animal Care and Use Committees (IACUCs). Animal protectionists wanted assurance that one of their own would serve on the IACUC as an animal advocate, and in the process revealed their deep ambivalence about laboratory animal veterinarians, wanting to trust them in the laboratories as the animals' allies, but remembering a long history of laboratory animal veterinarians' efforts to ally themselves with scientists. Chapter 8 reviews this contest for the moral authority to speak for animals.

Attention to animal pain combines expertise and advocacy, fact and value. But before we can attend to pain, we have to diagnose it, and that is not always so easy, especially with animal patients who do not speak our language. Chapter 9 is a case study of one hotly contested but largely unseen controversy: whether a particular method of killing rats, decapitation in a table-top guillotine, inflicts excruciatingly intense or totally negligible pain. What do we make of brain wave tracings from six rats, described but never shown in a 1975 research paper? It's a below-the-radar controversy that raises important questions: how much pain warrants a change in policy? How do we chart a course when the experts cannot agree on the meaning of the available data? Why such concern over half a minute of pain, when animals are being killed by the millions in laboratories? How has it come to be that animal pain counts for everything, while killing animals comes and goes as a matter of concern?

Should laboratory monkeys have a chance to socialize and play? Do laboratory dogs need, deserve, or even want to get out of their cages for exercise? Claiming a billion-dollar price tag for compliance, the biomedical research community reacted forcefully to two new provisions of the 1985 Animal Welfare Act amendment calling for exercise programs for dogs and for the psychological well-being of primates. Chapter 10 reviews this history, including a look at the scientific studies of dog exercise that were deployed to allay expensive exercise regulations, as veterinarian-scientists fought an uphill battle in convincing the USDA that despite what "everyone knows" about our best friends, they neither need nor choose more exercise than what they can get living alone in a small cage.

Chapter 11 is my look to the future. Animal research will end some day; how will our children's children judge what we did in our laboratories? Until they are all finally liberated, what goals should we have for the animals? More than ever, laboratory animal medicine is becoming mouse medicine, with the welfare challenge for veterinarians of treating hordes of tiny near-identical subjects as individual, sensitive patients with lives of their own. I have to believe we can succeed in this, else how can I justify the work I do in the animal laboratories?

Before we go further: A word about words

Language is powerful, and all modern writers face the dilemma of how to write in a language that presumes maleness in its pronouns. Should the default pronoun be he, they, s/he, or some random blend? I face an added dilemma—what to do about animals in a speciesist language that allows only for human and other? Except in direct quotes about them, I resist calling any animal "it." I have tried to avoid confusion in sentences occupied by both an animal and a person, but feel that the occasional small confusion is justified in my resistance to "de-animalizing" the animals. They are not objects, however inscrutable their subjectivity may sometimes be.

There are several other "de-animalizing" tactics beyond the choice of pronoun. Animals in laboratories are typically assigned numbers rather than names, a move resisted by many animal caregivers, at least for some animals. In scientific reports, they become "preparations," "models," "specimens," "tools," which further transforms the animal from subject to object. Indeed, so does generic reference to "the animal" rather than "animals" or "an animal" as in the first half of the preceding sentence. They are "supplies" in grant applications and "materials" in scientific publications (Arluke 1993). Animals are animals, and that is what I call them throughout. Humans are animals, too, of course, but I hope the reader can forgive me the shortcut of not always specifying "human animal" versus "nonhuman animal." Unless otherwise specified, when I say "animal" I mean "nonhuman animal."

The word "vivisection" is occasionally used by older researchers, but is currently mostly pejorative and used primarily against researchers, with torture and suffering implied. I avoid it. On the other hand, "antivivisectionists" actively choose that word to describe their political affiliation, and I see no reason to shy away from it. I use it in a narrow sense, to describe people who champion the near-total abolition of animal experimentation, not just its reform. Frequently, I place the abolitionist antivivisectionists and animal rights activists with the reformist animal welfare advocates as "animal protectionists," much though I cling to my belief that animal protection is also a top priority of most laboratory animal veterinarians and scientists.

I use the terms "pro-research" and "pro-animal" cautiously, and for lack of better terms, but they are problematic in several ways. For one thing, People for the Ethical Treatment of Animals and other antivivisectionist/abolitionist groups maintain a relatively low profile in the USDA correspondence of the 1980s, ceding that ground to those animal protection organizations who claimed that their stand was reformist and incrementalist, *not* antiresearch or abolitionist. Additionally, many of those who were arguing for the least restrictive regulations would vigorously resist any accusation that they were anti-animal. In fact, the major thrust of their argument has been that the USDA and the animal protectionists' agenda was not in fact pro-animal, despite good intentions, lacking the veterinarians' and the scientists' knowledge of animal biology and welfare.

Finally, the vast majority of animals in laboratories are *killed* when their usefulness has ended. "Sacrifice," "terminate," and "cull" are words that may blunt that reality, but in this context, they are all synonyms for "kill." "Euthanasia" is "mercy killing" in human medicine where one hopes the motive is to put the patient out of pain and misery. Not so in veterinary medicine: Euthanasia focuses on method (the ideal of pain- and stress-free killing) rather than motive in the animal business, and that is the sense in which I use that word in this book.

2

Life in the animal laboratory

IT DOES NOT SURPRISE ME THAT MOST PEOPLE HAVE NO DETAILED KNOWLEDGE OF what happens to animals in laboratories. Nor does it surprise me that so many have certain knowledge that it is cruel and must be stopped. But animal research will not end any time soon because far too many people are far too convinced of its necessity. That is why so many of us who care about animals devote our energies to reform and improvement, rather than lending support to abolitionist movements.

This book is about making life incrementally better for research animals. That requires the reader to have some basic familiarity with animals' lives in the laboratory. In this chapter, I describe what an animal experiment is, what kinds of animals are in laboratories, who the people are who work in animal laboratories, and what regulation and oversight they operate under. We'll start with the animals.

The animals in American laboratories

When you think of animals in laboratories, what images come to mind? The larger animal protection and animal rights organizations maintain websites and publish magazines showing the worst of animal research: the rabbits with caustic chemicals dripped in their eyes, the monkeys in restraint devices, the cats with brain electrodes. These are some of the images that come to people's minds when I confess to what I *really* do as a veterinarian. None of them is pretty (figure 2.1).

The terms "animal research" and "animal testing" span an array of activities. It is essential for any close examination of laboratory animal welfare policy to have an idea of the kinds of activities being regulated. Readers who have never set foot in an animal laboratory may recall dissecting various animals in biology class, but their direct familiarity with the enterprise ends there.

Thanks to the activism of the late Henry Spira, a civil rights activist who turned his attention to animal issues in the 1970s, many people outside of animal research now think first of toxicity testing when they think of laboratory animals. The two most common procedures that have found their way to the popular and animal protectionist press are the LD_{50} test and the Draize test. The LD_{50} test quantifies the acute toxicity of a substance in mice by administering increasing doses into cohorts of ten mice and finding the dose that kills half (thus, "lethal dose 50%") of a

23

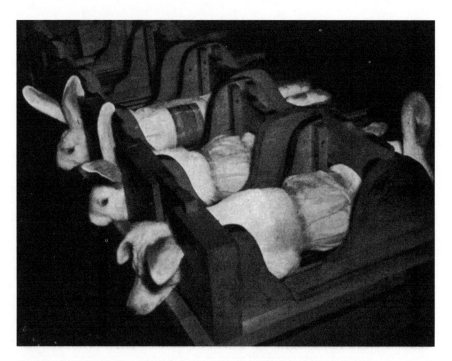

Fig. 2.1   Rabbits (and one dog) in stocks for contact-irritancy (Draize) testing.
REPRINTED FROM *The Journal of Pharmacology and Experimental Therapeutics.*

cohort. The Draize test quantifies contact toxicity in rabbits' eyes by immobilizing rabbits, instilling test substances into their eyes, and scoring the amount of damage and reaction (Draize et al. 1944).[1] These two painful and deadly tests were rendered even less tolerable by Spira's cannily linking them to the most trivial of purposes: testing new shades of eye makeup for their safety. On April 15, 1980, his Coalition to Stop the Draize Rabbit Blinding Test took out an ad in the *New York Times*, asking, "How many rabbits does Revlon blind for the sake of beauty" (Millennium Guild 1980)?

I've worked with laboratory rabbits for more than twenty years, and I have never seen a Draize test. American laboratories still use the Draize and other safety tests in animals, but it's not the sort of thing we do on college campuses. The Animal Welfare Act covers laboratory animals in teaching (classroom dissections), testing (such as the Draize test), and research. On university campuses, such as where I've practiced, animals are not used to test chemicals and cosmetics but to serve in research in the pursuit of new knowledge.

Research uses of animals vary widely. Some animals are used to produce cells or tissues for use in test tubes and tissue culture. This may be as simple as humanely euthanizing an animal to collect cells and organs. Or it could require several months of immunizing a rabbit to collect blood samples rich in antibodies. Some projects require complicated surgeries, as when surgeons and immunologists work together to develop organ transplant procedures or to study organ rejection. Some surgical projects may last for days while an anesthetized animal's body functions are studied; at the end of such a long procedure the animal may either be awakened from anesthesia or, more likely, euthanized. In some experiments, cancers, infection, or other diseases may be induced and treatments or vaccines studied. Some studies remove organs or specific cell types, so that their function may be learned by studying the resulting deficit.[2] Some animal research is as simple and noninvasive as taking to the field or sitting in the laboratory watching normal animal behavior.

It is impossible to understand the value and justification of animal research without considering the complex concept of animals as models. There are thousands of examples—thus the menagerie aspect of the modern animal laboratory. Songbirds show remarkable brain growth as they learn new songs, and so may also shed light on regeneration of central nervous system tissue after injury. Dogs and pigs are an ideal size for developing new techniques in cardiac surgery. Frog eggs provide large cell-membranes for the study of biochemical functions. Woodchucks carry a woodchuck hepatitis virus similar in many ways to the human hepatitis B virus, while the susceptibility of armadillos to leprosy has earned them a place in the laboratory. Rats are classic model animals in learning research.

Even a single area of inquiry can enlist a range of animal species. Take HIV research as an example. Cats or monkeys with the feline or the simian immunodeficiency virus (similar in many ways to humans with the human immune deficiency virus infection) are enlisted in the search for vaccines and antivirals. Chimpanzees have been infected with the actual human virus (Muchmore 2001), as have immune-deficient mice, who may receive both human immune cells and the human virus.[3] In support of these efforts, calf serum feeds human and animal cells grown and studied in tissue culture, while rabbits, goats, and mice produce the antibodies that are necessary for some assays.[4]

Model animals are not simply furry little homunculi with tails, nor is their utility easily faulted simply by finding differences between the animal model and the human. Sometimes, animal models are valuable precisely because they differ somehow from humans. How helpful it might be if chimpanzees or immune-deficient mice with HIV infection perfectly replicated AIDS in humans. We could then test all of our antiviral drugs and vaccines and treatments. And yet, if they don't, perhaps we can learn the source of their resistance and find our way out of this epidemic. The differences can be as powerful as the similarities in a well-characterized animal model. Thus cats and monkeys and horses and sheep, all with their own retroviruses more or less similar to HIV, are enrolled alongside the transgenic mice, the cells in tissue culture, and the human volunteers in the medical battle against AIDS.

Animal numbers

By all counts, American research laboratories employ a very large number of animals, but how many? An exact count is impossible. For starters, no government agency requires reporting of rat, mouse, fish, bird, frog, or invertebrate numbers.

Table 2.1 Estimates of animal numbers in American laboratories
in 1993 and 2001.

Animal species	1993	2001
Guinea pigs, hamster, and rabbits	1,136,900	690,800
Dogs	106,200	70,000
Primates	49,600	49,400
Cats	34,000	22,800
Farm animals	165,400	161,700
Other animals[a]	212,300	242,300
Mice and rats	11–19,000,000	80,000,000[b]

Adapted from Rowan et al. (1995), with permission of the Center for Animals and Public Policy, Tufts University School of Veterinary Medicine, with 2001 figures added from the USDA (2002). Where the two disagree, USDA numbers are used.
[a]Other species covered by the Animal Welfare Act include gerbils, ferrets, and zoo and wild mammals, but not fish, frogs, rats, mice, or birds.
[b]This is the author's estimate; the USDA does not count rats and mice, and Rowan et al.'s estimates only go up to 1993, before the widespread increase in use of transgenic rodents.

Moreover, many laboratories do not count baby animals until they have been weaned from their mother, and that number can be substantial in mouse research. Rowan, Loew, and Weer (1995) of the Tufts University Center for Animals and Public Policy make an admittedly rough estimate that some 14–21 million animals were used in American laboratories in 1992, down from an all-time high of 50 million or more in 1970 (p. 15). They provided a very rough estimate of annual animal use in the early 1990s by species, combed from various government and other sources. They did not count invertebrates such as shrimp or fruit flies, and they did not distinguish frogs, fish, or birds among "other animals" in their charts. Their tallies for 1993 are in table 2.1.

Since those 1993 estimates, USDA figures show a rough leveling, or slight decrease in use of the larger animals. Dog and cat numbers are down by a third, while monkey numbers are roughly stable or may even be increasing (USDA 2001).

Mouse and rat numbers, however, are booming. Since the development of transgenic technologies in the early 1990s, any possible trend toward decreasing numbers have been dramatically reversed. Most major campuses of which I am aware are frantically building new facilities to keep up with increasing demand for rodent housing. Absent any formal figures, surveys, or required reporting, I believe my own observations are as accurate an estimate as any, and I believe that there were surely 80–100 million laboratory rats and mice bred for research in the United States in 2002, and that number will continue to increase for several years. If that estimate is approximately correct, and the USDA's figures are accurate, then primates, dogs, and cats compose well under 1% of the mammals in American laboratories.

By comparison, and to put these numbers in a broader context, Peter Singer, in his best-selling book *Animal Liberation* (1990), reported some 5 billion animals killed for their meat each year in the United States in 1990. That number is surely dwarfed if one counts fish and invertebrates (shrimp and shellfish) as well, and has likely increased in the past decade. So, depending on how you count and define animals, there may be some 100 or more animals eaten for every laboratory animal used in America.

Of more concern than the raw numbers, of course, is what happens to those animals in the laboratories: their confinement, their pain and distress, their suffering, their deaths. Here the reader should start to appreciate the critical role of knowing the facts about animals' experiences in assessing the ethics and policy of animal research: How you feel about animal research probably reflects what you believe the animals feel in the laboratories.

As Congress reworked the Animal Welfare Act in 1970 to minimize the pain and distress of laboratory animals, it added reporting requirements to quantify how many animals of what species were undergoing painful research projects, and whether scientists were taking steps to treat pain and distress with anesthetics, painkillers, and tranquilizers. The USDA, charged with enforcing the act, developed a reporting scheme, revised in 1977, in which laboratories categorize the animal use they report as:

Category C: No pain or distress greater than minor or momentary,
Category D: Potentially painful or distressful animal experiments "for which appropriate anesthetic, analgesic, or tranquilizing drugs were used," or
Category E: Potentially painful or distressful animal experiments "for which the use of appropriate anesthetic, analgesic, or tranquilizing drugs would adversely affect the procedures, results or interpretation of the research" (U.S. Department of Agriculture 1977, p. 31026).

Just as we cannot get a precise count of how many animals are used in American laboratories, it is virtually impossible to quantify with any precision how much pain and suffering those animals experience. Mandatory self-reporting only applies to USDA-regulated species, and so it does not include rats or mice or birds or frogs. Moreover, this quantification of pain and distress depends on how the reporting facilities define, identify, and classify pain (or distress, which is part of the mandatory reporting system and is not separated from pain). Though the human experience of pain exists on a continuum (think of a broken bone versus a paper cut), for animal work the typical threshold for reporting is pain which is greater than "minor or momentary." A simple injection of a painless substance or collection of a blood sample are the paradigm examples of pain that need not be reported or treated. Anything more severe goes in the annual report, under either category D or E.

The American Medical Association (1992) finds comfort in the government's figures that only 8% of laboratory animals are in category E: "Most experiments today do not involve pain, most animals used in experiments do not suffer pain, and the degree of pain that is inflicted during some experiments has been greatly reduced through the establishment of rules for the humane conduct of experiments and the development of new types of instruments and techniques" (p.17).

The Humane Society of the United States counters that pain and distress are underestimated in laboratories' self-reporting (Stephens et al. 1998). The animals in category D, for instance, undergo invasive procedures and receive painkilling medications, but there is no guarantee that those drugs obliterate *all* pain. Animals may be reported in category D, for instance, if they are anesthetized for surgery, even if postoperative pain is left undiagnosed and untreated (Stephens et al. 1998). Indeed, the USDA gives little guidance on how to report animals on complicated studies. And if the AMA's and USDA's figures are accurate, along with my estimate of rodent numbers, then some 8 million animals per year would be category E animals, experiencing unrelieved pain and distress of varying severity.

I remain skeptical of anyone's efforts to quantify laboratory animal suffering nationwide with our current knowledge base and unclear criteria. Antivivisectionists want you to believe that most research animals experience severe and unremitting pain; research advocates would prefer you thought of the laboratory as a high-tech petting zoo where almost all the animals are almost always happy. Neither extreme seems an accurate portrayal to me, but I hope the intelligent reader will come to see that even in the middle zone, in which we assume that some animals experience some degree of pain and distress which must be attended to, questions of how to recognize, diagnose, and quantify animals' experiences loom large.

Searching for alternatives

So much animal suffering—aren't there alternatives? Yes, indeed, there are some, and federal law since 1986 requires that scientists "consider alternatives to any procedure likely to produce pain to or distress in an experimental animal" (U.S. Congress 1985a). Dating back to the work of William Russell and Rex Burch (1959), laboratory animal professionals and their external watchdogs discuss alternatives in the language of the "3Rs": replacement, reduction, and refinement.

Replacement alternatives are conceptually the most straightforward: find ways to generate research data without using animals at all. Candidates for consideration include studying cells in tissue culture (in vitro techniques), developing computer simulations, making better use of human epidemiological data and human volunteers, or using inanimate models in teaching. Scientists also seek to replace so-called higher animals when possible, by switching from dogs to mice, or from mice to fruit flies. In 1981, responding to Spira's criticisms, the Cosmetic, Toiletry, and Fragrance Association provided seed money to establish the Johns Hopkins Center for Alternatives to Animal Testing (CAAT). The CAAT provides grants, hosts conferences, and publishes reports to develop methods to replace animals in testing (Zurlo et al. 1994). Nonanimal replacements are often cheaper and easier than working with animals and may yield data that are cleaner and simpler to interpret. Most animal research groups with which I am familiar do indeed incorporate several nonanimal replacements but have not found they could yet wean

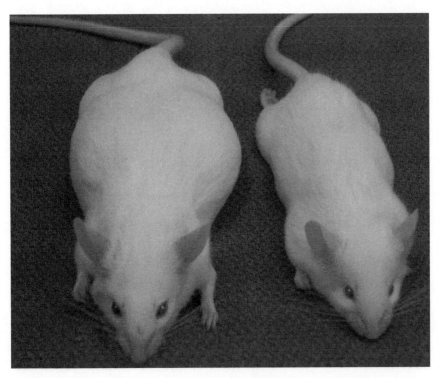

Fig. 2.2   The abdomen of the mouse on the left is distended from injected tumor cells, and the antibody-rich ascites fluid the cells produce. As fluid distention progresses, it debilitates and can kill the mouse. Cells grown in tissue culture have largely replaced this technique.

themselves totally from animals, if only as a source of cells for in vitro studies or for the serums and growth factors needed to nourish those cells.

One major limiting factor is technology, the lag in developing reliable non-animal alternatives. But the technologies are improving. When I started in laboratory animal care in the early 1980s, mice were essential for producing monoclonal antibodies. Tumor cells (hybridomas) injected into the mouse abdomen produced fluid (ascites) rich in antibodies, but at great discomfort to the mouse (figure 2.2). The cells could grow in culture, but not well enough to produce good yields of antibodies. But technology has developed, and it's rare to find a mouse on an ascites-production protocol now.[5]

Reduction is just as it sounds, it aims to lower the numbers of animals required. This often means rethinking statistical tests, to use just the number necessary for statistically valid results (Festing and Altman 2002). Reduction attempts may rely on refining the study, as when use of healthier, more genetically homogeneous animals lowers in-group variability. Sometimes, the move toward reduction can compete with other alternative approaches; switching from dogs to frogs, for instance, may increase several-fold the number of test animals for a study, if only

Table 2.2 Some refinement alternatives to reduce pain
            or distress in animal research.

Choice of experimental endpoints that precede onset of disease or mortality
Improved use of anesthetics and painkillers
Housing social animals in compatible groups
Using flexible tethers to replace rigid restraint devices
Replacing open surgery with endoscopic techniques
Providing supportive veterinary care
Maintaining infection-free animal colonies
Designing cages that allow animals to dig, run, climb, and hide
Training animals to cooperate with research procedures
Frequent monitoring of body weight or other indicators of well-being
Using positive reinforcement in behavioral studies
Killing animals using the least painful methods

---

because of their smaller size. Reducing the number of procedures per animal in a training course may increase the number of animals required; the result will be less pain per animal, and possibly less aggregate pain, but typically increased numbers of animals being killed.

Refinement alternatives are the core of this book: all the myriad ways to rethink animal care and use to reduce the potential for pain and distress. Scientists may seek humane endpoints, stopping tumor or toxicity studies before animals develop severe disease. They may expand their use of anesthetics and painkillers. They may develop assays that require smaller or less frequent blood samples. They may improve the housing for animals in their experiments. Table 2.2 lists more examples of ways of refining animal care and use.

Refinement is a team effort that enrolls several people's expertise and action. To illustrate the pursuit of refinement alternatives and to introduce the human dramatis personae of the animal laboratory, we'll consider the life of one experimental animal in detail.

The people in the animal laboratories

Figure 2.3 shows a common image from animal rights protests: a rhesus monkey with brain electrodes implanted for a neurology study. Monkeys account for a tiny proportion of laboratory animals, and only a small minority of them undergo this sort of research. The commonest application of this research method would be to implant electrodes into the monkey's brain. The electrodes serve not to shock the monkey, but to record the activity in individual brain cells as the animal performs a task for a reward (following a visual image across a screen, operating some computer equipment by hand, recognizing a specific sound). It's ugly to look at, but

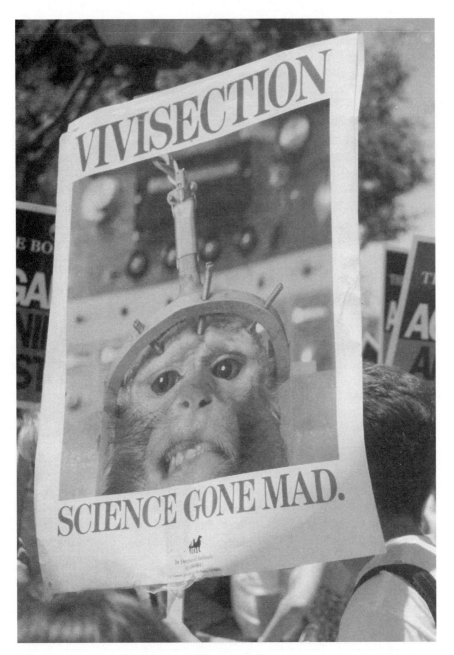

Fig. 2.3   The image of animal research. Poster of a monkey with brain electrodes implanted. PHOTO COURTESY OF HAL HERZOG.

the animal has larger concerns than her appearance. For this animal's sake, we need to overcome immediate revulsion and look closer at her life.

Months before the animal arrives at the campus, a scientist (the principal investigator) designs the experiment and writes the grant application, hoping to convince the National Institutes of Health or another funding agency of the novelty and value of the science. Final approval of the grant, as well as local permission to obtain animals, rests on approval by the IACUC of that university.

The IACUC is the in-house committee on animal care and use. Though most of its members may be faculty scientists on an academic campus, by law it must also include a veterinarian, a nonscientist, and at least one person whose only affiliation with the institution is as an IACUC member. Other members may include students or technical staff. The IACUC will not review the scientific detail so much as the efforts to minimize pain and distress, to seek alternatives to any potentially painful experiments, and to safeguard the monkey's welfare. The alternatives questions to ask in assessing the appropriateness of this research project include:

Why monkeys and not frogs, or cells in culture?
How many monkeys are absolutely required?
What pain management is used for the surgery and postsurgical care?
Must the animal be rigidly restrained during recording sessions?
Can the animal have in-cage companions and enrichments between sessions?
If the reward is food or fluid, how much must the animal be restricted beforehand to willingly work for such a reward?
How well trained are the people performing the various tasks of surgery, testing, health assessment, and animal care?
What criteria signal the time to call in veterinarians or to end the animal's enrollment in the study?

The staff veterinarian and his or her assistants examine the monkey upon her arrival. Unlike pet dogs and cats, rhesus monkeys must usually be anesthetized for physical examination or for blood collection. They are much too strong and wild to be handled safely without sedation; even administration of the sedative requires specialized caging, a "squeeze-cage" with a cage-back that can be pulled forward to immobilize the animal between the front and back cage walls. The veterinary staff turn her care over to the husbandry staff who will feed her, clean her cage, and make daily observations of her health and behavior.

On the morning of surgery, the monkey might see the animal caregiver early on, feeding the other animals in the room (though just like a human patient, she herself would not be allowed food so close to general anesthesia). One group of technicians or students or veterinarians might administer anesthesia during the procedure, while another will perform the surgical instrumentation. Anesthesia is monitored and delivered much as in human surgery; heart rate and body temperature and blood pressure and responsiveness are all monitored to ensure that the animal is deeply anesthetized enough not to feel anything, but not so deeply anesthetized as to threaten her life. Surgery requires the same scalpels and suture as in human surgery, and as in human brain surgery, holes will be drilled or a small square window cut into the bone of the skull to place the electrodes.

When the monkey awakens from anesthesia, she may be back in her home cage. Technicians will monitor her recovery, watch for signs of pain, and administer painkillers. After a few weeks, her convalescent period has ended and scientists will begin the actual experiment and data collection.

There is no requirement that a veterinarian be present during the surgery or anesthesia, but if things do not go well, back comes the vet to diagnose and treat, with painkillers, anti-inflammatory drugs, or antibiotics. A member of the behavior staff will assess how well this animal adapts to caged life and oversee efforts at pair-housing or enriching the environment with toys and treats. At any point during all of this, a veterinary inspector from the USDA may visit, inspect the animal and her quarters, and review her health and research records.

Not all animal projects pull in quite such a full cast. If this were a rat instead of a monkey, the committee would still review plans to work with her, but she would have no vet check on her arrival and she would be out of the USDA Animal Welfare Act inspector's jurisdiction. One graduate student working late into the night might simultaneously serve as her anesthetist, scrub nurse, surgeon, and recovery room nurse.

Few formal rules govern which individuals can perform different experimental procedures on animals. For example, there is no requirement that research surgeries on animals be performed by veterinarians (though there are such laws for therapeutic surgeries performed on pet and food animals). Instead, IACUCs review the qualifications and training of the specific individual for the task at hand. Much of research animal surgery and anesthesia is performed by technicians, undergraduates, graduate students, or faculty scientists (often quite competently, in my experience) with little or no training or oversight from veterinarians. The principal investigators may have medical training themselves (as physicians, psychiatrists, or dentists) and may see human patients as well as conduct research.

The dramatis personae of the animal laboratory include both the research scientist and staff, as well as the individuals I collectively refer to as laboratory animal professionals. In a large institution with centralized animal care, animal caregivers (also known, and professionally certified, as laboratory animal technicians) provide daily care, cleaning, and feeding for several researchers' animals. They may work one or several tiers below a director of animal care, often a veterinarian with academic faculty status. In some settings, animal caregivers may also perform research services. They collect animals' blood samples, feed them test diets, weigh them, and euthanize them. Or they may perform some medical care, report illnesses to the veterinary staff, and administer vaccinations and medications. In other settings, separate specialized groups of research technicians and veterinary assistants may perform these more technical but less frequent tasks. Curiously, though prominent actors in sociological studies of laboratory culture, animal caregivers and other technicians are virtually invisible in the policy discussions that I document throughout this book. Virtually no one, for instance, proposes a mandatory seat on IACUCs for the people who are with the animals all day long. As Arluke and Sanders (1996) have observed, however, animal technicians are the hands through which the institutional culture and the research programs are filtered, and their power, for better or worse, in the animals' lives is significant.

But the laboratory animal professionals who figure most prominently in this book are the laboratory animal veterinarians, like myself, who staff the animal facilities, oversee the animals' health care, and find themselves increasingly in regulatory, administrative, and oversight positions. Veterinarians did not always have a central place in animal research laboratories, but the 1980s round of legislative updates secured vets a role that had been expanding for half a century. No behind-the-scenes look at an animal laboratory is complete without looking at the development of these laws and the changes they have wrought.

Animal welfare rules and regulations

I write about regulations for two reasons. The first is that they are potentially powerful forces in the lives of the animals I have cared for. Though they must first be filtered, and sometimes dampened in the process through IACUCs, laboratory animal veterinarians, administrators, animal caregivers, and scientists, the regulations *do* trickle down with some impact on how people treat animals in the laboratory. They must house their animals in cages of a certain minimum size, spare them certain research procedures when possible, and meet standards of hygiene and medical care. As a laboratory animal veterinarian, it has been my responsibility to know these national standards for animal care and to strive to meet or exceed them for animals in my care.

I write about the regulations as well because periods of regulatory revision become a public stage on which to audition ideas of how to treat animals. In writing their letters to the USDA to shape the Animal Welfare Act regulations, scientists, animal protectionists, and veterinarians have described what they believe they know about animals and how they think that knowledge should balance against the needs of medical progress. They describe their values and their allegiances. They discuss their conceptions of animal welfare, which sorts of evidence count and which do not, in determining that a particular policy will hurt or harm the animals. This correspondence to the USDA is a matter of public record, and its review constituted much of my research for this book. Thus, rules and regulations are important in and of themselves for the effects they have, while their construction provides a window into the thinking of those who would speak for animals.

Most American laboratories operate under two main sets of animal welfare regulations, which I will refer to as the Animal Welfare Act and the NIH guidelines. The two have converged over three decades of convoluted history and are now virtually indistinguishable. They do, however, have important distinctions in their history, philosophical basis, and scope that the reader should appreciate. At the risk of gross oversimplification, I characterize the Animal Welfare Act as a "top-down" law, written by Congress in response to public pressure and imposed upon research laboratories. The NIH guidelines however, grew from a set of self-regulatory standards and guidance written for laboratory animals, later encoded, from the bottom up, as federal law. While the Animal Welfare Act represents what people want for animals, the NIH guidelines have been presented as expert information on what animals want and need.

Readers content to trust me with this oversimplification can look at tables 2.3 and 2.4 for comparison of these two regulations, and then move on to chapter 3. For more of the background on these regulations, and why I draw the distinction between their underlying philosophies, read on.

The United Kingdom passed its first law protecting laboratory animals in 1876 (Townsend and Morton 1995). Ninety years later, the United States followed suit. Several bills had been introduced over the years to regulate laboratory animal use in America at the federal level. In 1965, *Sports Illustrated* magazine ran a story on Pepper, a dalmatian strayed or stolen from her family and sold to a medical laboratory (Phinizy 1965). A few months later, *Life* magazine ran its exposé on dog dealers who sell to labs, full of disturbing pictures of the conditions there (figure 2.4; Silva 1966). The public response was overwhelming, and before long, Congress had passed the Laboratory Animal Welfare Act of 1966 (U.S. Congress 1966a).[6]

Born as an act of Congress in 1966, the Animal Welfare Act has been amended in 1970, 1976, 1985, 1990, and 2002. The act, in less than 3000 words, authorizes the USDA to write and enforce its 100+ pages of animal welfare regulations. The act gives some broad and some specific direction to the USDA on what to cover. The 1985 amendment resulted in a contentious period of USDA rules writing, finally completed in February 1991, over five years and two months after passage of the amended act. The controversies of this rule-writing period fill most of the remaining chapters of this book.

For present purposes, readers should understand the distinction between the *act*—the law as passed and amended by Congress—and the *regulations* as promulgated by the USDA. As with many other areas of regulation, Congress fleshes out a general law, empowering and funding a government agency to fill in and enforce the details. For instance, when Congress determined in 1985 that the secretary of agriculture should set standards giving laboratory dogs the "opportunity for exercise," it fell to the USDA to decide which dogs should get how much exercise and under whose direction—all points of contention as the USDA tried to finalize rules.

The Animal Welfare Act gets all the press, but the National Institutes of Health (NIH) has animal welfare requirements that are equally significant. The history of the Animal Welfare Act is fairly simple and public, explaining why most descriptions and analyses of the American regulatory scene focus mainly on the act. In contrast, the other set of rulebooks is an assortment of (1) self-regulatory professional standards written by laboratory animal veterinarians and scientists, (2) policies on grant administration within the NIH and its parent institution, the Public Health Service (PHS), (3) a voluntary program of accreditation, and (4) a congressional act of law, the Health Research Extension Act of 1985. Small wonder that so many discussions quickly skip over this complex with eyes averted, and stay

Table 2.3 Comparison of the Animal Welfare Act and the *Guide for the Care and Use of Laboratory Animals.*

	Animal Welfare Act and the USDA	NIH guidelines and the *Guide*
Who writes the rules	Congress passes the act; government veterinarians at the USDA write the regulations.	A veterinary association (the Animal Care Panel) wrote the first edition (1963). Subsequent editions by vets and others assembled by the National Academy of Science (nongovernmental, but with government funding).
Enforcement	Routine unannounced USDA inspections; self-reporting to the USDA.	Self-reporting to the NIH; NIH inspections if problems are suspected.
Species of research animals covered	Warm-blooded animals. Birds and lab mice and rats are excluded, as are farm animals on agricultural research projects.	All vertebrate animals
Regulates how animals are obtained	Yes, since its inception in 1966.	No, though "All animals must be acquired lawfully."
Regulates how animals are used in experiments	Mandates adequate vet care (including pain relief) since 1970. 1985: IACUC review required.	Has always contained some suggestions for animal use. Committee review first suggested in fourth edition (1972).
Exercise for dogs	Proposed in 1974; not mandated until 1985. Flexible "performance standards" with veterinarian overseeing an "appropriate plan to provide dogs with the opportunity for exercise."	Left to "professional judgment" in early editions. Dog pens encouraged for animals housed greater than three months. 1996: "Animals should have opportunities to exhibit species-typical activity" patterns.
Psychological well-being	Mandated for primates in 1985; flexible "performance standards" with veterinarian overseeing an "appropriate plan for environment enhancement adequate to promote the psychological well-being of nonhuman primates."	1985: "Consideration should also be given to enriching the environment as appropriate to the species, especially when animals will be held for long periods."

See text for specific references.

Table 2.4 Historical developments in the Animal Welfare Act and the *Guide for the Care and Use of Laboratory Animals.*

Year	Animal Welfare Act	*Guide*
1963		First edition; written by Animal Care Panel as *Guide for Laboratory Animal Facilities and Care*
1965		Second edition; written by Institute of Laboratory Animal Resources (as are all subsequent editions)
1966	Laboratory Animal Welfare Act, focus on animal acquisition	
1968		Third edition
1970	Amended: species coverage expanded to all warm-blooded animals (but USDA excludes mice and rats); provision for adequate vet care (including pain relief during experiments); annual report required on painful experiments and use of painkillers	
1972		Fourth edition; title changed to *Guide for the Care and Use of Laboratory Animals* to reflect expanded coverage of animal *use*
1974	USDA proposes dog exercise regulations, never adopted as final rules	
1976	Amended. Focus on animal transportation standards. No mention of 1974 exercise proposal	
1978		Fifth edition
1985	Amended. Provisions for IACUCs, psychological well-being of nonhuman primates, exercise for dogs.	Health Research Extension Act gives *Guide* the force of law; sixth edition of *Guide*
1990	Amended: Pet Protection Act	
1991	USDA finalizes rules subsequent to the 1985 amendment	
1996		Seventh edition; first with a non-scientist, nonveterinarian community representative
2002	Amended: Definition of "animal" amended to specifically exclude "birds, rats of the genus *Rattus* and mice of the genus *Mus,* bred for use in research"	

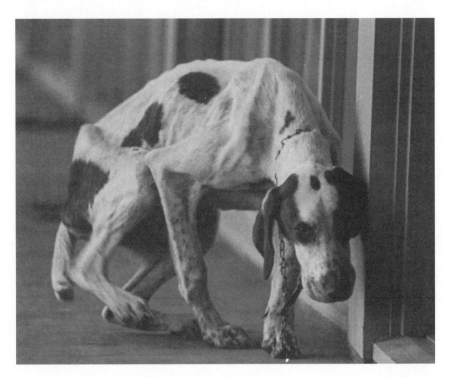

Fig. 2.4 "Concentration Camp for Dogs" was the title of the *Life* article on dog dealers. This malnourished dog was the lead photo. PHOTOGRAPH BY STAN WAYMAN, REPRINTED WITH PERMISSION.

focused instead on the Animal Welfare Act. But the differences between the two (including their different handling by historians and analysts) are important enough that it is worth trying to sort out this mishmash.[7]

The essential difference between the USDA and NIH approaches to animal welfare assurance is in their political genesis. Passage of the Animal Welfare Act followed years of lobbying from animal protection and antivivisection groups, with exposés of dog dealing providing the final spark. This was thrust upon the scientific community and their animal suppliers, with enforcement placed in the hands of the USDA's veterinarians rather than the NIH's scientists. The final form of act amendments and updated regulations are compromises of animal protectionist and research advocacy interests. Since passage of the Freedom of Information Act in 1976, much of the process of regulation writing has been public information— hence my easy access to the USDA correspondence of the late 1980s.

In contrast, the Animal Care Panel, a professional association of veterinarians and other laboratory animal professionals, wrote the first edition of the *Guide* in 1963 (Animal Care Panel 1963). The emphasis from the start was on flexible self-regulation by research facilities. A program for institutions to voluntarily seek accreditation by a body of their peers was established in 1964; since 1971 NIH has formally recognized such accreditation as assurance of compliance with their requirement for animal welfare programs for grant recipients. In 1985, a few months before a major overhaul of the Animal Welfare Act, the U.S. Congress granted this complex of self-regulatory policies, documents, and programs legal status. In that year, Congress included mandatory compliance with the Public Health Service Policy on Humane Care and Use of Laboratory Animals as part of the Health Research Extension Act (the bill that assures federal funding of the NIH).

The *Guide for the Care and Use of Laboratory Animals* is the centerpiece of the NIH's self-regulatory approach to laboratory animal welfare. Tables 2.3 and 2.4 focus on the *Guide* and the Animal Welfare Act, sacrificing some of the complexity of the system in favor of readability and clarity. Neither set of rules was born de novo, nor have they evolved independently. They followed a series of booklets of standards published by the *Guide's* publishers (the National Academy of Sciences' Institute of Laboratory Animal Resources), professional codes of various research societies (such as the American Physiological Society), or codes and guidelines promoted by animal protection organizations (such as the Animal Welfare Institute's *Comfortable Quarters,* first published in the late 1950s). These assorted documents, along with their various European counterparts, have provided a pool of ideas and standards that have been available to the authors of the *Guide* and the act, but in no way undermine the centrality and significance of these two documents.

The 1985 Animal Welfare Act contained several controversial provisions, such as the institution of animal care and use committees to review research proposals, exercise programs for dogs, and provisions for the psychological well-being of nonhuman primates. The USDA's regulations that followed contained their own controversial topics, including the continued exclusion of rats, mice, and birds from coverage, changes in mandated cage sizes, delineation of the attending laboratory animal veterinarian's role in research institutions, compliance with the American Veterinary Medical Association's recommendations on humane animal euthanasia, and a shift in regulatory philosophy toward flexible "performance standards." Tables 2.3 and 2.4 show just how long-standing some of these issues have been. Some appeared first in early editions of the *Guide,* as recommendations for good practice, before they found their way into the act as law. In other instances, as in the *Guide's* dismissal of public concerns for dog exercise programs in its earlier editions, the *Guide* stands as the professionals' corrective and resistance to what they saw as ill-informed agendas of protectionists and legislators.

The important distinction to reiterate here between the *Guide* (with its associated programs and policies) and the Animal Welfare Act is that the *Guide* is relatively closed to outsiders, both in its authorship and in its enforcement. I see three important differences between the two.

(1) *Who writes the rules.* Congress passed the Animal Welfare Act in 1966, with strong input from animal protection organizations, as well as from the scientific community (in government terms, the "regulated industry"), research advocacy organizations, and the NIH. This pattern continued with each amendment. Con-

gress passes the act, and USDA staff members (most of them veterinarians) write the regulations, but not without public input. The USDA publishes its proposed regulations in the *Federal Register,* solicits comments, and publicly summarizes and responds to those comments as it publishes its final rules.

In the late 1980s, the Animal Welfare Institute and other animal protection organizations stand out as prime players, carefully analyzing proposed regulations and mobilizing their memberships into letter-writing campaigns.[8] Concurrently, the National Association for Biomedical Research squared off against protectionists in its leadership role among researchers and research institutes. Most of the 1985 Animal Welfare Act regulations are a negotiated settlement between these two interest groups, along with less publicly visible efforts within government offices to harmonize the NIH and the USDA. The active role of the animal protectionists and the more-or-less transparent political process (with correspondence to Congress and the USDA matters of public record and fully accessible) have always kept the Animal Welfare Act a more visible document for historians and critics than the *Guide* has been.

In contrast, the *Guide for the Care and Use of Laboratory Animals* has always been portrayed as more a scientific/expert document than a political one. Its authors have primarily been laboratory animal veterinarians, though over the years other scientists have joined, and the 1996 edition included a nonscientist/nonveterinarian "community representative" as well. The authoring institutions, the Animal Care Panel in 1963, and later, the Institute of Laboratory Animal Resources (now renamed the Institute for Laboratory Animal Research), are technically nongovernmental and exempt from government's rules-writing regulations.[9] The authors can decide who will serve on the authoring panel, determine how much public input to solicit, send drafts for anonymous peer review, without publication of draft proposals in the *Federal Register.*

(2) *Enforcement approaches.* The USDA's reputation among the laboratory animal professionals I have spoken to has been one of rigid inflexibility, while the *Guide's* approach has been flexible self-regulation. This distinction, which may never have been as sharp as it has often been painted, blurred in the 1980s. The NIH approach took a turn for tighter control, with passage of the Health Research Extension Act. Meanwhile, the Animal Welfare Act's empowerment of IACUCs and of loosely articulated "performance standards," especially for newer provisions such as exercise plans for dogs and provision of environments that enhance the psychological well-being of primates, created a more flexible self-regulatory atmosphere.

The USDA approach has relied on USDA inspectors (most of them veterinarians) performing unannounced site visits and writing detailed citations that can lead to fines or even to criminal proceedings. Since passage of the Freedom of Information Act in 1976, a facility's Animal Welfare Act violations are publicly accessible. The NIH, in contrast, has relied on written assurances from institutions that their animal care program will conform to the *Guide,* with occasional "for-cause" inspections when NIH suspects something is amiss. The NIH likewise recognizes accreditation by the Association for the Assessment and Accreditation of Laboratory Animal Care (AAALAC) as evidence of compliance. Institutions seeking AAALAC accreditation submit a detailed description of their animal care program and host a prearranged triennial site visit by scientists and/or veterinarians associated with AAALAC. These veterinarians and scientists are peers based at other research institutions. An institution's written animal welfare assurances and accreditation status are accessible through NIH, but AAALAC accreditation and site visit reports are not government documents (AAALAC is a private organization) and are confidential.

The USDA's detailed rule book stands in contrast to the *Guide*'s emphasis on professional judgment tailored to the specific context. Research institutions voluntarily seek and pay for AAALAC accreditation, a collegial and confidential exercise in peer review and professional self-regulation. In contrast, the USDA shows up at the door, unannounced, often unwelcome, ready to inspect. AAALAC has relied primarily on senior laboratory animal veterinarians for its site visits, whereas the USDA started its inspection system by reassigning livestock health inspectors to go into the medical schools and pharmaceuticals firms and has only recently sought laboratory animal training for its animal welfare inspectors.

(3) *What the standards cover.* The Animal Welfare Act started life as an anti–pet-theft law in 1966. Its species coverage is restricted to warm-blooded animals (i.e., birds and mammals), but it excludes rats, mice, and birds.[10] The Public Health Service policy covers all vertebrate animals (i.e., fish, amphibians, reptiles, birds, and mammals), though only in institutions receiving federal funds. A private research or testing laboratory that receives no federal money and uses only mice and rats is thus exempt from the major laboratory animal welfare regulations.

The USDA's pet-theft/animal acquisition focus includes provisions for documenting legally sanctioned acquisition of dogs and cats, whereas the *Guide* simply states that animals must be acquired legally (i.e., in compliance with the Animal Welfare Act and other laws), without further elaboration. The Animal Welfare Act's 1970s amendments brought zoo animals, competitive dog fights, and animal transportation under its aegis—none of which I treat in depth here, and none of which appear in the *Guide*.

Ignoring dog theft as a cause for serious concern, the *Guide* and Public Health Service policy have always applied more directly to the research institution (rather than the animals' route thereto), with recommendations on how to staff an animal facility and how to treat animals during experiments. In contrast, Congress was always careful to emphasize that none of the Animal Welfare Act's provisions were to interfere with the design or conduct of research experiments. Even so, Congress overstepped that principle in 1970 and in 1985, authorizing first the attending veterinarian (in 1970), and later the IACUC (in 1985), to oversee researchers' efforts to minimize pain and distress of research animals, including during the conduct of experiments. IACUC oversight of animal use has become the strongest point of convergence and harmonization between the two regulatory approaches throughout the late 1980s and into the twenty-first century.

Both sets of regulations have a good deal to say about how to house and care for animals, with their strongest emphasis historically placed on what happens to animals before they are delivered to the laboratory. The USDA focused on getting animals legally; the *Guide* focused on getting them in good health. Throughout their histories, both have gingerly handled the possibility that animal experimentation may actually hurt and kill these initially healthy, legally acquired subjects or that improvements in animal welfare can cost considerable sums of time and money. Congress tried to avoid the subject altogether, preserving scientific freedom of inquiry with its insistence that the Animal Welfare Act not cover research design, but it then continually eroded that exemption with its provisions on pain control. Pushed further, and spurred no doubt by the exposés of two primate laboratories in the early 1980s, Congress and the USDA granted increased research oversight to IACUCs and laboratory animal veterinarians. Their approach followed the NIH's lead, requiring IACUC scrutiny, but also allowing that IACUCs could approve any "necessary" departures from animal welfare standards if experimental design dictated it.

The emerging consensus after thirty years of national animal welfare policy looks roughly like this: locally empowered review committees of scientists, veterinarians, and lay people should (1) oversee animal care programs that maintain fit animals in good psychological health and (2) monitor scientists' efforts to reduce unnecessary pain or distress to animals on experiment.

So why compare the two if they have been on this path of steady convergence? The convergence itself suggests some inexorable code of animal welfare ethics on which all reasonable people would agree, with the *Guide* and the act simply two routes to the same goal. The more-or-less democratic process by which the Animal Welfare Act balances protectionists' and researchers' priorities converges with the scientific authority of the *Guide* in this reasonable consensus. I want to challenge the presumption that these consensus standards and guidelines are natural and inevitable. People have actively chosen these standards out of a range of possible options, bringing their own assumptions about animals and their own balance of pro-animal and pro-research values to the table.

Conclusion

By anyone's count, very large numbers of animals live and die in American laboratories. The animal species are as varied as the types of research, and numbers shift over time as new technologies (such as genetic modification of mice) require more animals, or as alternatives (such as cell culture production of animals) replace or reduce animals. These animals see a variety of people, including scientists, animal caregivers, animal behavior specialists, students, IACUC committee members, veterinarians, and government inspectors.

The laws these people operate under shape animal care in important ways. Though the two main laws, the Animal Welfare Act and the NIH guidelines, have converged in important ways, their philosophical and historical roots are very different. The Animal Welfare Act is forced upon research institutions with little claim to expertise beyond what the American people want and what USDA inspectors' enforcement experience tells them. The NIH guidelines have trusted veterinarians and scientists to publish their professional expertise on what animals want and need. Put forth as a professional information rather than top-down regulation, the standards of *Guide for the Care and Use of Laboratory Animals* are seen to flow naturally from what experts know about animals, with no political agenda implied, and no public input sought.

3

Animal welfare: Philosophy meets science

AS A VETERINARIAN TRYING TO MAKE SENSE OF ANIMAL WELFARE PUBLIC POLICY, I have looked to philosophers of animal ethics for some guidance. And why not? Philosophers have published extensively on animals over the past twenty-five years, and their appearance at veterinary and laboratory animal conferences and in our journals has become a familiar sight. In this chapter, I guide a brief tour of select influential philosophical approaches to animal welfare, to see how they have and how they could enlighten animal welfare policy.

Peter Singer and Tom Regan have done the most to bring animal liberation philosophies to a broad audience, as well as pushing many philosophers to treat animals seriously. Between them, they have made a compelling case for either a strong recognition of animal rights (Regan) or for such a serious weighting of animal harm versus human benefit (Singer) as to both be near-abolitionists on the use of animals in research. Singer's 1975 *Animal Liberation* and Regan's 1983 *The Case for Animal Rights* are now essential reading for any serious student of animal ethics, if for no other reason than that their work is the starting point from which, or against which, so many other writers take off.[1]

Speciesism

Singer's concept of speciesism is compelling and something that all animal ethicists must grapple with. Speciesism is a concept that gets hopelessly muddled in some hands, and so I hope to clarify how I use the word and believe it should be used. "Speciesism" means basing moral distinction on species membership alone rather than on attributes of the members of a species.

Liberationists like Regan and Singer argue that there no morally relevant criteria shared by all humans and no nonhumans that could justify a sharp moral divide. On all attributes other than species membership—intelligence, ability to feel pain or fear or distress, consciousness—the differences may be more quantitative than qualitative, and there are at least some severely deficient humans with lower apparent cognitive ability than some highly functioning animals.

The best test of speciesist reasoning is the hypothetical moral status we would accord to a newly discovered species—an extraterrestrial, a marine mammal, a long-lost hominid, an android—who was like us (if we could ever really tell) in all those attributes to which some people grant moral significance: intelligence, self-consciousness, rational autonomy, moral sensibility, and so on. If we would still exclude such a race from our moral community simply because they are not one of us, then we are committing (guiltily? appropriately?) speciesism.

Singer (1975) argues that basing moral distinctions on species membership is really no different than basing such distinctions on any other taxonomy—on race, or gender, or on membership of any particular ethnic group. To my mind, no one has convincingly challenged this basic premise, deeply rooted though it may be in our thinking. No one has convinced me why species membership per se should be permissible as a moral boundary marker in a way that race would not. No one these days (I hope) would believe I would be justified to limit my moral concern only to Italian-Americans, simply because they are my closest living relatives; expanding my scope to all people of European origin is no better. To avoid charges of racism, I must expand my circle of concern to the entire species. But why stop there? Instead of species, why not set the moral-taxonomic boundary at the level of genus (which would include ancestral hominid species, were living representatives ever found), or family?[2]

Singer's anti-speciesism is not a claim of equal capacity, nor a call for total equality. He does not, for instance, call for giving dogs the vote. He calls, rather, for equal consideration of interests (recognizing the difficulty of divining another's interests): if a dog and a child have roughly similar interests in avoiding pain, then we have roughly similar obligations to avoid causing them pain.

Regan and Singer raise compelling arguments that must be entertained if we are to continue using animals in laboratories. Though a strong animal liberationist stance would radically change the lives we live—limiting or eliminating meat consumption, hunting, and animal research and testing—philosophers like Regan, Singer, and Bernard Rollin are quick to point to how very nonradical they believe their philosophy is. They take basic moral principles already established within moral discourse, ask why animals should be excluded, and argue that the truly rational, reasonable, and consistent position is to include animals in our moral sphere. To exclude them would be the radical and irrational position; it would be speciesism. Eventually, they may have their day, and people will look back in horror that we ever felt justified performing animal experimentation.

But animal research is here, now. Can we find an ethic that guides us toward better meeting ethical responsibilities to animals without jettisoning laboratory research altogether? Among veterinarians and animal researchers, the philosophies of Bernard Rollin (1992), Jerrold Tannenbaum (1986, 1995), and Andrew Rowan (1984) have found a wide audience in journals and at conferences; none of these three argues for abolition of animal research. In contrast to Singer and Regan's abolitionism, current public policy on laboratory animal welfare (as embodied, for instance, in the Animal Welfare Act and the NIH *Guide for the Care and Use of Laboratory Animals*) starts with the philosophical premise that animal use for human ends not only is justifiable, but that we may justifiably kill and hurt them in that use. Society's moral consensus, as summarized in 1990 by a working group at the Hastings Center, condones animal use, but nonetheless calls for some protection of some animals. Society's "troubled middle" and current public policy call for strong justification, but do not prohibit, the infliction of pain and suffering on animals (Donnelly 1990). It is precisely this balancing act of human interests and animal harm that stirs the most controversy in policy debates and is most in need of some sort of philosophical refinement.

Let me restate this, as it is roughly the consensus working ethic that guides most of us in animal research and as it underlies most of animal welfare policy: *It is wrong to inflict harm on individuals without strong justification.*

But the devil is in the details: whether "individuals" applies only to humans, to humans and some animals, to humans and all animals, and whether it applies equally to all; what to count as "harm" and how to recognize its presence; and how to assess the justification for harming another.

Every day in the animal research laboratory, laboratory animal professionals and IACUCs face large and small decisions about animal welfare. As a veterinarian working in research universities, I have often been involved in these decisions. What I am looking for from the philosophers is a practical and applied ethics that will help IACUCs, veterinarians, scientists, and regulators evaluate individual cases of animal research. Let's start with a case.

An animal care and use committee receives a protocol application for permission to use dogs to teach a class on surgery and anesthesia for medical students. The professor has done her best to assure that students develop competence using computer simulations of anesthetic responses and good psychomotor skills for suturing and tissue handling using nonliving animal models. Eventually, though, she believes her students develop their best skills by following all of this training with procedures performed on live animals. The committee must consider a host of questions that we won't go into here: choice of anesthetics; qualifications of lab instructors; how the animals will be housed; and many many others. Focus for now on the questions of what kind and how many animals the committee will allow. In the interest of reducing animal numbers, should the instructor allow animals to recover from anesthesia so that she may use a smaller number of animals a few times over? Or should she never allow the animals the potential pain of postsurgical recovery and euthanize them while still anesthetized on the surgery table even if that means using more animals?[3] Should she try to switch from dogs to "lower" animals? If so, are rats sufficiently "lower"? What if their smaller size would dictate using a larger number of rats, or made it more difficult to deliver adequate anesthesia and analgesia, or compromised what the students were able to learn from the lab? How much of an incremental increase in the students' learning justifies inflicting pain or death or both on animals?

These are the sorts of questions that animal care and use committees consider at their meetings, not the big question of whether people have any right to use animals in research and teaching. That big question is vitally important, but by the time we are determining cases, it has already been decided in favor of human priority. Yes, we will continue using animals for the foreseeable future; the question is not whether, but how. Can we find guidance from philosophers to help us decide when painless death is preferable to life with some potential pain, to rank species one above another, to rule whether more animals should experience low-level suffering so that a small number do not suffer greatly? Can we figure out which human needs and desires might justify inflicting pain or death on animals? Can we find guidance to make decisions for animals who cannot tell us their preferences and experiences directly? These are the kinds of questions for which we currently have but the crudest tools for crafting decisions.

In search of a useful applied ethic of animal welfare policy, some of my criteria are:

- Does it satisfactorily address questions of "drawing the line" between and among humans and other animals? Does it map well onto my conviction that there is a moral hierarchy with humans at or near the top, nonlife and bacteria at or near the bottom, and other plants and animals ranged in between? If not, does it convincingly challenge that conviction?
- Does it give some guidance in balancing human needs against animal welfare?
- Does it help us identify what makes for better or worse animal welfare?
- Does it harmonize with the best available information about animal biology and animal psychology?
- Does it answer whether painlessly killing an animal is an act of moral concern?

Animal minds and animal ethics

The philosopher David DeGrazia (1996, p. 76) writes, "The path to the ethical treatment of animals runs through their minds," emphasizing the importance of understanding the mental lives of animals—their sentience, intelligence, consciousness, self-consciousness, capacities for pleasure and pain—in judging animal ethics. If an animal's welfare resides in how she or he feels, and if those feelings are the function of the mind, then any serious ethical discussion of animal welfare must somehow account for what is in the animal's mind. As DeGrazia puts it, "What sorts of mental capacities we attribute to animals have a great deal to do with how we think they should be treated" (1996, p. 1).

DeGrazia's thesis (which I find quite convincing) raises two important and interrelated questions. First, is it true? Is there really a distinction to be drawn between the mental and the physical in animal welfare? Are welfare concerns such as hunger and pain really connected to animals' minds, or are they physical, or some combination of the two? The corollary question is, how do we read animals' minds, or their bodies for that matter, to assess the quality of their welfare?

I start with a few approaches to animal ethics that do *not* rely on assessing animals' mental capacities, to see how well they help with deciding particular cases of animal use.

Albert Schweitzer proposed reverence for life, the "ethic of love widened into universality," (quoted in Free 1982, p. 23), as a guiding principle for treating the world around us.[4] Here is his description of the ethical man: "He does not ask how far this or that life deserves sympathy as valuable in itself, nor how far it is capable of feeling. To him life as such is sacred. He shatters no ice crystal that sparkles in the sun, tears no leaf from its tress, breaks off no flower, and is careful not to crush any insect as he walks" (Free 1982, p. 28).

This is beautiful, but does it help make decisions about when and how to experiment on animals? If the "ethical man" shatters no ice crystal and crushes no insect, could he ethically harm animals in the laboratory? Apparently so, for Schweitzer was not a research abolitionist. He wrote:

> Those who experiment upon animals by surgery and drugs, or inoculate them with diseases in order to be able to help mankind by the results obtained, should never quiet their consciences with the conviction that their cruel action may in general have a worthy purpose. In every single instance they must consider whether it is really necessary to demand of an animal this sacrifice for men. And they must take anxious care that the pain be mitigated as much as possible. (Free 1982, p. 36)

Schweitzer felt that all life is sacred, regardless of its place on any human scale, and he claimed to worry as much for the worm on his hook as for the fish that he would catch. He nevertheless recognized the occasional need to make distinctions when to preserve one life and sacrifice another, but offered little guidance for such decisions. Indeed, "through this series of decisions [the truly ethical man] is conscious of acting on subjective grounds and arbitrarily" (Free 1982, p. 29).

By placing all of his emphasis on the qualities of the ethical man, rather than those to whom this man owes ethical consideration, Schweitzer gives us little help in facing cases. Does the ethical man find the "life" of an ice crystal comparable to the life of an insect, a flower, or a laboratory dog? If the distinction is so truly arbitrary and subjective, why does he make a special case for mitigating pain as much as possible in experimentation? Does he believe flowers and ice crystals and animals all feel pain, or all feel it equally, or does he in fact believe that we do have a criterion—sentience (i.e., the capacity to suffer)—that is not merely arbitrary?

Some other writers, working with a sociobiological perspective, similarly focus only on the qualities of human actors, and not on the animals acted upon. Curiously, my fellow veterinarians and other animal scientists often advance such positions; curious because their argument for a scientific approach to animal ethics requires none of the animal expertise that characterizes their professional lives, but rests instead on claims about human nature. Meat consumption is as often the context for this sort of reasoning, as is animal research, possibly reflecting the greater number of veterinarians working in food animal than in laboratory animal practice. "Man is a predatory species," wrote veterinarian Robert Miller, a self-professed animal lover, and so, like other predators, people "have an inherent right to utilize other animals to preserve their own existence" (Miller 1983, p. 21). In a paean to biological determinism, another veterinarian, Randall Ott, chides animal liberationists for their "unnatural beliefs" and writes: "Understanding of the behavior of the human animal is found in the study of social activity of other predators" (Ott 1995, p. 1029). Other veterinarians share this fascination with man as predator: "I have no rumen or cecum," writes David Smith, "I have a 'garbage gut' to eat anything, including meat, and would be flying in the face of evolution" to forsake eating meat (Smith 1990, p. 1738).

These veterinarians' statements reveal the difficult task of integrating facts (here, biological facts, if shaky ones, about human evolution) into morality. Notice in these statements, though, that these veterinarians' appeals to biology are all about *us* and nothing about animals. A man-as-predator morality seems to justify all meat eating equally, with no distinctions among different types of animals or different types of farming practices.

The sociobiological approach illustrates the different ways that facts of nature can be brought to bear on morality, but we must think carefully about which facts to consider for particular ethical issues. Consider again these treatments of meat consumption. Smith (1990) argues that the evolutionary fact of history as predators carries moral weight, it justifies killing and eating other animals. But what of other biological information, like the assessment that we can live very healthy lives without eating meat (American Dietetic Association 1997)? Is there nothing about the animals, about some animals, at least, that would set moral limits on this carnivory? And what of other evolutionary information, the skeletons in our closet of cannibalism, infanticide, violence toward other humans? Would it also "fly in the face of evolution" to denounce such acts as immoral?

Consider these two statements: (1) People evolved as predators, and therefore meat eating is morally justified and (2) people can live long and healthy lives as vegetarians, and therefore meat eating cannot be morally justified. Both contain facts about human beings, both of which could be simultaneously true, but they say nothing in detail about the animals we might eat. How do we reconcile the two claims?

Nor is this sort of pop sociobiology limited to questions of eating animals. In the right hands, even activities that might seem highly unnatural or even monstrous—experimenting on animals, swapping genes from one species to another—are really just "natural" expressions of basic instincts of predation, curiosity, and so on. Animals use members of other species in various ways, and predation is but one example. And so veterinarian and neurobiologist Adrian Morrison (1998) writes: "I believe animal use by humans is natural and no less appropriate in the scheme of things than animal use by other animals. Therefore, I reject as nonsense the notion of 'speciesism' that the animal rights movement promotes. It is a perversion of biology, not a principle. Vivisection fits into the category of appropriate uses" (p. 1). Not only is animal experimentation a "natural" human activity (Morrison uses cats to study sleep disorders), it is a moral imperative: "Indeed, increasing knowledge in all spheres, even if it requires the death of animals, is our obligation as the most intelligent species (by far) on earth" (p. 1).

These sociobiological attempts to justify human use of animals illustrate not just the challenge of relating facts to morality, but also (a vital concern of my work here) the devilish difficulty of defining the "facts" in the first place. Note how Morrison's defense of vivisection requires both establishing the "fact" that animal use is natural (are there predatory genes that somehow also encode for scientific curiosity?) as well as the argument (dismissed by David Hume, and later by G. E. Moore, who applied the term "naturalistic fallacy" [MacNabb 1967; Moore 1903]) that what is natural is what is moral.

I find little in either the all-inclusive Schweitzerian reverence for life ethic or in the all-exclusive sociobiological focus on human evolution that would help to prioritize and make sense of animal welfare policy. In both of these approaches, the facts about animals drop out as irrelevant, and there is no guidance as to which species get the greatest protections, or what sorts of protections they get. In contrast, most philosophers of animal ethics focus intently on what it is about animals that would determine their moral status.

Consider briefly two opposing groups of philosophers, the contractarians and the liberationists, who do incorporate animal capacities into their moral reasoning, but who set the bar either so low or so high that either all or no animals are included. On the one hand, we have the contractarian philosophers such as Peter Carruthers, Carl Cohen, and Michael A. Fox. All offer a version of the theory that rights are limited to members of a moral community of equals, who share an implicit contract to recognize each other's rights. Membership in such a moral community requires a pretty high level of cognitive functioning: the ability to think in moral, rational and abstract terms and to act intentionally, in other words, the capacity for autonomy (Carruthers 1992; Cohen 1986; M. A. Fox 1986).

For the contractarian philosophers, the basis of morality is the mutual respect of autonomous equals. Their bar is set quite high for nonhuman animals to gain access; so high, indeed, that most have simply stated it as axiomatic that animals fail to qualify. Others quickly dismiss contemporary studies of intelligence or language acquisition in great apes as uncertain or unconvincing. But even those of their challengers who take such studies seriously (David DeGrazia, for example, and many of the contributors to Paola Cavalieri and Peter Singer's Great Ape Project)[5] see only the smallest handful of nonhuman contenders (chimps, gorillas, bonobos, and maybe orangutans) as possibly autonomous enough to warrant rights within the contractarians' framework. You can see here a scientific question with important philosophical implications: how closely does ape intelligence equal ours?[6]

However, not everyone restricts morality to a contract among equals. Liberationist philosophers focus not on a creature's capacity to engage in moral behavior, but on his or her capacity to suffer from the immoral behavior of others. In other words, you need not believe that dogs are capable of acting as your equal in a moral capacity to believe that how you treat them can be very much a question of morality. This passage from the eighteenth-century philosopher Jeremy Bentham has been quoted to the point of cliché, but it is still a powerful articulation of the basis of (some) animal liberationist thought:

> The day has been, I grieve to say in many places it is not yet past, in which the greater part of the species, under the denomination of slaves, have been treated by the law exactly upon the same footing as, in England for example, the inferior races of animals are still. The day *may come,* when the rest of animal creation may acquire those rights which never could have been withholden from them but by the hand of tyranny. The French have already discovered that the blackness of the skin is no reason why a human being should be abandoned without redress to the caprice of a tormentor. It may come one day to be recognized that the number of the legs, or the villosity of the skin, or the termination of the *os sacrum,* are reasons equally insufficient for abandoning a sensitive being to the same fate. What else is it that should trace the insuperable line? Is it the faculty of reason, or, perhaps, the faculty of discourse? But a full-grown horse or dog is beyond comparison a more rational, as well as a more conversable animal, than an infant of a day, or a week, or even a month, old. But suppose they were otherwise, what would it avail? the question is not, Can they *reason?* nor, Can they *talk?* but, Can they *suffer?* (Bentham 1789, p. 311)

The key concept of animal liberationist philosophy is that creatures incapable of acting as moral agents may nevertheless be objects of moral concern. But neither sidestepping the question of animals' intellectual equality, nor granting human superiority on this measure, excuses the liberationists from considering of the mental capacities of animals.

For Singer (1990), for instance, the most minimal capacity for pleasure and pain is sufficient to warrant equal consideration of sentient animals' interests. Demonstrate (or assume) that animals suffer when in pain, and you have demonstrated a moral obligation to spare them pain as you would a similarly afflicted human.

For his part, Regan focuses on consciousness, though not the high-level self-reflexive consciousness that is the province of the contractarians' autonomous rational agents. Most adult mammals, Regan contends, have sufficient consciousness to make them "the experiencing subject of a life." Their lives matter to them. They are not merely some bit of protoplasm reacting to external forces, but individuals possessed of some level of awareness. Such a level of consciousness is sufficient, in Regan's mind, to make them rights holders. As rights holders, humans and other animals must never be used simply as the means to another's ends, no matter how benign that use may seem.

Rollin has been particularly influential among veterinarians, scientists, and policy-makers. Rather than focus on sentience (like Singer) or consciousness (like Regan), Rollin finds the case for animal rights in the interests that their lives give them, their "functional nature," to which he applies the Greek word *telos.* Their *telos* is inherent in their being, not imposed from outside of themselves. A car has a telos or purpose, but one imposed on it by its human manufacturers. In contrast, a spider "has an intrinsic nature, one that requires it to be alive . . . its life consists precisely in the struggle to perform these [life] functions, to actualize this nature, to fulfill these needs, to maintain this life . . . to preserve its integrity and unity" (Rollin 1992, pp. 75–76). It has a *telos*, born of its evolution and genes, not imposed from without. Whereas Regan and Singer seem to have excluded spiders from their moral sphere, Rollin argues that any creature with evidence of interests, whether or not that creature has evident sentience or the capacity to suffer, "is worthy of being an object of moral concern." As he points out, a frequent characterization of cruel and sadistic people is that "they would pull the wings off of flies" (p. 96).

Because Rollin focuses more on an animal's *telos* than on sentience, the rights he would recognize go beyond mere pleasure and pain, cruelty and kindness. He urges us to give animals lives in which they can "flourish after their kind," and do the things that they are designed by their genetic constitution to do. "Fish gotta swim and birds gotta fly," he says (Rollin 1995, p. 17). He looks to ethologists, carefully studying the behavior of the wild and domestic animals around us, to tell us what the rest of animalkind "gotta do."

Marginal cases and drawing the line

Just as controversy studies provide sociologists and historians a window into how scientists evaluate, endorse, accept, or reject claims of scientific fact, so "marginal cases" illuminate philosophers' reasoning. Both the proponents and opponents of expanded moral protections for animals have marginal case considerations to address. How they handle them depends greatly on what they claim to know about animals and how they claim to know it.

Contractarians who exclude animals as incapable of being fully autonomous participants in the moral community face the marginal case of humans who are similarly deficient (especially if we accept as fact that a severely deficient human is less rational, conscious, and autonomous than a fully functioning adult dog, dolphin, monkey, or ape). This is the point where Cohen (1986) drops his call for limiting rights to the autonomous and retreats to species-based arguments: infants and the severely retarded get rights because their close relatives, their species-mates (i.e., normal adult humans), do on the whole meet his criteria for morally autonomous rights holders. So just when his contractarian reasoning might really help us analyze cases, he drops it, and in the process, undermines contractarianism as a useful tool in animal ethics.[7]

Animal liberationists like Regan, Singer, and Rollin have a different set of marginal cases to worry about, and this is where assessment of animal minds really starts to become important. Erasing the line between human and nonhuman is only half of Regan's and Singer's projects. Those who would erase, or at least, smudge, the line between humans and animals face the inevitable question, Where *do* we draw the line? If we include dogs and monkeys in our moral sphere, why not fish? Amoebas? It's a question familiar to vegetarians, what I call the "how can you kill broccoli?" challenge.

The line-drawing question of which species deserve moral protections is paramount in animal welfare public policy. The major federal policies regulating animal use are quite explicit in their inclusions and exclusions, and animal protectionists have devoted enormous resources throughout the 1990s to expanding Animal Welfare Act coverage to rats, mice, and birds. Moreover, part of the Animal Welfare Act's mandate to consider alternatives to painful uses of experimental animals can include replacement of some animals with plants, cell cultures, microorganisms or other "lower" animal species.

The point bears repeating, as it is the central concern of this book: What we humans do about animals depends on what we know (or think we know) about them. And the central fact we want to know about animals in this context is how their minds are working. If we choose to follow Singer's prescription in our practical decisions about animals' lives, we must have some idea of which animals are capable of experiencing pleasures and pains, which animals have the capacity to suffer. If we are moved by Regan's arguments, we must have some sense of which animals are sufficiently conscious to be subjects of their lives.

Because drawing the line is currently so important in public policy, and because it is an illustrative example of philosophers' relationship with knowledge about animals, let us take a closer look at how some current philosophers handle the issue. Many current animal ethicists are explicitly political and fully recognize and encourage potential links between their academic work and public policy. As such, they draw a distinction between the philosophical implications of their work and the immediate pragmatic political implications. How they prioritize their political goals is one more reflection of how they draw the line among species.

"Ought implies can," says Rollin (1992, p. 138), borrowing from and building on Kant; it is not for the moral philosopher to prescribe action that cannot be realized. Rollin is deeply pragmatic and realizes our society is not about to turn away from eating meat or from potentially beneficial animal research any too quickly. Like Singer, he sees enough that is clearly wrong with present practice and feels little need to belabor the subtleties, the marginal cases, as he rolls up his sleeves to get down to cases. His generous inclusion of protozoa and flatworms as creatures deserving of moral concern loses some of its radical flavor in the face of his concern with animal *pain* (and to a slightly lesser degree, animal death), especially the pain of those animals least foreign to the human observer, the vertebrates (Rollin 1992).

Regan, too, proposes a pragmatic first step in line drawing that may not map precisely onto his philosophical argument. Regan's focus is on those animals with sufficient consciousness to be the subjects of their own lives. He writes as though there is indeed in nature a sharp divide between those creatures who have this consciousness and those who do not. Among those who have it, they have it equally; they are equal rights holders deserving equal consideration. To deny them this is an immoral act. But what creatures have this consciousness, where to draw the line? Regan is not entirely sure, but assumes that most normally functioning adult mammals over the age of one year meet his criteria. Freely admitting that this agenda for action, especially the one year criterion, is arbitrary, he claims that it is less arbitrary than considering two-month-old human infants to be full rights holders while excluding adult dogs. While the jury (of philosophers? of scientists?) is out, he is content to propose this political readjustment, giving the benefit of the doubt to some marginal cases—younger mammals, frogs, *maybe* snails (Regan 1983).

Singer's approach to line drawing is illustrative, as he explains his shift from the first to the second edition of *Animal Liberation* (1990) on the moral status of oysters. For Singer, sentience (particularly sensitivity to pain) is the focus, rather than subjectivity, consciousness, or *telos*. Singer argues that behavior, neural anatomy/ physiology, and evolutionary arguments all converge on the certainty that vertebrate animals do feel pain more or less similarly to the way that humans do. And as for invertebrates, Singer suggested in 1975 a divide between the crustacea (shrimp, lobsters) and the neurologically less sophisticated mollusks (at least the clams and oysters, though probably not their remarkable cousin, the octopus). In 1990 he is less convinced. Once outside of his moral compass, oysters have now acquired benefit-of-the-doubt status. Oysters are hardly an essential of anyone's nutrition, and so in the face of uncertainty about their possible sentience, Singer refrains from eating them. Whether he would find their use as a research substitute for mammals acceptable is left unstated (Singer 1990). Perhaps because he is not strongly defending this particular boundary between animals of moral concern and those outside, Singer leaves it as a change of heart (and diet) based on conversations with another philosopher rather than new data or theoretical advances in cognitive psychology of oysters.

Like Regan and Singer, Rollin also prioritizes among animals when his philosophy waxes political. A spider is his illustrative case of an animal with a *telos* to respect, but he does draw a line, as he quickly dismisses plants, bacteria, viruses, and cells in culture, though alive, as insufficiently aware or conscious to have interests that would merit moral concern. And though spiders warrant his concern on paper, in actual fact they have received little of his political attention; he has pragmatically set aside the marginal cases as he has testified before legislatures on behalf of stronger standards for laboratory animal care (Rollin 1992, p. 96).

For the most part, contractarians and liberationists can work with precisely the same assessment of animal mental capacities and come out with vastly different prescriptions on animal experimentation (or any other exploitation or harm of animals). A few wrinkles notwithstanding (cognitive studies of great apes that suggest something close to human autonomy; Carruthers's and some other philosophers' insistence that animals do not have sufficient consciousness even to merit concern in Singer's sentience-based ethics), both camps agree that (some) animals are capable of feeling pleasure and pain and that few if any count as autonomous rational agents. They treat the large majority of research animal species (sentient vertebrate fish and frogs and mammals and birds, who nonetheless cannot count as autonomous) differently not because of epistemological differences in what they believe to be true about these animals but because of differing ethical prescriptions of what should count in granting someone moral consideration.

But these liberationist and antiliberationist philosophers really are working at opposite extremes. For the most part, those who are working directly on policy and regulatory questions, those making decisions about individual animals living in laboratories, occupy a middle zone in which epistemological assessments about animals make all the difference.

The central importance of who knows what about animals will be especially crucial as we look more closely at policy debates: Do dogs need exercise? When should research animals get painkillers? Must guinea pigs get bigger cages? Can nonscientists contribute to the review of animal research proposals? Who should have the authority to make these determinations, or, in short, who shall have the authority to speak for the animals?

Cost and benefit in animal research ethics

Between the extremes of abolitionism and laissez-faire, any foray into research animal ethics and policy requires some sort of assessment and weighing of costs (especially the costs to animal welfare) and benefits (in gains in knowledge important to humans). This is true no matter what your philosophical basis for believing that animal welfare warrants consideration.

Those writing for a scientific or veterinary audience have tended to reduce moral philosophy to utilitarian/consequentialist versus deontological/rights-based ethical theories, a legacy of the historical influence of Singer's and Regan's writing. I find little use in overplaying the distinction in most applications of ethics to specific animal research questions and believe that utilitarianism, rights-based approaches, and any others all require some assessment of consequences for their application in this sphere.

Utilitarians, by definition, assess the costs and benefits, pleasures and pains, goods and harms associated with any proposed act in deciding its morality. The extension of utilitarianism to animals is the central thesis of Singer's work and requires that harm to animals be included in deciding the morality of a proposed research project. While Singer believes the animal suffering in vivisection to be so extensive as to rule out most experiments, others find the benefits of research so overwhelming as to overshadow any attendant animal suffering (Robb 1991).

Utilitarianism, especially its simplest form, act utilitarianism, has certain problems that are imported with it when applying it to animal ethics. Act utilitarianism risks riding roughshod over individuals if that will sufficiently advance the common good, a concern that requires modifying the theory somewhat, or tempering it with a rightslike focus on what happens to individuals. It can be incredibly arduous trying to calculate all the costs and benefits every time a decision is made, a process made simpler in some modifications of the theory, such as rule utilitarianism, developing rules, which, if adopted, would maximize good consequences.

An essential concern about utilitarian approaches to animal welfare issues is that costs and benefits, pleasures and pains, must somehow be quantified. Patrick Bateson (1986), for instance, develops an intriguing three-dimensional decision model for deciding when the quality of a project and the probability of generating important research results are high enough to warrant inflicting a certain level of animal suffering. The enormous difficulty of making those calculations fit into the model is of vital importance; rights-based theories offer a way around that challenge, but not successfully.

Deontological rights-based theories are often found at the two extremes of abolition or of laissez-faire. They are congenial to antivivisectionist positions, if (like Regan and unlike Cohen) one does not restrict rights to those autonomous agents who are capable of respecting the rights of others. On the other hand, the contractarian rights theorists like Cohen make just the opposite case by restricting rights to humans. But many rights theorists occupy that middle ground; they would recognize rights for animals and still see justification for some animal research. Tannenbaum (1986), for instance, links rights to "welfare interests," which he argues animals possess. He differs from the animal liberationists in believing that some pressing human interests (including our search for medical knowledge through animal research) could justifiably override these rights and interests of animals. But he carefully accepts the notion of rights to suggest that "there are some ways of treating animals that are beyond the moral pale because of basic claims that animals have" (p. 1259).

Barbara Orlans and colleagues (1998) make a similar point in their discussion of thresholds in the justification of animal research, whether generally or for specific projects: "It is also unclear whether research that exceeds a certain threshold or upper limit of pain, suffering, anxiety, fear, and distress can be justified" (pp. 32–33). They point out the convention in use of human subjects in research of incorporating some balancing of benefits and potential costs as well as insisting on thresholds, "for example, upper levels of risk, pain, and discomfort" (p. 33).

Orlans et al. (1998) also worry that a cost-benefit approach to animal ethics will frequently underrepresent animals' interests, and they note that, in animal research, "Humans receive the benefits, animals the costs. Animals are subjects or objects of sacrifice; humans are not," and they go on to argue, "Cost-benefit analysis is an essential tool of public policy, but deciding issues of animal welfare through cost-benefit tradeoffs may be morally less satisfactory than looking directly and sympathetically at the suffering involved by animals and placing a limit on that suffering through [setting] thresholds [beyond which animals should not be harmed]" (pp. 35, 36).

But notice here that shifting from a straightforward, utilitarian cost-benefit scheme to a consideration of thresholds does nothing to deliver us from the major challenge of utilitarian animal welfare: the need to assess what animals are feeling. My conclusion is that no matter how we phrase it, if we are going to use animals in research but hope to set some moral limits on that use, we are committed to somehow assessing the quality and quantity of animal pain, distress, happiness, boredom, joy, loneliness, fear, and so on, that make up animal welfare. And we somehow need to assess the quality and quantity of benefit (including potential, future benefit) to be drawn from a particular research program.

Many of these philosophers write as though assessing animal welfare costs is a pretty straightforward business, or at the worst, a technical challenge that animal welfare scientists are on their way to solving. As Jane Smith and Kenneth Boyd (1991) point out, "It might be argued that weighing as suggested here is not possible, since there are no units of human (or animal) benefit and of cost to animals which could make these commensurable" (p. 140). But this is precisely what IACUCs somehow do, day in and day out. Smith and Boyd write, "Certainly, if weighing is thought of in terms of a mathematical calculus, this is correct. In everyday life, however, personal, professional and political judgments on moral issues normally require the weighing of factors and considerations which cannot be quantified with mathematical precision" (p. 140).

Smith and Boyd (1991) offer a scheme for scoring just this sort of rough assessment of animal research costs and benefits. Theirs is a three-dimensional decision model with potential benefits (the value of the hoped-for outcome), likelihood of achieving those benefits in a particular laboratory or experiment, and animal suffering represented on its three axes. Their working ethic is not so controversial: "Research involving more than mild animal suffering ought not to proceed unless there is the likelihood that significant benefit will result" (pp. 140–141). They offer scales to quantify animal suffering and likelihood of significant benefit but offer no magic key to tell how to weight one against the other.

Boundary work: Philosophy + science = animal welfare

At this point, I hope you agree that there is much more to laboratory animal welfare policy than the polarized yes–no big question of whether to allow animal research. The consensus position throughout the late twentieth century, reflected in American public policy, is that animal research is justifiable and allowable, while simultaneously animal welfare must be protected. If that ethical consensus continues, then we must address the questions of how to assess animal welfare, how to assess the benefits of animal research, and how to balance one against the other. My focus in this book is on the first of those three needs: the assessment of animal welfare.

Before we leave this chapter's visit to the pristine world of the philosopher for our examination of philosophy-in-action (i.e., politics and policy making), it is worthwhile to focus on those philosophers who have devoted some attention to a muddy area where science and philosophy intersect: animal welfare studies.

Moral philosophers have really just four options about what to do with the facts about animals as they weave their animal ethic. The first, characterized by the sociobiological and the reverence-for-life approaches that try to ignore animals' natures entirely, is untenable in its failure to distinguish among animals. The second option is to work entirely with common sense and armchair knowledge of animals, to take as the starting assumption that animals do feel pain, that they are clearly our intellectual inferiors, and that they do not have true languages. Connections among these facts (such as that animals, lacking language, cannot be conscious or rational, or conversely, that animals showing strong social or maternal behaviors must have strong moral sense) may be logically compelling, but if the assumptions are put to the test and fail, so does the philosophy.

And what better way to put assumptions about animals to the test than through scientific study? Thus, virtually all current, in-depth treatments of animal ethics engage scientific information about animals, such as studies of language use in apes, but especially studies of pain perception in animals. And here we find philosophers' two remaining options. Do they politely respect the boundary between science and philosophy, leave fact making to the scientists, and then use those facts in their philosophizing? Or do they muddy the water, challenge the professional boundaries, and encroach on scientists' professional jurisdiction of making and certifying scientific knowledge?

Singer does a little of both. Let's look again at Singer's shifting ruling on the ethics of eating oysters. In the fifteen years between the two editions of *Animal Liberation,* he did not change his basic philosophy that similar interests of sentient beings deserve equal consideration regardless of what species those beings belong to. "Sentient beings" are pretty much those capable of suffering from the perception of pain. Rather than simply rest on the common-sense presumption that animals (at least, the familiar mammals and birds) obviously are capable of pain perception, Singer lines up his allies among scientists. He cites neurologists, animal behaviorists, and "three separate expert government committees on matters related to animals," to add legitimacy to the claim that animals perceive pain, as well as fear, anxiety, and stress (Singer 1990, p. 13). It is then his purview as philosopher to put that scientific fact into its moral context.

Because part of Singer's project is replacing the line that separates human from nonhuman with a line between sentient and nonsentient, he must consider his marginal cases, where to draw that line. In updating *Animal Liberation* for the 1990 edition, Singer strengthens his case for the inclusion of crustaceans with the experimental observations of the impressively credentialed John Baker, a zoologist at the University of Oxford and a fellow of the Royal Society, who concludes, to the ethical diner's dismay, that lobsters do, indeed, feel pain (Baker and Dolan 1977). Oysters remain an uncertain case for Singer, though he has shifted to giving them more the benefit of the doubt; however, for this change of mind he does not cite scientists' data on oyster neurophysiology but rather his private conversations with another philosopher.

Recall, however, that Singer is not an all-inclusive reverence-for-life advocate, but limits his sphere of moral concern to those creatures who are sentient: "If a being is not capable of suffering, or of enjoyment, there is nothing to take into account" (1990, p. 171). So ethical people do not eat sentient animals and they give oysters the benefit of the doubt; what about plants? As Singer notes, implicit in the call to vegetarianism is the acceptance of killing and eating plants. Noting that some have proposed some pain sensation even in plants, he dismisses the possibility, not by addressing the data head-on, but by dismissing the credibility of the relevant studies because they were "not carried out at serious research institutions" and attempts by "researchers in major universities" failed to find evidence of sentience in plants (p. 235).

So Singer picks and chooses his scientific citations as a trial lawyer might pick his expert witnesses, building the case that animals, including lobsters, feel pain while plants do not; on this he can base his moral prescriptions for vegetarianism. But note that he does not engage the data directly. He does not prescribe how scientists *ought* to study pain sensation in lobsters, plants, and oysters, what experiments they should run, or how they should analyze their data. He leaves that to their discretion, while still not treating all scientists or all scientific data as equally valid. He respects their control, as a professional group, over the jurisdiction of fact making. He justifies his preference for one scientist's work over another's through the external indicators of their own regard for each other's status: membership in the Royal Society, participation on government-sanctioned expert committees, employment at serious or less serious universities and research institutions.

An attorney, ethicist, and professor of veterinary ethics, Tannenbaum takes a different approach to the demarcation between science and philosophy, between fact and value. He carves out a place for philosophy and value inquiry in the study of animal welfare, even as he reinforces the separate domain of scientists. Like Rollin, Tannenbaum has published extensively in veterinary texts and journals and taught ethics at veterinary colleges. Both have argued for an expanded moral concern for animals, for moving beyond issues of animal health and disease (especially health and disease conceived of as purely physical phenomena). Both Tannenbaum (1986) and Rollin (1995) espouse a notion of animal rights that still allows for human use of animals for food or experimentation, and both have urged veterinarians to distance themselves somewhat from the more extreme wing of the animal rights movement.

Of course, we will want to know which animal species might have rights and strong welfare interests, where to draw the line. That is not Tannenbaum's project, and he does not voice a strong opinion on that. He excludes inanimate objects such as buildings, statues, rocks, and rivers, but he does not elaborate on whether it would be similarly nonsensical to speak of plants having interests, or where insects or even fish might fit in. For discussions and examples, Tannenbaum restricts himself almost exclusively to mammals (1995).

Regardless of who is admitted to our circle of concern, we also want to know what composes animals' welfare, bringing us once again to our central concern: Who knows what about animals' minds? Throughout his work, Tannenbaum displays great respect to veterinarians and to scientists. He writes with them as a primary audience and urges them to high standards, clear thinking, to recognition of the value of their work. Nevertheless, he does not cede the recognition of animal welfare totally to veterinarians or to "animal welfare scientists." In particular, Tannenbaum critiques what he calls the "pure science" model of animal welfare studies, the idea that welfare is a scientific concept that can be separated from values and ethics: "Adherents of the pure science model all insist that deciding what conditions are relevant to animal welfare and determining whether such states are present, is a purely factual, descriptive task that does not involve making value judgments" (Tannenbaum 1995, p. 153).

Tannenbaum points out the value-laden nature of decisions about animal welfare research, such as which animals, which issues to study and fund, or how to use our findings. "The choice of which animals' welfare is worth understanding reflects value judgments about which animals *ought* to be protected or helped. For example, there exist in most cities large numbers of rats, which can be quite dangerous to people and other animals. Few but the hardiest animal activists would suggest that we should worry about these animals' general welfare" (1995, p. 155).

However, the expectation that some studies will not attract funding or that their results would be ignored in practice does not in itself undermine the theoretical possibility that welfare can be cast as a purely empirical question. Wisely, Tannenbaum takes it further than that.

What is animal welfare? Tannenbaum (1995) catalogs a "tower of Babel" of welfare definitions gleaned from several animal welfare scientists. Here are a few candidates: absence of suffering; mental well-being; physical well-being; freedom from pain and suffering; absence of stress or distress; complete harmony with the environment; fulfillment of needs; and physiological systems that allow survival or reproduction. These definitions are not mutually exclusive.

If some or all of these definitions of welfare are correct, they lend themselves to scientific measurement through a variety of methodologies: preference studies, pathological examination (including psychopathology), assessment of reproductive parameters, analysis of stress hormone levels, and immune function assays. If these definitions are correct, then animal welfare scientists might draw boundaries around their nascent discipline that exclude nonscientific voices, whether the reasoned and respectful Tannenbaum or the rowdy animal rights activists carrying placards on the streets.

Tannenbaum points out, I think quite correctly, that it is not how we prioritize welfare (which projects we fund, which species we favor) that undermines the "pure science" model, but how we *define* welfare. For example, a point I will explore more fully when we look at dog exercise regulations, "someone who defines welfare in terms of the fulfillment of needs will not recognize as independently relevant to welfare the fulfillment of what might better be termed 'wants'" (Tannenbaum 1995, p. 162). Tannenbaum hints at something DeGrazia develops more formally, that there is a philosophical question of how we balance subjective theories of value or welfare (such as what an animal *wants* or how an animal *feels*) and objective theories (such as what promotes good health or what is good for the animal). Absent a shared commitment to some value-theory–based definition of welfare, scientists cannot resolve their controversy of how to measure it.

If Tannenbaum can successfully establish an intrinsic component of values and ethics into the definition of welfare, then he would have grounds to challenge

ANIMAL WELFARE: PHILOSOPHY MEETS SCIENCE

the boundaries drawn by any welfare scientists who would exclude him. He would have full right to discuss not just which of their projects to fund, or what to do with their results, but how to conceive of their research questions, interpret their data, frame their hypotheses, and construct their facts, for there is then no part of welfare that is the exclusive domain of scientists.

Tannenbaum stops short of this more radical conclusion. He does not demolish the boundary between scientific empirical study on the one hand and philosophical inquiry on the other. Rather, he simply moves that boundary, with apparent faith that science does indeed produce some facts that are not value laden. Perhaps that is why he finds such a ready readership among veterinarians. The problem as Tannenbaum presents it is not so much with a pure science conception of science itself; the problem is trying to slip a bit too much (in this case, the concept of welfare) into the domain of pure science. Indeed, he details a catalog of "scientific issues" or "unresolved factual issues" about laboratory animals— questions relating to pain and other "negative mental states"—in need of further study, all phrased in perfect harmony with a pure science paradigm (Tannenbaum 1995, p. 478).

Tannenbaum leaves the scientists' jurisdiction intact, smaller perhaps than they might originally have staked it, but sovereign nonetheless. He leaves the study of pain to scientists, with his agenda of "unresolved factual issues" about laboratory animals for them to resolve, while policy makers work out a regulatory definition of pain (that would standardize reporting to the USDA, for instance) and philosophers discuss whether it "may sometimes be preferable to cause more *total* pain if doing so will cause less pain to each individual animal" (Tannenbaum 1995, p. 477).

This sort of boundary redrawing, and respect for the boundaries drawn, allows ethicists and scientists to have their own jurisdictions. Respecting each other's turf, scientists and ethicists may talk congenially to one another, even if sometimes they may just talk past each other.

Much less inclined to let scientists have their private jurisdiction is the ethicist Rollin. His *The Unheeded Cry* (1989) is a probing examination of how scientific ideology can create scientific facts with profound animal welfare implications. Rollin examines how the psychological school of behaviorism, born of an era when physics ruled the sciences and rigor was equated with reductionism, led to a conception of animals as mindless automata, a scientific milieu in which it was always inappropriate to speculate on animals' minds or feelings. Mindless automata do not have interests; they do not suffer in a meaningful way. As René Descartes did centuries ago for the physiologists, twentieth-century behaviorists did for experimental biologists: they gave philosophical (though packaged as scientific) permission to discount whatever animal pain or suffering their experiments might cause (Rollin 1989).[8]

Rollin has relentlessly challenged the boundaries among philosophy and science and politics. He has found a wide audience among research scientists, veterinarians, ranchers, and other animal users. He has testified before the U.S. Congress and has consulted for several governments on animal welfare policy matters. He has edited a two-volume technical text on research animal care and use and several articles in veterinary, animal science, and agricultural journals (Rollin and Kesel 1990, 1995). His work has been overtly political and has successfully influenced policy and how people treat animals.

Rollin's castigation of behaviorists is not an indictment of scientists generally. Rejecting psychological behaviorism, for example, he embraces ethology, naturalistic studies of animal behavior.[9] He has evident faith in the wisdom of ethology and urges faculties to teach it in introductory biology classes. "In the final analysis, we can understand the wants, needs, desires, and interests of other creatures. Perhaps in a deep sense we can understand those better than we can understand the needs of other humans despite language, because there are apparently so few layers of deception in animals" (Rollin 1992, p. 94).

Beyond Tannenbaum's suggested list of questions about animal pain in need of further scientific study, Rollin would prescribe not just the topics but the method of science used. Is it that ethologists are less tainted by ideology than the behaviorists are? Or simply that if ethologists have embedded value biases in their science, they are values that Rollin finds more correct?

Rollin (1995) offers guidance to the sorts of empirical studies—both the questions to address as well as the methodologies—needed to better characterize animal pain and suffering. As he sees it, animal welfare research should not rely too heavily on some of its traditional methodologies, such as measuring the stress hormone cortisol or quantifying abnormal and stereotypical behaviors.[10] The critical public, he asserts, will not tolerate research if they cannot see its relationship to how animals feel. Nor will they accept the thesis that stereotypic behaviors are coping methods that make bad situations tolerable; if situations are bad enough to elicit such pathological coping measurements, they are beyond the pale of public tolerance. Rollin's public (not always clearly defined, but evidently a reasonable, morally virtuous majority who are neither animal-using professionals [farmers, scientists] nor extreme animal rights proponents) will not tolerate research that flies in the face of common sense or that merely proves what we all already know (such as that animals are indeed capable of perceiving pain).

Though Rollin is savvy to public perceptions, he is not interested merely in window dressing, in advising researchers, for example, how to mollify an uneasy public while proceeding with their research business-as-usual. Rather, Rollin's focus on public perception reflects both his ideological commitment to the validity of common-sense knowledge and his political conviction that meaningful change does not come from the fringes but from some common ground. Faith in common-sense knowledge allows him to assess without intimidation the work of animal welfare scientists, veterinarians, agriculturalists, and others who would speak for animals under the mantle of expert knowledge.

Rollin's forays into biology and animal behavior are impressive, and his work has provided much of the inspiration for my current efforts. Rollin and I part in our views of much of the more controversial cases in animal welfare science. Controversy studies have been a crucial concern of sociologists and philosophers of science, especially those inclined toward "social constructivism" as an explanatory framework. Rollin shows little patience for scientists who would hide behind controversial knowledge claims to avoid changing their treatment of animals—common sense alone tells us that many current scientific uses of animals cause them great pain and distress. But whereas Rollin may tend to downplay controversial and competing interpretations of animal welfare data, I have found the controversial questions to be important windows into seeing how decisions are made.

Consider Rollin's (1992) discussion of the Draize test, that now-notorious test of ocular toxicity in which toxicologists instill test substances into the eyes of conscious, restrained rabbits. Lab personnel score the irritancy to rabbit eyes, and regulators read in this a measure of potential safety for human eyes. No one seems to particularly like the Draize test, but its use persists. Rollin points to controversy in the validity of the test. While one author claims that rabbit eyes are less sensitive to irritants than are human eyes (in which case a toxic substance could slip through undetected), "other 'experts' claim the opposite . . . identifying irritants that would not affect human eyes!" (Rollin 1992, p.147).

What Rollin fails to address in his consideration of the Draize test, however, is *how* experts could disagree on such a point. And this is important, I would argue, for not every controversial assessment of what animals might feel will be swept away with wholesale condemnation of the practice under question. Rollin is so quick to dismiss some scientists' efforts as stupid, illogical, redundant, or otherwise discordant with common sense that one is left hungry for the scientists' version of why they would resort to such mindless chicanery. Scientists may require different standards of evidence, trust one type of research over another, or (just like Singer's condemnation of studies of plants' putative sentience) trust some scientists and institutions and journals more than others. Does this mean that they are only "experts" in quotes? Or does it mean simply that experts can interpret data differently, with real-world implications for practice? Either way, developing animal welfare policy that truly reflects what is best for animals will require navigating among competing claims of expert knowledge that neither embrace all claims as equally valid nor reject them all as equally specious.

Finally, let us come back to the philosopher DeGrazia's (1996) claim that "The path to the ethical treatment of animals runs through their minds" (p. 76). This is not precisely equal to saying that animal welfare is determined by how animals feel. (Well, it is, actually, but only with the stipulation that *where* animals feel, in a morally relevant way, is in their minds.) DeGrazia convincingly argues that the kind of animal feelings that call for moral attention from people are those that are sufficiently conscious, sufficiently present in an animal's awareness, to meaningfully warrant words such as "suffering." This is how DeGrazia deals with the marginal case issue: he would treat similar interests similarly pretty much regardless of species membership, but he believes that only individuals of a certain level of consciousness can reasonably be said to have interests. You may destroy a plant's life in harvesting it for dinner, but the plant presumably does not have sufficient (if any) consciousness to have what could reasonably be called an interest in avoiding this destruction.

Like many philosophers working with an eye to modern evolutionary biology, where specifically DeGrazia draws the line is not all that specific. To the extent that some type of self-awareness confers enhanced moral status, he writes: "Our inevitable conclusion is that *self-awareness is not all-or-nothing but comes in degrees and in different forms*" (1996, p. 182, emphasis in original). He would erase the "thick ontological line between humans and other animals" (p. 182). Not only does he see the biopsychological capacities (like self-awareness) that confer moral status as existing on a continuum (with corresponding degrees of moral consideration due), but also he sees a complex web of morally significant capacities that interact with each other. The abilities to perceive pain, distress, fear, and anxiety may all be morally significant, but present in varying degrees in various animals: "That fish can have anxious states is much less firmly established . . . and it is conceivable that some animals, maybe fish, can experience pain and distress, yet not suffer, because their pain and distress never gets very intense" (p. 128).[11]

This complexity in DeGrazia's philosophy, in which various capacities have both physical and mental components, are present to varying degrees in various animals, and are only indirectly knowable, foreshadow the complexity we will see in the historical development of animal welfare policy.

Take animal pain, for example, a concern that runs through decades of welfare policy debates. Really, if inflicting pain on animals is not a moral issue, then what of animal ethics could possibly be? But if DeGrazia is correct that the locus of animal welfare is in animals' minds, how does the intensely physical experience of pain fit in? DeGrazia follows Rollin in drawing ethical distinctions between nociception (the neurophysiology or "hardware" of pain perception, the wiring that gets pain impulses from throughout the body into the brain) and the mind's conscious perception of pain as an emotionally unpleasant experience. It is conceivable that some animals (insects, perhaps) might have nociceptive capabilities, can detect and respond to what we might class as noxious or potentially damaging stimuli, without having the sophisticated mental apparatus for consciously unpleasant pain perception. Furthermore, some animals (sharks, for instance) may have the capacity for both nociception and pain, but do not have much capacity to experience anxiety, blunting some of the intense displeasure of pain and in the process reducing their pain's moral significance.

If the moral significance of physical/emotional hybrid phenomena such as pain and anxiety depends on knowing which animals have them in which form and to what extent, it is no surprise to find disagreement among those who would speak for animals in the policy arena. Is it the neuropharmacologists and neurophysiologists who study such things as pain pathways and anxiety centers? The ethologists who study behavioral manifestations that presumably flow from these internal states? The veterinarians who treat the animal body with painkillers and the animal mind with tranquilizers? Or the mass of untrained nonexperts who find their common-sense intuition largely vindicated by the scientists' discoveries:

that animals are a jumble of physical and mental experiences arranged roughly along some sort of evolutionary hierarchy that warrants differing but substantial moral consideration?

Conclusion

In this chapter, I have looked at the animal ethics philosophies that might inform and shape our treatment of animals. The review has not been exhaustive; that would require a book in itself, of which several already exist.[12] Moreover, I have steered clear of the big question of animal rights. In our current society, we do indeed allow some quite frightening uses of animals, but we nonetheless hope to contain them within some ethical bounds. The abolitionist position of a strong animal rights philosophy does not require policy-related questions about animal welfare: how to recognize it, how to respect it. Incrementalist and reformist approaches to laboratory animal policy cannot ignore those questions.

Any ethical framework that allows some limited use of animals for human ends requires some sort of comparison of costs and benefits. Even those who would grant limited rights to animals allow that human interests will sometimes overrule those rights. The challenge is not just how to estimate benefits in advance of a research project yet to be done, but how to evaluate the costs to animals. In most instances, this requires some sort of assessment of how different types of animals feel under different sorts of conditions.

Many philosophers rest their animal ethics arguments on facts about animal minds: some are drawn from common sense and observation; some are feats of logic; some are drawn from the scientific literature. Some of these facts are more controversial than others. "Making facts" is a job of scientists that some philosophers have challenged and others have left intact as they navigate the boundary between their disciplines. By allowing scientists their own jurisdiction of fact making, philosophers are able to focus on their own efforts (politely waiting while scientists fill in the knowledge gaps) and can expect a reciprocal respect for their own profession.

Despite Descartes's assertion of centuries ago, the dualism between mind and body may just not hold up in the light of twenty-first-century biopsychology, where the most esoteric mental functions appear to be cerebral, in both the intellectual and neuroanatomical senses of that word. Materialist philosophy and neuropsychology merge in the conclusion that all mental functions (emotions, thought, consciousness, anxiety, etc.) rest on the physical functioning of the body—mostly, but not exclusively, the brain and the nervous system. Russell and Burch, writing in 1959 about alternatives to painful animal experimentation, brought the word "psychosomiasis" into the animal ethicist's vocabulary, emphasizing the role of animals' mental well-being on their physiology and health. The interdigitation of mind and body may be neither complete nor symmetrical, however, and the possibility that some animals have physical states (such as nociception) without higher cognitive components that true suffering would require further complicate questions of what animals get what sorts of considerations and of who is competent to de-cide. And so we find no shortage of experts arguing about what is true about ani-mals' minds and bodies, what are the best ways to know these truths with cer-tainty, and how these truths should be reflected in animal welfare policy.

In the coming chapters, I examine several of the animal welfare issues that were prominent during the 1980s update of the American Animal Welfare Act: species to include or exclude; roles for veterinarians and lay people in reviewing science; and special provisions for dog and monkey housing. I emphasize the use of facts in policy arguments and examine where those facts came from. Contrary to the scientists' and some philosophers' assumptions that scientific facts are un-problematic statements of how the world works, I emphasize the very human hand (political, philosophical, and social) that shapes the facts that shape the way we think about and speak for what animals want.

4

A rat is a pig: The significance of species

The adaptable dog . . . can be happy whether maintained in a cage or running over tracts of land . . . He can live alone or with a group . . . All he asks is food, sanitation, freedom from parasites and disease; with these, he makes a good and faithful servant, a willing and eager slave. In return for his service, he deserves all the comfort we can afford him.
—Leon Whitney, in *The Care and Breeding of Laboratory Animals*, p. 182

A standardized animal is needed, for a standardized animal is to the biologist what the pure chemical is to the chemist . . . The animal is a very sensitive bit of apparatus.
—Edmond Farris, *The Care and Breeding of Laboratory Animals*, pp. x–xi

On the day a primate animal is introduced into the laboratory, changes and new responsibilities come not only to those in the animal room . . . a minor disturbance is revealed to the observant person—[a health report on a monkey is] a far cry from the finality of the report, "A mouse dead in cage ten." The whole new attitude can be summed up, perhaps, by saying that it is the importance of the individual animal, a primate animal whose needs and wishes we can better understand, whose actions fascinate and sometimes revolt, whose intelligence and emotional life demand a special care lest an injury to the psyche reflect on the soma. And above all, this is an animal of man's own order . . .
—G. Van Wagenen, in *The Care and Breeding of Laboratory Animals*, p. 1

AN ANIMAL'S FATE IN THE LABORATORY HAS A GREAT DEAL TO DO WITH HIS OR HER species. Formally, different species enjoy different levels of protection in federal animal welfare policies. Informally, as the above quotes from a 1950s publication illustrate, different animals do elicit different responses, and nearly all of us who work with laboratory animals will admit to differing levels of care for different species. We treat species differently because they *are* different, but what are those differences, how do we learn about them, and how much differential treatment do they really warrant?

The different species receive different types of treatment not just in the laboratory, but in the rhetorical contests to shape that treatment. In this chapter I describe the central role that dogs played in early efforts to legislate animal experimentation in the United States, the spotlight monkeys and apes were under in the 1980s, and the curious status of rats and mice, numerically most prevalent in the laboratories, but actively excluded from Animal Welfare Act coverage for decades. In the process I show how different species of animals lend themselves to different ethical frameworks and different rhetorical and propagandist strategies.

"All animals are created equal," George Orwell wrote in *Animal Farm* in 1945, "but some are more equal than others." It was true on the animal farm of his novel, and true as well in animal welfare policy.

An animal species' moral and legal status in the laboratory rests on several factors: is it an endangered species? Does it have a backbone? Is it warm-blooded? Is it a farm species or a pet species? Is it domestic or wild? Does it have the mental capacity to experience pain and distress? Is it a member of the order Primates or of the order Rodentia? Is it cute and cuddly?

Within a species, an individual animal's moral and legal status can vary with where she came from and why she's in the lab. Is she a "purpose-bred" or "random source" dog or cat or mouse or rat? Is she a farm animal on agricultural or on biomedical research? Is she an unwanted intruder, a vermin, scurrying in the corners? Is she on a federally funded research program?

We have separate rules in American animal welfare policy for all of these different categories of animals.[1] The rules are important for the animals who are in the laboratories today, but also for how they reflect what we think about animals—their capacities, their needs, their desserts, and our obligations.

Speciesism and species hierarchies

Human or nonhuman: that remains the most important distinction in current policy. In important ways, a chimpanzee, despite what genetic similarities might predict, is closer in legal standing to a mouse, a fish, or even a mosquito than he is to his human cousins. Some animal interests may be protected in various ways by cruelty, welfare, and environmental regulations, but the animals have no legal standing in courts; are property of individuals, organizations, or the state; and may be extensively used as means to human ends. Even laws that protect animals are generally written to promote human interests, as when the Congress finds that the Animal Welfare Act is necessary not because animals matter in and of themselves, but because "measures which help meet the public concern for laboratory animal care and treatment are important in assuring that research will continue to progress" (U.S. Congress 1985a).

Under the provisions of the Animal Welfare Act and the NIH's *Guide for the Care and Use of Laboratory Animals,* not all animal interests lose out to all human interests, but they come pretty close. Both sets of rules are quick to assert that virtually any procedure can be performed on any experimental animal if it is scientifically justified. Still, there are some brakes on the use of laboratory animals, especially potentially painful uses. Under these rules, scientists should assure that their research is not unnecessarily duplicative, and they should consider nonanimal and nonpainful alternatives. They should think long and hard before inflicting pain on animals and should consult with their veterinarian and their IACUC before proceeding. However, the continued practice of painful and distressing experiments too numerous to catalog—toxicity trials and infectious disease experiments and burn studies and others—are testimony to the priority we give human interests over animal interests.

Despite the legal chasm between humans and others, the Animal Welfare Act and the *Guide* do entail sufficient protections for animals to fuel protectionists' efforts to broaden their umbrella over more animal species. Both documents, for example, assert that cost savings alone is not sufficient justification for some practices—the performance of multiple surgeries on a single animal, for instance. And the need for "scientific justification," though left discretely vague in national policy, can yet be a powerful tool for animal welfare in the hands of a conscientious IACUC.

Some animal rights activists dismiss the Animal Welfare Act as limited, useless, or worse (Francione 1995). Others believe it is the closest thing they have to the protections they seek for animals. Because of this, the USDA's exclusion of mice, rats, and birds from Animal Welfare Act coverage generated more mail in the late 1980s than almost any other aspect of the regulations and became the focus of a lawsuit brought forth by the Animal Legal Defense Fund and the Humane Society of the United States in 1990 (Shalev 1994a) and of court cases and special legislative actions at the turn of the millennium.

Backbones and warm blood

Anatomy and physiology confer moral and legal status, but only as proxies for what people seem to care most about: sentience. Despite the warnings of some philosophers of overreliance on such a criterion (Beauchamp 1992; Linzey 1998), public policy focuses heavily on pleasure and pain and suffering and distress as the locus of moral concern for animals. Anatomy and physiology—the possession of a backbone, the ability to regulate one's own body temperature—correlate, very roughly, perhaps, with the subjective mental and emotional experiences people seem to care about safeguarding.

Philosophers look to traits such as sentience and autonomy to draw their moral lines around species. Policy makers also draw lines, though the two major sets of American laboratory animal policies use two different criteria of which animals count. For the NIH, backbones confer legal status.[2] Of far greater concern to animal protectionists than the *Guide* has been the Animal Welfare Act's definition of "animal" over the years. In 1966, the Laboratory Animal Welfare Act was mostly a pet protection law focused on dogs and cats, though with some provisions for other animals. As Congress saw it at the time, "The term 'animal' means live dogs, cats, monkeys (nonhuman primate mammals), guinea pigs, hamsters, and rabbits" (U.S. Congress 1966a). Four years later, it expanded its definition, and things started to get confusing:

> The term "animal" means any live or dead dog, cat, monkey (nonhuman primate mammal), guinea pig, hamster, rabbit, or such other warm-blooded animal, as the Secretary may determine is being used, or is intended for use, for research, testing, experimentation, or exhibition purposes, or as a pet; but such term excludes horses not used for research purposes and other farm animals, such as but not limited to livestock or poultry used or intended for use for improving animal nutrition, breeding, management, or production efficiency, or for improving the quality of food or fiber. (U.S. Congress 1970a)

Allow me to translate. In amending the Animal Welfare Act in 1970, Congress was particularly concerned to add zoo animals, but under no circumstances was it prepared to regulate farming practices. This opened the door for the Secretary of Agriculture and the USDA to regulate sheep and other farm animal species in the laboratory (though not on the farm). The USDA received some criticism for the decades it took to start inspecting and regulating pigs on heart transplant projects, but nothing like the response it has had over excluding the far more numerous mice, rats, and birds. Is a mouse, rat, or bird the kind of animal that the Secretary of Agriculture might "determine is being used, or is intended for use, for research, testing, experimentation, or exhibition purposes"? Given that they account for some 90% of research animals in America, it would seem hard to determine otherwise (Office of Technology Assessment 1986). And yet, three decades after the congressional redefinition of "animal" and despite rodents' inclusion in the *Guide,* these animals have remained outside of USDA's coverage.

In 1970, Congress gave the USDA the authority, though not the resources, to expand Animal Welfare Act coverage to mice and rats. The USDA declined, defining "animal" in its regulations to exclude "birds, aquatic animals, rats and mice, and horses and other farm animals, such as but not limited to livestock or poultry" (Animal and Plant Health Service 1971). The USDA defended this exclusion primarily for lack of manpower and money, though conceding that rats and mice are the animals used in greatest quantity in the United States. But more, in its internal discussions, it "felt that perhaps with these particular species of animals there was not any great inhumane care in handling" (Schwindaman et al. 1973). That's a curious conclusion to draw. Mice and rats at the time were certainly used in the same sorts of toxicity tests and infectious disease studies that contemporaneous hamsters and guinea pigs (who did receive Animal Welfare Act coverage) were experiencing, and yet, somehow, hamsters got in the door while mice stayed outside.

Warm blood, beady eyes

In subsequent amendments to the Animal Welfare Act, Congress continued to give the USDA the leeway to determine whether rats and mice were warm-blooded animals used or intended for use in research. The public record through the 1970s shows little evidence that this was much of a cause of concern for animal protection groups. The USDA continued to decline the opportunity, though in the late 1980s it refined the definition of animal somewhat, specifying that only laboratory-bred species of *Mus* and *Rattus* were excluded, while free-living house mice (*Mus musculus*), Norway rats (*Rattus norvegicus*), black rats (*R. rattus*), and other wild mice and rats would be covered, as are other wild mammals (Animal and Plant Health Inspection Service 1987). This time around, the USDA explained it not as a lack of resources (though that must surely have been a significant factor), nor because lab-bred rodents' risk of inhumane treatment was so low, but because of the major and lengthy process that would delay release of proposed regulations affecting other species. Though it was already into the fourth year of regulation-writing following passage of the 1985 act at this point, and though the USDA had been mandated to harmonize its regulations with the NIH (which had a well-established, detailed set of standards covering rats and mice), it could nevertheless say that "we do not believe it would be in the best interests of animal welfare in general" if it took the time to develop standards for the two species that compose a good 95% of mammals in American research laboratories (Animal and Plant Health Inspection Service 1989a).

No doubt the USDA has always seen the task of regulating mouse and rat use as overwhelming. Their inclusion would not just increase the number of animals to inspect at institutions already being regulated, but would dramatically increase the number of facilities inspected, for there are many laboratories that work with these two species exclusively (possibly, at least in part, to avoid USDA inspections in the first place). On the other hand, if cats or dogs predominated in American laboratories, it is hard to imagine the USDA excluding them for lack of resources.

And so it is worth considering how rodents could continually be excluded by the USDA, why Congress waited until 2002 to address the situation, and how animal protectionists took this up as a cause in the late 1980s, rather than in 1970. This political situation is only tenable so long as rats and mice are excluded from serious moral concern in the public eye. Congress has long tried to strike a political balance between the need for research and the public concern for animals. Rats and mice have long lacked the political capital to warrant inclusion under the Animal Welfare Act, as evidence of public concern for their welfare has been lacking. This situation began to change as protectionists adopted the concept of animal rights to frame their political agenda.

At any point, but especially with the Animal Welfare Act amendments of 1976, 1985, or 1990, Congress could have overruled the USDA and stipulated that mice and rats were specifically covered by the act. It did not. Clearly, at no point had mice, rats, or birds been a high enough priority for either the USDA or the Congress to assure coverage under the Animal Welfare Act. Rounding out efforts to grant mice and rats some legal protection was the Animal Legal Defense Fund's 1990 lawsuit against the USDA, a suit it eventually lost for lack of legal standing to sue on either their own or the rodents' behalf. Finally, in 1998, the Alternatives Research and Development Foundation petitioned for coverage, a federal judge upheld the suit, and the USDA settled out of court in 2000, with plans to publish proposed rodent standards for public comment. Within days, Congress moved to block the USDA from spending any federal funds to "change or modify the definition of 'animal' in existing regulations pursuant to the Animal Welfare Act" (Nolen 2000, p. 1607). This one-year restriction was extended for another year in 2001. In 2002, Congress finally voted to amend the act and exclude these animals (U.S. Congress 2002).[3]

Imagine the public outcry at the exclusion of so many animals from Animal Welfare Act protections. After all, by the most conservative counts, rats and mice must account for some 15 million research animals in the United States annually, and I believe there are at least five times that number. That public outcry, however, at least as reflected in pressure on the USDA to change the situation, was apparently quite muted between 1970 and 1985. In 1971, the USDA reported *no* public response to its proposed exclusion of rats and mice from legal protections. Likewise, in 1977, when it updated regulations following the 1976 Animal Welfare Act amendment, there was no public response.[4]

Whatever the animal protection organizations were thinking among themselves, they were not aggressively pushing inclusion of rats and mice as a political strategy in the 1970s. The USDA was well aware of some interest in including rats and mice under Animal Welfare Act coverage as early as 1970, but it was not until the late 1980s that the animal protection organizations mobilized the support of their general membership on this issue. The 1985 Animal Welfare Act amendment generated a flood of mail to the USDA, and much of that was on behalf of the rodents. In March 1989, the USDA reported receiving more than 1000 public comments (991 from the "general public" and 24 from the "research community") calling for inclusion of rats and mice, and only 322 (25 from the "general public" and 297 from the "research community") agreeing with the USDA's exclusion (Animal and Plant Health Inspection Service 1989b, p. 10823). This correspondence continued after the USDA had set its final rule on the definition of "animal" (in March 1989).

Efforts on the behalf of rats and mice were not limited to the animal protectionist organizations. As the USDA reported, some individual scientists and laboratory animal veterinarians also wanted rats and mice included, as did the National Association for Biomedical Research (though it switched its position on this as time went by, citing the USDA's lack of enforcement resources). No research institutions called for such an increase in USDA jurisdiction—quite the contrary: the National Institute of Mental Health suggested that the exclusion of rats and mice should be extended to exclusion of guinea pigs and hamsters as well.

As literature on laboratory animal welfare grew though the 1980s, so too did attention to the second-class status of rats and mice. Prominent animal protectionists such as Andrew Rowan (1984) and Michael W. Fox (1986), writing before the 1985 amendment took effect, did not make much of the exclusion. After that, it is rare to find any later books on laboratory animals that do not call attention to this omission (Francione 1995; Orlans 1993).

Thus, over about twenty years, rats and mice went from obscurity and exclusion to having their day in court and in the halls of Congress. How this happened has everything to do with the public image of rodents among the human species and with a shift in the philosophical bases for animal welfare protections.

Species images in politics and propaganda

Rats and mice have long had a rocky relationship with the human species. Long detested for their invasion of human food stores, their standing could only suffer as their connection with plague, typhoid, and other human diseases became evident. Far from claiming a role as "man's best friend," they have been reviled. Just picture them, skulking around in dark corners at night, their beady, expressionless eyes, their long naked tails, their eerie squeaks and squeals. Now try generating public sympathy for their laboratory counterparts, giving their all to the human species in their service to science.

There is a propaganda war afoot over the use of animals in research, and it has been going on for some time. My laboratory insider's perspective is that it's just not fair. Antivivisectionists have the easy message: that animal research is bad because it hurts animals and it must be stopped. Even a child can understand that. Research defenders have the more complex and difficult message: that animal research is good enough to outweigh whatever animal suffering it may entail. That message could strike even a child, especially one growing up in a world largely rid of childhood's traditional scourges, as morally suspect: good ends do not justify bad means. How to convey that complicated message in a sound bite in an intellectually honest way?

Scientists have defended animal experimentation on many grounds. For some, the list of benefits is so long and vital, growing with every day, almost to need no justification. Still, it helps to justify the ends if the means can be presented as benignly as possible. As we will see in a later chapter, one way to do this is through veterinarians' testimonials that little pain or distress occurs in the research laboratory. Another approach has been to "spin" the species involved in the science, something both sides in the propaganda wars have been doing for well over a century now.

"Most vivisection," wrote Samuel Wilks in 1881, "is nothing more than pricking mice with the point of a needle" (p. 937). Forget for a moment what toxins might be in the needle; reflect instead on how easy it is to dismiss a mouse as an animal of concern. Why worry about mice, when nineteenth-century vivisectors were strapping conscious dogs to tables, exposing their organs in public dissections and demonstrations? Yes, dogs, our best friends. John Vyvyan (1969) places the birth of the antivivisection movement in Frances Power Cobbes's 1863 petition against the Florentine laboratory of a Professor Schiff, and the "'nuisances' of the moaning dogs" there. Time and again, the public censure of vivisectionists in the eighteenth and nineteenth centuries focused on dogs as science's victims. "Least of all is it proof that someone has the skill to cure people for he has the heart to torment dogs," wrote mathematician Abraham Kastner in 1800 (quoted in Rupke 1987, p. 36). Shifting public attention from dogs to rodents and back again has long been a strategy in the debates about animal research.

Research advocates' deflection from dogs to rodents has continued throughout the twentieth century, while antivivisectionists have often used the opposite ploy. Randolph Hearst, for example, was an ardent antivivisectionist in the early part of the century, and the newspapers in his chain focused heavily on the use of dogs, especially the use of stolen pet dogs. In response to such coverage, and to antivivisectionists' tactics of quoting passages from scientific research reports to depict the worst of animal experimentation, journal editors such as Francis Peyton Rous at the *Journal of Experimental Medicine* carefully reviewed articles for potentially inflammatory descriptions or depictions of experiments. In addition to his focus on animal numbers, source of animals, and mention of anesthesia, Rous took pains to eliminate dogs from his publication whenever possible, not by refusing to publish research on canine subjects, but through transforming "dog" to "animal" in journal articles (Lederer 1992).

More recent pro-research materials also highlight the fact that rodents vastly outnumber dogs and cats and monkeys in laboratories. The Foundation for Biomedical Research and the National Academy of Sciences have both publicized the Office of Technology Assessment's 1986 estimate that rodents compose 85–90% of American research animals. No one would emphasize this statistic if the general public cared equally about all species of animals (Committee on the Use of Laboratory Animals in Biomedical and Behavioral Research 1988; Foundation for Biomedical Research 1990).

As in print, so with pictures: it is not just what is said and shown about animal research, but the animal species itself that carries the message. In an 1882 painting entitled *Vivisection—The Last Appeal,* a small dog sits up in a begging posture (figure 4.1). A scientist approaches him, holding a jar (of ether? chloroform?) behind his back. The picture works on what we all presume to know about dogs: a good dog will accept whatever fate the scientist has in store for her; the dog's posture, upright, front paws raised together, is universally read as begging for something.

It is not just that pictures are more powerful than words; we all already know that. Of note here is that different species do not just receive different treatment; they call for different treatments. Each species has its own persona, its public identity, in our culture. We share certain assumptions, for instance, of how to read dogs' minds and bodies, what the nature of our interspecies relationship with dogs is all about. Imagery is powerful, but the specific animal in the image defines that power.

Try substituting the dog in the painting with a rat, or a group of mice. If they're sitting uncaged on a tabletop in a laboratory, they must be vermin that have gotten in somehow where they don't belong. What sort of moral obligations, if any, do we have to them if that is the case? What does it mean when they rise up on their haunches? Are they just sniffing the air—for food, for danger—their squinty, pink eyes all but useless in the glare of the laboratory? This simple switch of species can radically change the audience's perceptions and response. Picture the next step: Will a rodent willingly, tragically, submit to chloroform in a jar, or must he be seized, forcibly sacrificed for the progress of science? Embedded in our cultural

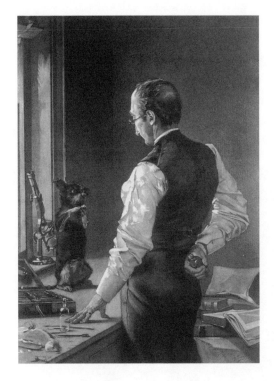

Fig. 4.1 *Vivisection* engraving by John McLure Hamilton, 1883, after a painting by Charles John Tomkins, 1882. THE WELLCOME LIBRARY, LONDON.

identities of dog and rat is the certain knowledge, regardless of any data an animal behaviorist might produce, that the dog will cooperate while the rat must be forced.

The same species politics work just as well for modern audiences. In 1965, *Sports Illustrated* magazine dramatized its exposé of pet theft for laboratory use with the tale of Pepper, an affectionate family dog stolen from a farm in Pennsylvania, dead nine days later in a laboratory in New York City's Montefiore Hospital (Phinizy 1965). Three months later, *Life* magazine published its own exposé of dog trafficking (figure 2.4, Silva 1966). "Concentration Camp for Dogs" was short on text and rich with photographs: a half-starved dog hunched over in obvious distress; dogs chained up amidst junked cars and old lumber, looking dolefully into the camera lens; a dead dog who has frozen solid in the Pennsylvania winter. These articles, and the canine victims they portrayed, are widely credited with securing passage of the Laboratory Animal Welfare Act following years of unsuccessful legislative initiatives.[5]

Twenty years later, animal protectionists agitated to update the Animal Welfare Act, or to abolish vivisection altogether, and the choice of species remained important. In one widely used poster, People for the Ethical Treatment of Animals (PETA) used a photograph of a monkey, Domitian, in a restraint chair (figure 4.2). He looks at you in despair, the twisting of his limbs suggesting his struggles to escape. The caption reads, "This is vivisection. Don't let anyone tell you different." In

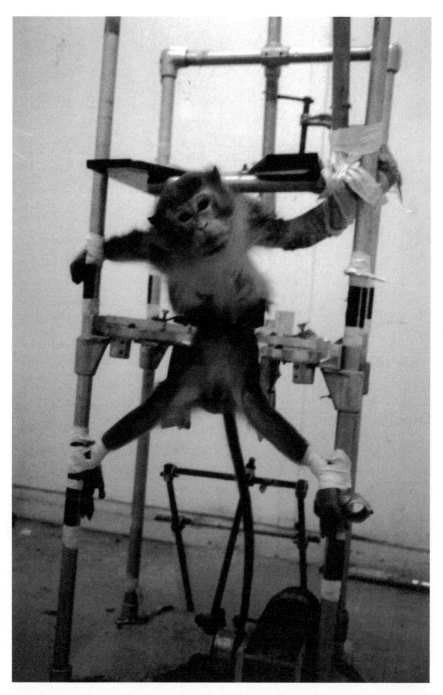

Fig. 4.2   People for the Ethical Treatment of Animals used this picture of one of the "Silver Spring monkeys" widely with the caption, "This is vivisection. Don't let anyone tell you different." COURTESY OF PEOPLE FOR THE ETHICAL TREATMENT OF ANIMALS.

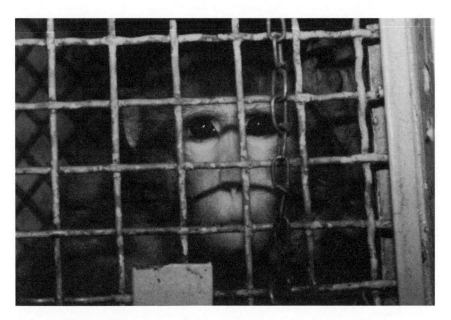

Fig. 4.3   What does this monkey's face tell you about animal research? COURTESY OF
PEOPLE FOR THE ETHICAL TREATMENT OF ANIMALS.

another PETA image, printed on T-shirts, monkey Sarah looks forlornly into the
camera lens through the bars of a cage (figure 4.3). Forlorn? Possibly. Curious and
watchful that there is a camera in her face? Expectant of some treat to follow? How
many of us know monkey faces well enough to read her snapshot look? I am not
at all sure that I do.[6]

While research advocates emphasize the preponderance of rodents in research
laboratories, the imagery in antivivisectionist materials tells a different story. In a
primer on animal rights, for example, Amy Blount Achor (1996) does indeed mention the high percentage of laboratory rodents in her call for their protection under
the Animal Welfare Act, but her text does not match her images. Far out of proportion to their numbers in laboratories, she shows five primate photos, two rabbits, two cats (one with the caption "Cats and dogs are often the animals of choice
for medical research and training," p. 121), and one lone photo of a laboratory rat.

Meanwhile, no grimacing monkeys or starving dogs appear in pro-research
campaigns, of course. If animals are pictured, they are frequently rats and mice,
with no research manipulations in progress for the camera's eye, and no individual animal's name in the caption. Two sleek white rats grace a Foundation for Biomedical Research poster promoting animal research; the caption: "They've saved
more lives than 911." No cage, no laboratory equipment, no white coats, just the
rats and their résumé.

Though not usually a pro-research lobby institution, the National Institute of
Environmental Health Sciences (NIEHS) produced a glossy booklet in 1989 promoting animal research in environmental toxicology. Heading the description of

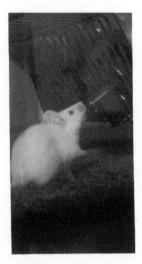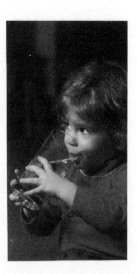

Water of Life

Fig. 4.4 Using mice in studies of water safety, from a 1989 pamphlet. FROM THE NATIONAL INSTITUTE OF ENVIRONMENTAL HEALTH SCIENCES.

the need for animal studies of water pollution are two photographs: on the left, a white mouse sips from the tube of her water bottle which may be full of carcinogens and toxins; on the right, a child drinks from a glass of water (figure 4.4). Three other mice are the only other research animals pictured in the booklet, though on the cover, the family dog stands watchful as a toddler drinks from a water fountain. Nothing in the text suggests that any animals other than rodents find their way into NIEHS studies. And even though it's only rodents, the booklet dispels the myth that rodents have no federal protection, pointing out that the Public Health Service guidelines that cover them apply to a good 40% of American laboratories (without mentioning that the Animal Welfare Act exclusion of rats and mice leaves them unprotected in many American laboratories [National Institute of Environmental Health Sciences 1989]).

The pro-research movement has also used pet and companion animals as "spokespersons" for animal research. It is rare to find pro-research materials from the mid-1980s on that do not include mention of animals as the beneficiaries of medical progress. In a curious twist on species chauvinism, they reach out to those people who might not support animal research for human benefit but would support it for animals.

For children, the North Carolina Association for Biomedical Research encodes laboratory animal messages in their choice of animal species for the 1991 coloring book *The Lucky Puppy*. In this book, Mary and her brother Matt learn about animal research from their veterinarian. Children can color in the picture of a scientist cradling a laboratory mouse in her hand, or connect the dots to reveal a picture of a mouse eating mouse chow. They can color the dancing mice, who are happy because their group got the right dose of experimental medicine and did not get sick. "Hooray!" cries Matt, the young animal lover, "I'm going to be a veterinarian when I grow up." Mary speaks up that she loves animals, too, as well as people, so she will become a research scientist one day. And the lucky puppy? He is not a laboratory dog, but Mary and Matt's pet, made better with the pills that had been tested on the dancing mice (North Carolina Association for Biomedical Research 1991).

One of the most ambitious efforts along this line is a 1993 booklet from the Foundation for Biomedical Research. Perhaps laboratory dogs themselves should feel some relief knowing their own species benefits from their travails in the laboratory, but in this publication, the whole animal kingdom pitches together to help each other out. The animals seem to recognize the moral hierarchy among their kind. Heartwarming pictures of baby eagles and baby elephants, whales, horses, dogs, cats, and sheep accompany a text that describes the various medical advances from which these animals have benefited. Eight generations of "Lassie" incarnations have taken heartworm medications and vaccines developed through the generosity of uncounted, unnamed, and unpictured laboratory animals. It is a curious world, in which distinctions between individuals and species continually blur, in which altruistic animal subjects seem somehow to benefit if their species (or perhaps any nonhuman species) benefits.

Rodents are listed throughout the Foundation for Biomedical Research book as important servants to research for other animals' benefit, but they remain discreetly behind the scenes, not a single rat or mouse in view. Nor are they featured as beneficiaries of medical progress. Animal lovers are called on to support animal research, for human and animal benefit, and assured again (one of the "Research facts you should know!") that most of this research is done on rats and mice. The species is the message (Foundation for Biomedical Research 1993).

It takes the right photo or painting to transform these scurrying vermin into objects of public sympathy, to stir empathetic feelings of relationship on the part of the human observer. Their eyes, for instance, are set on the sides of their head (the better to scan for predators with); they cannot look into the camera face-on as dogs and cats and people do. And then that naked scaly tail: time and again people have resisted my suggestion of rats as children's pets solely because of their tails (naked tails may help to regulate body temperature, but they have little value in eliciting human sympathies). If a transformation has succeeded at all, it may be more due to Mickey Mouse, Stuart Little, and Tom and Jerry, and other children's cartoons than to any successes on the part of antivivisectionists. Ironically, such anthropomorphic projections may end up being the most effective way to convey the information on which most behaviorists seem to have converged (apparent from watching the live animals, but only if one takes the time) that rats and mice are sentient and intelligent creatures in their own right.

Occasionally, the two sides switch their choice of research animal species, as scientists enlist dogs to defend animal research, or antivivisectionists shine their activist light on rodents. In these cases, what is happening to the animals competes with the choice of species to modulate the typical message. Research advocates

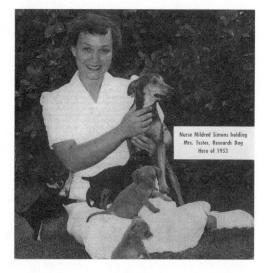

Nurse Mildred Simons holding
Mrs. Tester, Research Dog
Hero of 1953

Fig. 4.5 In the 1950s, research advocates could portray dogs as willing participants in animal research. For a while, the National Society for Medical Research publicized its research dog heroes program. COURTESY OF THE FOUNDATION FOR BIOMEDICAL RESEARCH.

show happy laboratory dogs while antivivisectionists show mice being bullied and poisoned in toxicology labs.

In the 1940s and 1950s, the National Society for Medical Research featured dogs with people on the cover of several issues of its *Bulletin,* even instituting a "Research Dog Hero" award. Almost always, dog and human are posing together with no research activity shown (figure 4.5). Several *Bulletin* articles during this period focus on the ways that pounds condemn unwanted dogs to meaningless lives and deaths, while life in the laboratory allows dogs some meaningful service to their human friends (National Society for Medical Research 1947, 1949, 1954). The message was not then "it's only rodents," but rather something like "dogs live to serve people," though at bottom it remains "animal research must remain free from restrictions."

Antivivisectionists have also varied their choice of animal images from time to time, despite occasional charges that they care only, inconsistently, about high-profile cute and friendly species. In the original 1975 edition of *Animal Liberation,* Peter Singer includes five images of research animals: two of rabbits in eye irritancy (Draize) tests, and three of monkeys, restrained against their will. But for the 1990 edition, he brought in a mouse as well, and the mouse is being force-fed some substance for a toxicity trial. In pictures like this, the small size of rodents serves to dramatize better than images of dogs, cats, or monkeys the "might makes right" ethic that antivivisectionists deplore: that we do what we do to animals because we *can* (Singer 1975, 1990).

The mainstream media do their share to perpetuate the coded information that accompanies the choice of species. Want to talk about the power of scientific research? Illustrate it with a picture of some clean white rats in their cage, and the focus stays on the science, not the animals. On the other hand, monkeys in cages and cats with electrode caps on their heads, photos that may be years old and gleaned from antivivisectionists' materials, lead the reader to feel sorrow for the plight of laboratory animals. The more a magazine tries to show the complexity of the issue, the more mixed the images: dogs and cats and lowly rodents, some actively engaged in laboratory work, others in obvious peace and contentment. In such articles, mixed species of animals are juxtaposed against mixed "species" of humans: playing with animals or experimenting on them; patients who have benefited from medical research; doctors and scientists in their authoritative white coats; sincere animal protectionists gently cradling a dog; crazy radicals dressed as lobsters or mice or pigs for their latest protest (Cowley et al. 1988; Reed and Carswell 1993; Rosenberger 1990).

The images of humans vary as much as the images of animals. In one Foundation for Biomedical Research poster, a young child looks into the camera from her hospital bed, surrounded by her stuffed animals. "It's the animals you don't see that really helped her recover." Fragile innocence is protected by medical miracles, impossible if animal research is shackled. Images of children are rare, however, in antivivisectionist materials, though beautiful people abound. A healthy, clear-skinned white woman poses with a fluffy white rabbit to encourage consumers to buy "cruelty-free" cosmetics that have not been tested on animals. Health equals beauty equals compassion in a benign and affluent world where disease never threatens to intrude.

And then there are the celebrities. Nothing brightens the pro-research and pro-animal campaigns more than genuine celebrities, most with no pretense of expertise. Resourceful lobbyists and advocacy groups line up their arrays of supportive movie stars, while they accuse each other of sensationalizing their issues and of feeding the public untruths and half-truths. They spotlight their dueling heartthrobs from the silver screen: actor Patrick Swayze poses on his horse for the Foundation for Biomedical Research's book on *Research Helping Animals* (1993), while actor Alec Baldwin has become a prominent supporter of People for the Ethical Treatment of Animals. Actress Kim Basinger is visible in her antivivisectionism, while Debbye Turner (Miss America 1990, and now a veterinarian) speaks up for research. Actor Charlton Heston speaks on behalf of The Incurably Ill for Animal Research, while the Doris Day Animal League has supported animal rights and animal protection legislation since 1987.

Movie stars are high-profile celebrities who grab public attention, but other celebrities can also serve, lending legitimacy to the cause as well as their flair. Celebrity-experts are more readily available for the pro-research campaign than for the antivivisectionists. C. Everett Koop, for instance, Surgeon General under Ronald Reagan, is featured in several pro-research pamphlets of the 1990s. This stern and serious physician looks the reader in the eye and says in plain language: "Without the use of animals in this research, continued medical milestones will be stifled" (Foundation for Biomedical Research 1990). Though several philosophers take strong pro-animal positions, they are rarely mediagenic celebrity-experts (Peter Singer seems to come the closest to this status, though his visage is hardly familiar in most households). The pro-research lobby ends up relying more heavily on images of experts for their campaigns than do the animal protectionists, just as they are better able to use images of patients, particularly children (Kruse 1998).

Arluke and Groves (1998) describe how pro- and anti-research propagandists both rely on images of innocent victims (children and animals, respectively) to promote their cause. There is more to it than that, however, for not all animal species read equally well as innocents. Animal-related propaganda plays on a range of stereotypes of animals, some of which have evolved through the years. Dogs and cats have steadfastly remained human companions in iconography, never the dangerous or aggressive animal that veterinarians and others sometimes work with. Thus their public identity relative to animal research ranges from victims to partners to beneficiaries. Rodents are often encoded as below moral concern, unable to generate the pathos of a dog or cat, the piddling price of lifesaving medicine for your child. But they have also been recast: in children's cartoons as underdogs in age-old cat-and-mouse struggles, and as the tiny innocents of the toxicology lab. Meanwhile, primates have a range of public identities, from clown, sometimes loveable, sometimes grotesque, to the highly intelligent and social human cousin, at home in the pristine beauty of equatorial jungles. Research advocates have been hard-put to enlist monkeys, either to cast them as willing partners in research or as happy beneficiaries of medical advances. And they have so far not developed an alternative primate image—smelly and violent and full of deadly infections—that might diminish their appeal to the sentiments. Those of us who work with them know there is some truth in the latter characterization, but it is not part of the current social identity of nonhuman primates.

The stereotypes of different animals mesh better or worse with different ethical frameworks for thinking about animals, frameworks that have shifted in their power and appeal throughout time. Contractarian and "humane" ethics were prominent a few decades back, but rights theories have come into vogue in recent years, and feminist ethics of care have gained increased respectability. As we will now see, different species (or different conceptions of a species) best fit these different ethical frameworks.

Philosophies of interspecies ethics I: Contract ethics

Philosophers seek a unifying ethical theory that will guide human interactions with animals. In practice, people use a plurality of ethical approaches in different situations, depending on the species and the issue, often changing over time. Animal protectionists blend contractarian, caring, and rights-based moralities as they argue for greater protections for animals, but which one they emphasize has varied with the era, the issue, and with different species "constituencies."

Dogs have been central since the early days of antivivisectionism, despite the range of species to be found in Victorian era experiments and dissections. This reflects both a genuine concern (and species bias) for dogs among Victorian antivivisectionists, as well as the strategic knowledge that the wide appeal of dogs could sway a larger audience. Victorian-era paintings and prints depict dogs as the scientist's animal of choice, rarely to the scientists' credit. But why should dogs figure so prominently as the classic victim of science? Are they so much more sensitive to pain and suffering than other animals? Is it because they are small? Innocent? Powerless? But other animals are as well. In the case of dogs, I suggest that it is not their sentience or their size so much as their long-standing symbiotic relationship with our own species that counts for so much.

We have a social contract with dogs, a covenant forged some 14,000 years ago or more. As far as we know, dogs chose domestication every bit as much as our ancestors chose to domesticate them, willingly hanging around human settlements and scavenging for food and handouts much as raccoons, pigeons, mice, and other animals do today. Whatever the precise history of how our two species developed their bond, the dog has become the archetypal domestic animal, at least in modern Western minds. Kept as pets, they are unlike birds or rabbits or goats, who must be caged or fenced to stay on human premises. Ethologists tell us with some specificity what most of us know in general terms: given minimal exposure to humans at the crucial period of puppyhood, dogs actively socialize to human beings and seek out our company (Fox and Bekoff 1975). Dogs are programmed—genetically—to fit into human society, given just the slightest encouragement. We readily become part of each other's social sphere, part of each other's family.

Dogs and humans have lived symbiotically for eons, protecting each other, hunting together, eating together, playing together. Symbiosis does not mean equality, however, and in veterinary medicine and in medical research, the symbiosis is asymmetrical. As a veterinarian, I have vaccinated puppies, treated their infections, X-rayed their limping legs, and sutured their wounds. They have not reciprocated—at least, not those individuals. Some dogs lick the hand that heals them; others bite it. Conversely, dogs have given their lives by the millions for medical research, or, rather, we have taken their lives, typically at their prime. We have developed surgical and anesthetic techniques using dogs as models, and we have trained generations of human and veterinary surgeons on their bodies. We have used dogs to study aging, hemophilia, shock, diabetes, and a host of other diseases (Gay 1984). Some of this knowledge trickles back down to veterinary health care for dogs, even for the dogs in the laboratories; that, after all, is the basis of the laboratory animal medicine that I have practiced for two decades. Much of it, however, does not; most dogs in laboratories are there for their role as models of human diseases.

What moral implications does this long coevolution entail? Does it entail special obligations to dogs that other animals do not merit? It does not, in the eyes of many of the major philosophers writing about animals: it makes them no more or less sentient than other animals (Singer's criterion for moral standing [1990]), no more or less the subject of their own lives (sensu Tom Regan [1990]), and gives them no more or less of a *telos* (sensu Bernard Rollin [1992]). Nor does it even give them rights in the eyes of contractarian philosophers like Cohen, because the contract only counts when it is based on rational autonomy, not tainted by genes and

instinct and evolution (Cohen 1986). But in the public eye, the symbiotic relationship of dogs with humans definitely calls forth a special ethic. "'A dog is man's
best friend' is an adage the defendants have either forgotten or decided to ignore,"
wrote Judge Charles Richey in his 1993 court opinion, chiding the USDA for its
failure to adequately define dog exercise standards in its Animal Welfare Act regulations (quoted in Labaton 1993). For antivivisectionists, use of dogs in laboratories—any dogs, not just strays and lost pets—is a breach of that contract.

The social contract ethic has existed alongside what is variously called a humane
or anticruelty ethic, in which the power imbalance between people and animals
engenders human obligations: noblesse oblige. The power of canine imagery in
antivivisectionist campaigns is that dogs fit both ethical sentiments so well: Laboratory dogs are easily portrayed both as helpless victim and as betrayed ally. The
little pup sitting up in the *Vivisection—The Last Appeal* painting is in a pitiable position, and his innocence and small size will not spare him. But neither will his loyalty. He knows what is coming, but does not run away. He stays. He begs. Those are
the things that good dogs do.

But just as it works against the dog in the painting, the human–canine contract can work to justify canine vivisection more generally. In 1926, Walter Brad-
ford Cannon, one-time chair of the American Medical Association's Council on
the Defense of Medical Research, published an article in *Hygeia* magazine extolling the dog's role in medical research. In the early part of the twentieth century,
legislation was introduced in both Britain and the United States to eliminate the
use of dogs in animal research. Cannon readily acknowledged dogs' "special place
in man's affection" (p. 2), and praised their important service during the World
War. But the medical profession was engaged in an even greater war, in which dogs
had been serving well and admirably for 300 years, and in which dogs stood alongside humans as beneficiaries as well. "The loyalty, devotion and self-sacrifice of the
dog have been emphasized; these noble qualities have their loftiest and most perfect expression when life itself is surrendered for the sake of the object worshiped,"
he wrote, and went on to quote William James: "If his poor, benighted mind could
only be made to catch a glimpse of the human intentions, all that is heroic in him
would religiously acquiesce" (p. 8).

Research advocates have continued to assert that the chance to serve as a laboratory subject gives meaning to a dog's life. Challenging animal protectionists' efforts against the use of pound animals in research, physician Glenn Geelhoed
wrote: "It is the researcher, not the activist, who assigns the greater value to those
lives. What an enormous legacy from the pound dog used in the lab, as compared
to fifteen million of its mates [who are simply killed in pounds and incinerated
every year]" (Geelhoed 1987, p. 77).

Without doubt, the most contentious long-standing issue in laboratory dog
welfare is the use of impounded and "random source" dogs for research. In brief,
should pounds and shelters be required or forbidden to send stray and unwanted
animals to research? This was only tangentially an issue in the 1985 Animal Welfare Act amendment (in which "Class B dealers" were allowed to continue buying

and selling dogs for laboratories with but a few added restrictions), but through the years, it has continued to keep proponents and opponents exercised. Much of the political animal welfare activity in the 1930s and 1940s, and again in the 1990s, has been focused on sources of dogs for laboratories.[7]

As befits a seventy-year-old debate, arguments and counter-arguments have proliferated. Much of the discussion about restricting the sources of laboratory dogs focus on dogs as human property (hence the antitheft focus of the early Laboratory Animal Welfare Act), or on dogs as expensive commodities to be conserved, or on weighing harms to dogs: Does buying purpose-bred dogs from well-run commercial dog farms, when unwanted dogs are being killed in animal shelters and pounds, simply double our country's canine death toll, or does it spare lost pets and street strays the added stress, transportation, cage restraint, pain, and death of a trip to the laboratory? Do laboratories compete with adoption programs for the friendliest and most handleable dogs in the shelter, or are they truly only taking dogs otherwise headed for euthanasia and disposal?

Debates about appropriate sources of laboratory dogs go far beyond questions of the well-being of individual animals or concerns to maximize human utility and reflect much of what we think about the relationship between our two species. Orlans and colleagues (1998) explain why pet dogs might engender greater human obligations than do purpose-bred dogs, and they may be entirely correct about obligations between individual humans and the individual dogs they have taken into their homes. Part of the problem, as Orlans et al. point out, is the disagreement about whether dogs in pounds should be considered pets (though lost, abandoned, former pets) or non-pets.

A shelter population includes a mix of truly feral dogs who have never known much human contact, loved pets who have gotten lost, unloved pets who were too rambunctious or otherwise problematic, litters of mongrel puppies for whom no homes have been found, biting dogs and abused dogs who have been confiscated from their humans, and others. The ethical/policy question arises: Do we have special obligations to these dogs from random sources (even totally sidestepping the prospects of pet theft associated with random-source dog dealers), and particularly, is there something about The Dog as a domestic pet species that should translate to *these* dogs, as would-be, could-be, former, or never-were individual pets?

Some people believe that domesticity itself gives people certain rights over animals. Budiansky (1992) has popularized the theory that domestication is best seen as a coevolutionary process in which animals chose to associate with people. The "choice" is largely the evolutionary process by which certain species have come closer and closer into the human fold, with those most genetically fit for coexistence with humans favored in evolutionary processes of natural selection. In Budiansky's hands, however, language of consciousness and volition keep creeping in, competing with the impersonal language of natural selection that he tries to maintain. Cautioning against the sentimental excesses of city-dwelling animal rights activists who have never hunted, have never slaughtered their own dinner, the evolutionary covenant he describes places strong restrictions on what animals can expect from domesticity. In this contract between equals, domestic species fare far better than in the wild, but they must pay the price. They must "expect" to be eaten, and in modern times, they must expect to be research subjects as well.

Budiansky's (1992) coevolutionary theory of domestication does not result in a very different moral status for animals than many who see domestication as a solely human invention would grant. If Man created domestic animals, then he should have dominion over their fates, as God expected dominion over the humans he created. I hear this sentiment most often expressed relative to food animals: meat-eating keeps domestic food animal species like cattle from extinction, for why else would we maintain them, and how could they survive on their own? It is a moral obligation, the reasoning goes, to save these man-made species from extinction by continuing to breed and eat them.

"Purpose-bred" dogs, such as beagles and others bred by the thousands on commercial farms solely for sale for research, can likewise be cast as man made. But purpose-bred dogs derive not from some anonymous wild animal, but from our domestic familiars. Nonetheless, they seem to give up the rights and privileges of pets, once they've been packaged as purpose bred. Many of the arguments against using pound dogs seem not to apply to them. I've talked to researchers and facility managers about exercise, socialization, and adoption programs for such purpose-bred dogs and come up against a contractarian wall: these dogs were bred for research and would not otherwise be alive; they have no claim to the niceties that pet dogs might expect (Carbone 1997b). While shelter and pound dogs without human ties still claim some of the contractual, if limited, benefits of the pet category, that remains a more difficult claim for purpose-bred dogs to sustain, even though regulations and guidelines see little distinction on paper between the two classes of dogs once they're in the research facility.

Contractarian language is not the only language that applies to dogs, nor is it applied exclusively to dogs. Any situation in which people believe they have "given life" to animals raises the prospect of reciprocity—not just meat or milk or wool or leather, but research service as well. In a 1956 *Reader's Digest* article, for example, Hector the rat, Powder Puff the pigeon, and Coconut the monkey ("with a radio antenna built into his head") all pitch in at the NIH to advance the cause for medical research (Harkness and Harkness 1956). As David del Mar (1998) describes, popular press descriptions of animals in the 1950s often based their admiration of animals on their service to humanity, service due to the benefits they received in turn from association with humans. Dogs, of course, figured prominently, but even wild animals benefited from human kindness and were expected to return something—often saving human lives with sacrificial devotion, or giving their lives to reverential hunters.

Laboratory rodents join in, too: an experiment in which rats are held at "slow-starvation levels" was described in *Reader's Digest* as an example of "man and animal joining together" (quoted in del Mar 1998). Certainly one of the hottest trends in animal research since the 1980s has been the propagation of mutant strains and the creation of transgenic laboratory rodents, whose opportunities for service are enhanced with genetic selection for immune system failures, propensity for assorted disorders, or the introduction of genes for cystic fibrosis, mammary gland tumors, and other diseases. Perhaps this creation entails reciprocal response on the part of the mice, yielding data as their part of the contract. On the other hand, it may be that this profound manipulation of animal nature creates an obligation of care best articulated through a different approach to moral thinking, feminist bioethics.

Philosophies of interspecies ethics II: Ethics of care

Contractarian theories of moral obligation and moral rights have figured prominently in discussions of animal welfare. They give animal protectionists some ground for their case, especially when they fight on behalf of "man's best friend," but they are limited. After all, why should humans honor a contract in which nothing is expected in return? Why should we feed and provide for dogs if their traditional forms of reciprocation—herding, guarding, hunting—are on the wane? Do they owe us nothing in return? And especially if we are willing to blur the distinctions between individuals and species, we see that research is not just a chance for dogs to give something back for what humans have given them, but a chance to better their own (or, rather, their own species') medical care. But contract theories have had a limited place for another reason: they are hard, masculinist, and impersonal theories in an animal protectionist movement in which women have long been prominent.

Women have been leaders of antivivisection and animal protectionist movements throughout the past century. Frances Power Cobbes in Britain and Caroline Earle White in Philadelphia were important leaders in the nineteenth century, while Christine Stevens, Ingrid Newkirk, and Barbara Orlans took up the cause a century later.[8] Surveys of rank-and-file members of protectionist movements in current times reveal a preponderance of women working on animal issues (Herzog 1998; Jamison and Lunch 1992). Long before Carol Gilligan, Annette Baier, and others had articulated feminist "ethics of care," these activist women were talking in terms that were anything but contractual (Baier 1985; Gilligan 1982). The work of modern feminist theorists, though few of them focus on animals, gives some framework for the sentiments that women (though not exclusively women) had been expressing for decades.

As Baier, feminist animal-rights theorist Carol Adams, and others see it, contractarian and rights theories, with their emphasis on justice, law, and free choice may work well for equals. However, the feminist emphasis on obligations to care, and relationships among *unequals* may be particularly suited for human–animal interactions (Adams 1990). The animals and people who share the medical laboratory hardly share power and privilege equally, and that differential may engender different sorts of responsibilities. The emphasis on the power differential is trivialized by masculinist rights-theorists as a "be kind to dumb animals" ethic, but it captures an important aspect of human–animal relations that rights and contract theories tend to overlook. The very power we have over animals calls for restraint of that power. This approach has the potential to open concern to a far greater range of animals than the domestication contract approach does, for obligation comes not from a centuries-old association between species but from the relationship-defining act of placing an individual animal under our control.

Despite the proliferation of philosophical treatments of animal ethics since 1975, there have been disappointingly few developing a feminist perspective. This is disappointing in two ways. First, much of the historical antivivisectionist movement has included elements that today would fit well within feminist theory and could be reconsidered more respectfully with this theoretical support. Second, much of the future of animal ethics may lie in feminist approaches. Whereas the past two decades have been dominated by the Regan/Singer challenges to presumed inequalities between human and nonhuman, those inequalities persist (if in no place other than the imbalance of who holds the keys to the laboratory door), and careful thought from more feminist voices could prove valuable.

The feminist emphasis on responsibility to powerless others explains much of the iconography of early antivivisectionist materials, images that emphasize the powerless circumstance of laboratory animals. And yet, despite how broadly the philosophical ethic might apply, not all species fit so easily into this rhetorical and visual mold. Dogs and cats certainly do, at least in modern Western cultures: just look at the begging pup in the *Vivisection—The Last Appeal* painting. Mice and rats remain a harder sell, though they are certainly as powerless in the laboratory as any dog or cat. The power imbalance is ripe for a feminist consideration, but rats and mice live a life largely independent of human warmth and of human exploitation: "pet" and "laboratory subject" are minor roles for them compared with their status as vermin. Secretive, nocturnal, and spreaders of infection and disease, rodents maintain a stubborn and even hostile independence that resists easy compartmentalization into the role of powerless victim. Even cleaned up for the laboratory—bred for pink-eyed, white-coated albinism—rats and mice face public relations challenges. It is still a much safer advertising gambit to plug a pink-eyed albino rabbit into advertisements for "cruelty-free" cosmetics.

Feminist ethics of care fit most comfortably only with certain species, at least when activists try to popularize their ethics and bring them into public policy. But feminist approaches have had other political limitations as well, and they have long been denigrated as, well, feminine, in the face of an overwhelmingly male population of scientists, doctors, lawmakers, and philosophers. Even the careful articulation of feminist philosophy of the 1970s and later has not always been sufficient to rescue caring from the appearance of "mere sentiment." Before then, that distinction was extremely unlikely. In 1909 and 1910, neurologist Charles Dana and psychologist James Warbasse medicalized the situation: women who doted on useless dogs and worried about them in laboratories out of proportion to their numbers were manifesting symptoms of "zoophilic psychosis" (Dana 1909; Warbasse 1910). Six decades later, on the eve of passage of the Laboratory Animal Welfare Act of 1966, surgeon Clarence Dennis of the National Society for

Medical Research revived the diagnosis, applying it retrospectively to Queen Victoria as well as to contemporary antivivisectionists, warning that political initiatives were threatening to "emasculate" research (Dennis 1966).

As the USDA sought public comments on Animal Welfare Act regulations in the late 1980s, the contractarian significance of domestication remained minor. Feminist and other ethics of care informed much of the correspondence but provided little detail in how to shape specific regulations. Writers invoked the special responsibilities of USDA staff as veterinarians and, rarely, religious concerns, in urging compassion and decency toward animals.[9] But in the face of the scientific community's increasing calls for science-based regulations, a different language and philosophy of animal protection gained currency. That language was the language of rights, and the animal standard-bearers for this new language were not so much our domestic familiars as our exotic relatives—the primates.

Philosophies of interspecies ethics III: Animal rights

The 1966 Laboratory Animal Welfare Act was consistent with respect for the interspecies contract of domestication. Crafted largely in response to exposés of dog trafficking, it codified into law an ethical focus on the mutual interactions between the human and canine species, with some spillover to a small coterie of other animal species. The law centered on protecting the interspecies bond, both by safeguarding family pets and by setting standards for trade in dogs from other sources. It complemented caring-based humane and anticruelty laws, even as it exempted scientists and their experiments from these laws. But the 1980s expansion of the Animal Welfare Act into the research laboratory, and calls for inclusion of rats and mice under its coverage, required the development of philosophical and political movements focused on animal rights.

As formulated in the 1970s and 1980s by philosophers such as Regan and Singer, the locus of animal liberationist and animal rights is with the individual, not with the species, and certainly not with the species' relationship with other species, including our own. In contrast to feminist bioethics, in which ethics flows from relationship, in animal-rights theory, ethics precedes, or even precludes, relationship. Rejecting both contractarian and feminist ethical bases, these philosophies do not privilege dogs, cats, and pet animals for their history of association with people, do not distinguish a priori between individual dogs from different sources, and generally foster a hands-off rather than a "be kind" relationship with nonhumans. Theoretically, they include all of those animals that meet their cognitive criteria (sentience for Singer, subjective consciousness for Regan), yielding a pool of species that will be larger than for most contractarians and may be larger or smaller than feminists might include.[10]

As with the other philosophical bases for animal protectionism, there is a species gap between theoretical concern and the rhetorical role of different species in the political sphere. Monkeys and other nonhuman primates have been particularly attractive canvasses onto which to paint animal rights campaign slogans, and that is precisely what happened in the early 1980s. Dogs brought a properly domestic face to popular press exposés of the mid-1960s: faithful but betrayed. In the 1980s, monkeys had their day.

In 1981, Alex Pacheco, cofounder of PETA, took a volunteer position in the laboratory of Dr. Edward Taub in Silver Spring, Maryland. Taub had surgically severed the sensory nerve supply to the arms of several macaque monkeys as a model to study long-term healing of the central nervous system after injury or stroke. Though the work was peer-reviewed and funded by NIH, the institute had never conducted animal welfare site visits at the laboratory. Pacheco brought in veterinarians, animal behaviorists, and the Maryland police, alleging cruelty and lack of veterinary care in the postoperative management of the monkeys. One hundred fourteen cruelty charges were whittled down to one, failure to provide adequate veterinary care to one animal, which was later overturned in a court ruling that Maryland anticruelty law did not cover federally funded laboratories. Taub lost his NIH funding over the incident, and the animal protectionists gained an important case for their legislative agenda (Rowan 1998). The "Silver Spring Monkeys Case" took center stage in 1981 congressional hearings as momentum gathered to update and expand the Animal Welfare Act. As the congressional committee investigated how the NIH and USDA had both failed to stop Taub's work, Pacheco had his day to testify. His monkey exposé got him in the door; once there, he testified to the need to extend the Animal Welfare Act to rats, mice, frogs, and all sentient animals (Subcommittee on Science, Research, and Technology 1981).

Shortly after the Silver Spring case worked its way through NIH peer review, congressional hearings, and the Maryland court system, a second exposé, also in a primate laboratory, hit the news. In 1984, five members of the clandestine Animal Liberation Front raided a laboratory at the University of Pennsylvania, stealing videotapes of experiments in progress. Dr. Thomas Gennarelli studied head injury in his laboratory by placing baboons in a device to stimulate the head trauma of sudden impacts, such as in automobile crashes. Several hours of purloined tapes were edited down to the twenty-minute *Unnecessary Fuss*, which was then distributed to congressional offices throughout Washington. The edited film shows researchers strapping baboons into the device and then operating it, laughing, smoking, acting disrespectful all the while, at one point commenting to each other that one of the baboons was awake prior to the head injury (despite protocol provisions for anesthesia for the procedure) (People for the Ethical Treatment of Animals 1984).

Though NIH had reacted quickly in the Silver Spring case, eventually removing Taub's funding, they were more conservative in handling the Pennsylvania case. A year after the raid, the NIH planned to renew Gennarelli's grant for another five years. After a four-day sit-in at NIH by animal protectionists and a petition signed by sixty members of Congress, Secretary of Health and Human Services Margaret Heckler instructed the NIH to suspend funding. The USDA, which had found only four minor violations days before the raid, later found 74, and ended up fining the university $4000. Within months, President Reagan signed the Improved Standards for Laboratory Animals (the Animal Welfare Act amendment of

1985) and the Health Research Extension Act (which codifies NIH animal welfare policies as federal law in federally funded research).

These two cases are significant in several ways: They taught the animal liberationists that direct (including illegal) action works; they highlighted the limits of regulatory protection of animals on experiment; and they resulted in two major pieces of federal animal welfare legislation. In addition, they shifted the spotlight from our best friends, the dogs, to our close cousins, the nonhuman primates, and from kindness and humane care to rights and abolitionism.

Monkeys and apes had been American research labs for decades, but their use (despite the millions sacrificed in the development of polio vaccines in the 1950s) was relatively limited. Their primary sources were the forests and plains of Africa, Asia, and Latin America, sources that were politically unreliable, and which yielded wild animals with an array of infections, parasites, capture injuries, and transport stresses that could make pound dogs seem like pampered nobility by comparison.[11] The NIH in the 1970s established a system of national primate centers to develop monkeys as research subjects: studying their captive needs, breeding them as research resources, and hosting research projects for scientists with insufficient facilities at their home institutions.

The 1966 Laboratory Animal Welfare Act included nonhuman primates, but with its focus on dog theft, and its exclusion of animals while on experimentation, that coverage was necessarily limited. Primate centers could further limit USDA inspections by considering all animals within a facility to be "on experiment," as part of the reason for the existence of such centers was researching how to maintain monkeys. In the 1960s when "be kind to animals" and "concentration camps for pets" were the phrases of the day, monkeys neither had much claim to a social contract with humans (at least, not in the United States, where they do not exist as free-living animals and would typically only be encountered in zoos or on television), nor might they elicit the protective impulses that kittens and puppies can stir. But monkeys fit perfectly with the animal liberationist and animal rights rhetoric of the 1970s and 1980s.

Primates are striking not in their social ties to people, but in their similarity. That similarity explains the extent of primate research, for otherwise they have little to recommend them as research subjects over dogs or rats or pigs: they are messy, expensive, and dangerous animals to work with. Most require sedation for a simple blood sample or physical examination. Some carry herpes viruses and other infections potentially fatal to people. But physiologically, behaviorally, and phylogenetically they are the closest there is to a human subject in the animal laboratory. Some nonhuman primate species, for instance, are about the only animals that will harbor and grow certain infections (hepatitis B and C viruses, for example) of human medical concern (Bennett et al. 1995; Bowden and Johnson-Delaney 1996).

Most animal rights and liberation philosophers stress mental criteria (sentience, subjectivity) as the basis for moral status for animals, and primates make the strongest claim to these criteria, dangerously eroding the human/animal divide that justifies animal experimentation. Language reflects some of the shifting cultural place of our simian relations: early laboratory animal literature refers to "subhuman" and "infrahuman" primates, while later work (including the text of the Animal Welfare Act) replaces "sub" with "non." Separate but equal? Judge Charles Richey went a step further: in deciding against the USDA's provisions for standards for nonhuman primates, he chose the phrase "near-human" instead (quoted in Labaton 1993).

Nonhuman primates then become separate nations, commanding a different type of respect than the obligations our loyal subjects and faithful allies, the dogs and the cats, engender. Rights replaced kindness as the language of animal protection in the 1980s, with monkeys and apes far more apt standard-bearers than dogs, mice, or other animals could be. Rights concerns were not limited to primates— witness the Animal Legal Defense Fund's pursuit in court of rodent rights and dog exercise standards in the Animal Welfare Act and PETA cofounder Ingrid Newkirk's assertion: "When it comes to having a central nervous system and the ability to experience pain, hunger, and thirst, a rat is a pig is a dog is a boy" (Newkirk 1992). But primates, with their intelligent, inquisitive, challenging eyes, buttress the use of rights and liberation languages as the ethical vocabulary for our duties to all sentient animals. They offer no loyalty, beg no mercy. "Keep your hands off me" could well be their motto.

Species specificity in public policy

How we treat members of different species depends not just on what we think different types of animals want, but also on our moral basis for considering animal welfare at all. The Dog, for instance, fits well with an interspecies social contract ethic, as well as with a feminist ethic of care. Other powerless animals, including those with less claim to a social contract of domesticity, may still fit well in an ethic of care or of humane kindness. The Monkey, on the other hand, neither loyal like The Dog nor cuddly like The Bunny, has fit well with a rhetoric and ethic of rights, an ethic that has covered, though erratically, other species as well.

Just as different species of animals and the public personae we construct for them play different rhetorical roles in vivisection debates, so, too, do they secure different protections in animal welfare policy. Dogs, and dogs alone, are singled out in the 1985 Animal Welfare Act for the opportunity for exercise, after decades of debate as to whether that was a necessary provision. Did Congress somehow find that dogs, but dogs alone, needed extra exercise? What about cats? Rabbits? Or did it just decide that our best friends, more than any other species in the laboratory, deserved this perquisite? Likewise, primates were singled out in the 1985 act as the recipients of environments that promote their psychological well-being. Only rarely in these controversies did anyone, animal protectionist or research defender, ask why other animals were not offered these special treatments.

Mice and rats have played the most ambivalent role: though easily the most numerous of mammals in the research laboratory, they scurry in and out of public concern, excluded from one set of protections, second-class citizens in another. There are good mice and bad mice, Herzog (1989) writes, vermin to be exterminated and laboratory subjects to be coddled (well, coddled within limits). Thousands of people petitioned the rodents' case before the USDA, and a federal judge ruled in their favor, while at the same time, research advocates can allay people's fears about the realities of vivisection, for mostly, it is just "pricking mice with the point of a needle" (Wilks 1881, p. 937).

Though mice and rats have been excluded from the Animal Welfare Act, they have been included in the *Guide for the Care and Use of Laboratory Animals* through most of its history. Though most of the *Guide* is written in general enough language to apply to many species, some earlier editions singled out rodents as requiring lower standards of sterility for surgery than for other animals (ILAR 1972). Why should rodents receive a lower level of sterility in research surgeries than other classes of animals receive? The reason could be ethical (we care less about them than we do about other types of animals), biological (their immune systems are more robust and ward off infections better), economical (equipment for instrument sterilization, personnel to support fully aseptic procedures, separate operating suites all add up when you consider the numbers of rodents in laboratories), or logistical (it is easier to do sterile surgery on tiny patients with tiny incisions, and thereby avoid infections), or, of course, some combination of all of these. A reflection of the uncertain basis of the differential treatment leads to confusion in what is required for other, perhaps less common, animals. Does a woodchuck's size mean that he receives the standard of care of similarly sized animals (cats, rabbits), or does his classification as Rodent carry the day? And how about birds and frogs? The *Guide* specifically singles out rodents for differential handling. If size or moral concern are the issue, then birds and frogs might be lumped with rodents. But if immune competence is the issue, then they need to be examined as separate cases and with some nod to the empirical literature on species-differences in immune function.

As with surgical standards, rodents have occupied a shifting and uncertain status in discussions of alternatives. "Alternatives" was a buzz word of 1980s animal welfare policy debates, with the 1985 Animal Welfare Act mandate "that the principal investigator considers alternatives to any procedure likely to produce pain to or distress in an experimental animal." As developed in the 1950s, by Russell and Burch (1959), and later elaborated on by Rowan (1984) and others, the word "alternatives" encompasses a broad array of approaches to minimize research animals' pain and distress. The "three R's" of alternatives include *replacement* of animals in research altogether (using computer simulations, epidemiological studies of human populations, microbiological and tissue culture systems, "lower" animals), *reduction* in the number of animals in a given study, and *refinement* of experimental procedures to minimize pain and distress (Rowan 1984; Russell and Burch 1959). The sticking point for mice and rats (and much more so for frogs, fish, and octopuses) is who constitutes a "lower animal" for replacement considerations. Do mice have some cause for hope that fish are being recruited to take their place in laboratories? Or are mice the "lower animals" that will replace others?

Experience with animal care and use committees reveals that species biases do indeed affect decisions about research proposals, though in ways that are difficult to document and quantify. Most IACUCs use the same form to review their investigators' proposals, regardless of species and experiment. Scientists milking cows, conducting brain surgeries on cats, watching birds through binoculars, or catching and killing fish are all reviewed by their campus IACUC. All are asked to think about alternatives to painful procedures, regardless of the vertebrate species involved (most committees do not review use of invertebrates). And the committees I have worked with take their work very seriously, regardless of the species in question, though monkey protocols always raise a red flag of special concern.

A handful of researchers have made an attempt to characterize the factors that influence IACUC reviews. Frans Stafleu (1994) and Rebecca Dresser (1989) have both conducted cross-institutional studies, asking scientists, IACUC members, and other subjects to review mock animal-use protocols.[12] Both Dresser and Stafleu found species bias in their respondents. Dresser found that "Committees tended to express more reservations and recommend more modifications as the experimental species changed from mice to rats, rats to cats, and cats to monkeys" (1989, p. 1189). Of course, some of this could be an artifact of the procedures associated with each species (production of ascites fluid in mice versus induction of stress ulcers in rats). In Stafleu's studies, Dutch scientists rated the "ethical acceptability," the balance of scientific gain against costs to animals, of hypothetical animal experiments. As long as the scientific merit of the studies seemed at all reasonable (and the scientists were apparently not quick to rate the hypothetical protocols as having high merit), they needed to perceive a very high level of animal discomfort, and then only for monkeys, not for rats, before it affected their ethical acceptability rating (Stafleu 1994; Stafleu et al. 1994).

Conclusion

Animal species are the dramatis personae of the vivisection debate, co-stars with the animal protectionists and the defenders of research. The Rat, The Pig, The Dog: each species has its own character, an amalgam of their histories of interaction with people, their behaviors, their size, their appearance, and all that we project onto them in our cultural forms. Frequently, the type (or the stereotype) stands for the individual. Each species plays its own role in the rhetoric, icons and propaganda for or against animal research, and each elicits its own pattern of ethical responses. Any attempt to craft an animal welfare policy that truly addresses an individual animal's needs will be done in a context in which species weighs heavily. Years of accumulated assumptions, observations, interactions, and beliefs about the type, the species, form the lens through which we look at any individual.

The language and philosophies of animal rights have gained momentum in the past two decades as a unifying theory that includes a wide range of sentient and/or conscious species. Animal rights exists alongside other ethical systems and values, sometimes in harmony, sometimes in competition, which elevate other characteristics of animals for moral consideration: the domestic contract, dependency and connection, species' conservation status, individual history, and source.

Actual practice, as in IACUC reviews of animal uses, reflects public opinion and the evolution-conscious philosophies of some writers. Rather than a sharp line dividing rights holders from those who are not rights holders, with rights holders egalitarians within their camps, people work with gradations and hierarchies of moral concern. Species may even be split within some of these hierarchies, depending on the individual's history, as in the case of pound versus purpose-bred dogs, or wild mice (vermin) versus laboratory mice (excluded from the Animal Welfare Act) versus wild mice in laboratory experiments (included under the Animal Welfare Act).

Monolithic philosophical systems do not match the current political reality. We do not have a system in which only humans count, in which all animals are excluded equally. Nor do we a have a system in which all animals are included equally. The hierarchies we have are shaped by what we know about animals through our human lens: who's conscious, who's intelligent, who's domestic, and who suffers boredom, anxiety, fear, or pain in laboratory experiments. The lens is not infinitely flexible—the animals' realities do place some constraints—but it is powerful and always present. As we further examine in the coming chapters how animal welfare policy has been crafted, we will see the power of being the person to speak for animals and what they want, of being the person to apply the lens of scientific studies, common sense, empathy, personal connection with individual animals, or other ways of knowing animals.

5

Performance standards: How big is your guinea pig's house?

NEW TO THE PRACTICE OF LABORATORY ANIMAL MEDICINE, I SOMETIMES ACCOM-
panied our Department of Agriculture veterinarian on her animal welfare inspections of our campus. One day we visited a rabbit room together. The rabbits were
large and looked very healthy. As caged animals will do, they sat quietly and
watched what we were up to. Often, USDA inspectors would get so absorbed in
looking for cracks in floors and walls, for dirt in corners, or for rust on cages, that
they seemed not to notice the actual animals that were present. This time, the inspector admired the rabbits' large size and robust health. I explained why we liked
that strain, and that we raised them on campus in our own breeding colony. But
then she started looking for her tape measure, asked the caretaker to find her a
scale. Before we knew it, we had an Animal Welfare Act violation in our record.
Laboratory rabbits larger than 11.9 pounds must never be housed in a 4-square-
foot cage, and this rabbit was several ounces over that limit (Animal and Plant
Health Inspection Service 1990b).

Minor USDA violations come with a thirty-day period in which to correct the
problem. We had thirty days to find a bigger cage, put the rabbit on a weight-loss
diet, or "remove" him—most probably through euthanasia. If we euthanized or
relocated him on the spot, our USDA record would still contain the citation, but
with the face-saving note "corrected at time of inspection." The USDA inspector
did not like the idea of euthanizing the rabbit simply to avoid the citation, and at
any rate, it was too late not to cite our violation—the rabbit had been weighed, the
cage had been measured. We indeed found a cage in storage large enough to meet
the USDA's standards for large rabbits: 3 inches longer and 4 inches deeper than
his original cage, and he now had the full 5 square feet required by law.

My guess is that the improvement in his welfare was as modest as the increase
in his cage size: he still could not hop or burrow, and his fate in the experiment
would not change. But my campus was now in compliance with the law.

When Congress amended the Animal Welfare Act in 1985 and the USDA set
about writing regulations, this was the scenario research advocates feared, that
minor changes in regulations—an additional inch of cage height for guinea pigs,
an added half square foot of floor space for cats—would result in expensive, in-
flexible rules. The USDA had a history of writing what we currently call "design"

or "engineering" standards: rigid specifications of cage sizes, room temperatures, and fence heights. A cage a few inches too small or an animal a few ounces over-weight could result in citations and, eventually, if left uncorrected, fines. Given the cost of stainless-steel animal caging (a rack of six 4-square-foot rabbit cages could cost more than $3000 in 2003) and qualified, trained, animal care technicians, in-cremental cage-size increases in the name of animal welfare could come at quite an expense.

As an alternative to such rigid regulation, many research advocates in the 1980s called for a more flexible regulatory approach, the adoption of "perform-ance standards." Whereas engineering or design standards prescribe a specific set of rules, performance standards instead describe desired outcomes and leave it to the regulated party to devise their own way of meeting those outcomes.

"Performance standards" became the catchphrase of the 1980s in animal wel-fare discussions, but it had different meanings for different people. Research advo-cates focused on the flexibility of allowing institutions to develop their own ways of meeting animal welfare standards. Animal protectionists focused on enforce-ability during USDA inspections. The debate over government intrusiveness versus efficacy and flexibility versus enforceability masked the fact that animal protection-ists and research advocates were often calling for substantively different standards.

This chapter examines debates about cage-size regulations, both for how they illustrate the standards issue and because they have been such a prominent con-troversy over several decades of animal care policy. A simple question whether, for example, guinea pigs in breeding groups require more space per animal than singly caged guinea pigs contains questions of expertise (how we know what guinea pigs need or want) and ethics (how we balance their essential needs and additional desires against the economic cost of providing them). And it begs the question; how could this issue garner so much detailed attention while the use of these ani-mals in toxicity trials and other painful experiments was excluded for years from government oversight? I focus on the first question in this chapter: How do we measure animal welfare in writing and enforcing policy? The next chapter pro-vides a historical look at the reasons animal *care* concerns (such as how to house animals) so overshadowed regulation of animal *use* in experiments.

Performance standards in animal welfare policy

Congress passed the Animal Welfare Act amendment, Improved Standards for Laboratory Animals, in 1985, instructing the USDA to write new regulations for research animal care and use. This included writing standards for programs to give dogs the opportunity for exercise and primates a "physical environment adequate to promote the psychological well-being," along with placing responsibilities on researchers to minimize animal pain and distress and to consider alternatives to painful experiments.

The amendment reflected Congress's intent, following exposés in two primate laboratories, that better enforcement of the act was needed. The USDA shared this sense and embarked on an ambitious effort to revamp all existing Animal Welfare Act standards, not just those singled out by Congress. Animal protection and research advocacy groups geared up for a major political struggle, with the result that it took USDA more than five years to finalize the regulations. In the process, USDA published proposed rules in March 1986, in March 1987, in March and again in August 1989, and in July and August 1990, with some parts of the rules finalized along the way. Having counted some 36,000 public comments on its proposals, it finalized the last section on February 15, 1991.[1]

The scientific community united in its opposition to new, rigid, and expensive regulations that they feared could price science out of business. In 1987, the National Association for Biomedical Research (NABR) estimated cost of compliance nationwide would exceed $500 million, even before potentially costly USDA proposals for dog and monkey exercise and psychological well-being were published. A year later, the USDA factored in dog and monkey regulatory proposals in its regulatory impact analysis and more than doubled NABR's estimate (Holden 1988).

Seeking relief from this regulatory burden, research advocates argued for self-regulation and flexible standards and called on the USDA to base any new rules on scientific data. Midway through the rule-writing period, the research community found and promoted the concept of "performance standards," a phrase that has stayed with this community for well over a decade. The 1996 *Guide for the Care and Use of Laboratory Animals,* for example, promotes the concept in its Introduction, for the first time in its seven editions (ILAR 1996). I have not found this phrase in the laboratory animal literature prior to 1989.

The Reagan-Bush administration embraced performance standards as the antidote to business-stifling overregulation. "Health, safety, and environmental regulations should address ends rather than means," wrote a presidential task force in 1983. "To the degree that performance can be measured or reasonably imputed, a standard based on this level of performance is always superior to more means-oriented regulation" (Presidential Task Force on Regulatory Relief 1983, p. 34). Environmental regulation is the paradigm. We have a goal to minimize harmful pollution. On one hand, a design or engineering standard might prescribe a very specific technique or piece of equipment for treating emissions, thereby reducing release of some particular pollutant. A performance standard, on the other hand, would establish levels of the pollutant that may be released but leave it to the individual factory how to meet that goal. If the factory finds cheaper or better routes to compliance, so be it. Research advocates hoped to apply the concept to animal welfare as well.

Think of performance and design standards as two extreme ends of a continuum of regulatory possibilities, one with maximal flexibility, the other with ease of enforcement, with ongoing tension between the two (Breyer 1982). The design standard is easier to enforce, as an inspector can see whether the prescribed system is in place or not, but it is not very flexible when cheaper or more effective techniques are developed. In contrast, unless the standard is easily and unambiguously measurable, not some vague exhortation to "minimize harmful pollution," for example, the performance standard may be difficult to enforce. Note in the pollution example that the regulatory standard is chosen *after* the trade-off is negotiated to allow some release of polluting emissions that would be prohibitively expensive to eliminate entirely; the choice of regulatory strategy is not the same as the choice of regulatory goal.

One opening for the use of performance standards was the new mandate for dog exercise programs. Though on the table for two decades, Senator Robert Dole finally included a mandate for dog exercise in the 1985 Animal Welfare Act amendment. Much of the subsequent contention over exercise standards was a performance versus design debate: should the USDA dictate the frequency, duration, and type of exercise periods dogs receive, or could a performance criterion be articulated? Cage size standards were likewise open to performance/design decisions in the 1980s, though in this case, their inclusion in the Animal Welfare Act regulations and in the *Guide* predated the vogue for performance standards by two decades. At stake for animal protectionists' interests was the chance to expand the minimum mandated cage sizes for the various species of laboratory animals, most of which had been set in the 1960s with minimal subsequent revision. At risk for the research advocates was the prospect of scrapping their present cages, many of them made of expensive, heavy-gauge stainless steel and sized to just barely meet then-existing regulations, and replacing them with new, larger, and even more expensive cages, a capital outlay estimated in the hundreds of millions of dollars nationwide.

Cage sizes

From its first edition in 1963, the *Guide for Laboratory Animals Facilities and Care* had included a chart of cage-size prescriptions. Its veterinarian authors insisted that the chart was just a guide, not a regulation, and that their recommendations were "arbitrary," though at the same time representative of "the best judgment of experienced animal-care workers as to a reasonable space allocation" (Animal Care Panel 1963). Congress followed suit; the 1966 Laboratory Animal Welfare Act directed the secretary of agriculture to promulgate standards for humane animal care including "minimum requirements with respect to the housing" of the animals (U.S. Congress 1966a). The USDA responded with design standards: the mandated minimum requirements with respect to the housing became detailed cage-size prescriptions for the six animal types covered by the act (dog, cat, rabbit, hamster, guinea pig, and nonhuman primates).

The USDA in 1966 modeled its cage-size prescriptions roughly on the *Guide for Laboratory Animals Facilities and Care*. Harmonization between the two sets of recommendations was spotty over the years, though each clearly had its eye on the other, with the USDA adopting some of the *Guide*'s recommendation verbatim, and some editions of the *Guide* including USDA cage sizes as an appendix. Both the USDA and the *Guide* based their cage sizes for a species on the size of the individual animal. Comparison is not easy, as they used different animal-size group-

Table 5.1 1960s and 1980s cage sizes in the Animal Welfare Act (USDA)
and the NIH's *Guide for the Care and Use of Laboratory Animals.*

Species	USDA proposal, 1966	USDA final, 1967	1965 *Guide*
General	"Sufficient space for the animals to make normal postural adjustments with adequate freedom of movement"	"Sufficient space to allow each dog and cat to turn about freely and to easily stand, sit and lie in a normal position"	"Sufficient space to assure freedom of movement"
Dog	6 in. longer than the dog and 6 in. higher than shoulder Up to 10 per enclosure No additional exercise	Same, but no height specified Up to 12 per enclosure Same	Based on weight, not body length Supplemental exercise left to "professional judgment"
Cat, 9 lb.	3 ft.^{2} per adult 2 ft. high Up to 10 per enclosure	2.5 ft.^{2} per adult No height requirement Up to 12 per enclosure	3 ft.^{2} per adult 2 ft. high Up to 6 per cage
Rabbit, 10 lb.	5 ft.^{2} (less if grouped) No height specified	3.75 ft.^{2} No height specified	3 ft.^{2} 16 in. high (reduced to 14 in. 1972)
Guinea pig, 351 g	45 in.^{2} 10 in. high	90 in.^{2} 6.5 in. high	72–100 in.^{2} 8 in.

See text for specific references.

ings for some species, while for dogs and monkeys, the USDA based cage size on body length rather than on body weight, as found in the *Guide*.

An important trend in these early days of regulation was that the *Guide*'s self-imposed but nonbinding recommendations were consistently more spacious for the animals than were the USDA's legally binding minimum requirements. Hamsters, for example, got taller cages (8 inches as opposed to 5.5) and more leg room (16–96 square inches per animal as opposed to 15). The *Guide* offered cats 3 square feet apiece, while the USDA cut that down to 2.5, a little less than four 8.5 × 11 inch sheets of paper laid out together for a grown cat (ILAR 1968; Irving 1967). In table 5.1, I list cage-size recommendations, proposals, and requirements in the 1960s and 1980s in the Animal Welfare Act proposed and final rules and in the *Guide* for four representative animals.

The *Guide* took on more of a regulatory role as the NIH began to use it as the standard for animal welfare in the 1970s. Though the *Guide* authors continued their insistence that its cage-size recommendations were simply guidelines for

USDA proposal, 1989	USDA final, 1991	1985 *Guide*
"Sufficient space to allow each dog and cat to turn about freely and to easily stand, sit and lie in a normal position and to walk in a normal manner"	"Sufficient space to allow each dog and cat to turn about freely and to easily stand, sit and lie in a normal position and to walk in a normal manner"	"The housing system should provide space that is adequate, permits freedom of movement and normal postural adjustments, and has a resting place appropriate to the species"
No change in cage floor size	Same 6 in. higher than head	Based on weight
Must be 6 in. higher than highest point (erect ears) No group maximum for "conditioned" dogs	Same	
Exercise requirements: 30 minutes per day in 80 ft.² pen	Performance standard: facility must develop an exercise plan	Dog pens encouraged instead of ages for occupancy > 3 months
4 ft.² 2 ft. high	4 ft.² 2 ft. high	4 ft.² 2 ft. high
4 ft.² 14 in. high	4 ft.² 14 in. high	4 ft.² 14 in. high
101 in.² 7 in. high	101 in.² 7 in. high	101 in. 7 in. high

flexible interpretation, the table of recommendations came to look less so, and in my work as a laboratory animal technician in the early 1980s, we slavishly weighed animals and measured cages with a precision that gave no nod to "professional judgment." As the table became more precise and the spirit of flexibility harder to sustain, rabbits and rodents lost some cage space, while cats and larger monkeys gained.

Thus, the *Guide* shifted in its recommendations as its use as a rule book shifted: The more spacious recommendations during its days as ideal, if flexible, guidelines became the more modest standards to which institutions might actually be held. The *Guide's* increasing use as a rule book meant that any change in its table of cage-size recommendations became a de facto mandate for expensive cage replacements for institutions hoping to maintain their accreditation status. Since so many of the *Guide's* authors were themselves laboratory animal veterinarians managing large animal care programs, they could hardly be unaware of the expense they would create—for their own institutions and for their peers—if they progressively increased cage sizes with each *Guide* update. Subsequent editions of the *Guide* in 1978, 1985, and 1996 have contained virtually no changes in the table of cage-size recommendations (Committee on Laboratory Animal Housing 1976; Committee on Rodents 1996; ILAR 1965, 1985).

Cage sizes evolved even more slowly under the Animal Welfare Act provisions, with no congressional amendments specifically calling for them and few independent initiatives in that direction on the part of the USDA. In 1985, Congress ordered the USDA to consult with NIH in writing new animal welfare regulations, and for the most part, the USDA sought to harmonize the two sets of cage-size specifications. Floor areas were increased for guinea pigs, hamsters, and rabbits, in harmony with the *Guide*. Cat cages were expanded, as the USDA proposed replacing their 2.5-square-foot requirement for an adult cat with the *Guide*'s 3 square feet for small cats and a full 4 square feet for cats weighing more than 4 kilograms (8.8 pounds), and with a required 2 feet of headroom. Half an inch was added to cage heights for both guinea pigs and hamsters to match the *Guide*'s cage heights (Animal and Plant Health Inspection Service 1999).

Raising the roof by half an inch for hamsters and guinea pigs struck many people as absurd. Was there a scientific reason? Could the animals appreciate the difference? Though research advocates themselves had called for harmonization with the *Guide*, the bible of laboratory animal care, they did not see the *Guide*'s table of cage-size recommendations as sufficient justification for the expensive change. No one provided the USDA with testimony that their own institution would feel the financial impact. Presumably, most academic research institutions were already complying with the *Guide*'s standards if they were receiving NIH research grants, and the *Guide* had been calling for 7-inch-high guinea pig cages since 1972 (having reduced them to 7 inches from the earlier editions' 8-inch recommendation). Nonetheless, concern ran high. As the American Veterinary Medical Association wrote the USDA in 1989: "It would be a travesty if even a single young scientist were denied the opportunity to pursue biomedical research because an institution could not afford new cages to comply with the additional 1/2-inch height requirement for its guinea pigs" (Regulatory Analysis and Development 1989). Even the Animal Legal Defense Fund, one of the most active animal protection organizations at the time, agreed with the research advocacy groups; though continually pushing for the greatest changes in standards, they saw no reason for institutions to scrap 6.5-inch cages, suggesting instead that such new standards only apply to new cage purchases (Regulatory Analysis and Development 1989).

The USDA stayed with its 1989 proposal to increase hamster, guinea pig, rabbit, and cat cages, despite the protests. When the *Guide* has made changes to its table of cage-size recommendations, its authors have neither called the reader's attention to the change, nor defended or explained the change. But the USDA's rules writers are bound by federal policies to announce proposed regulation changes in the *Federal Register*, solicit public comments, and respond to them in publishing their final rule. Ordered by Congress to consult with NIH when writing new standards, they overruled dissenting voices and simply adopted the *Guide*'s cage sizes without further comment (Animal and Plant Health Inspection Service 1990b).

Only in one instance, the case of breeding cages for guinea pigs with litters, did the USDA provide a reason (in addition to harmonization with the *Guide*) for changing its cage-size requirements. In 1989, the USDA moved to delete its twenty-two-year-old provision of extra space for breeding guinea pigs, one of the few standards in which Animal Welfare Act requirements had exceeded *Guide* recommendations for cage space (Animal and Plant Health Inspection Service 1989b).

Defining standards in animal housing

A performance standard articulates a measurable outcome for a regulated practice. It may well be the same outcome that is sought in a design standard, but it allows the regulated entity to decide how to meet it. From the start, animal welfare regulations have contained explicit cage-size charts (engineering standards) alongside a version of performance standards. Consider the USDA's thirty-five-year-old formula for dog cages, phrased though it is in the most complicated way possible: "Each dog housed in any primary enclosure shall be provided a minimum square footage of floor space equal to the mathematical square of the sum of the length of the dog in inches, as measured from the tip of its nose to the base of the tail, plus 6 inches, expressed in square feet" (Irving 1967, p. 3274).

In other words, in a roughly square cage, picture your own dog, minus her tail, in a cage that is six inches longer on each side than her body. That is the size cage she would receive under Animal Welfare Act regulations. Engineering standards for cats' cages were roughly comparable in pre-1990 Animal Welfare Act regulations: a 2.5-square-foot cage is approximately 19 inches on each side (for a square cage), not much longer than most cats. Or consider rabbits: if a 10-pound rabbit occupies a 4-square-foot cage, that's a square 24 inches long on each wall for an animal almost 20 inches long, *if* she keeps her feet tucked under her in a standing position. If that 10-pound rabbit attempts to stretch out her hind legs in a resting position, she'll be closer to 25 inches long and will need to stretch out diagonally in the cage. To do that, the rabbit must forsake another favored behavior of lying in contact with a secure cage wall; rarely have we seen them do this (Kalagassy et al. 1999).

The engineering standard in the regulations' charts produces this performance outcome: animal cages should be a few inches bigger on a side than is the animal, when standing or lying in a more-or-less compact position.

Both the Animal Welfare Act regulations and the *Guide* have implied this pattern as a performance standard since long before that phrase became the vogue. They have stated the standard both as explanation of where the numbers in their tables originate and to have some parameters for housing those species (gerbils, wild mammals, frogs, and others) that do not get explicit mention in the cage-size tables.

Take a look at how this performance standard for cage sizes is articulated in the *Guide* and the Animal Welfare Act, both before and after the phrase took center stage. In the 1960s: "Primary enclosures shall . . . provide sufficient space to allow each dog and cat to turn about freely and to easily stand, sit and lie in a normal position" (Irving 1967, p. 3274). "The caging or housing system . . . should be designed with the animal's physical comfort as a primary consideration . . . providing sufficient space to assure freedom of movement" (ILAR 1965, p. 3). In the late 1980s and early 1990s, the USDA increased its design standard cage sizes for cats, rabbits, guinea pigs, and hamsters. USDA also updated its performance standards, with a new stipulation that dogs and cats be able to "walk in a normal manner."

The animal welfare regulations state a performance standard for what a dog must be able to do in a cage, as well as an engineering standard of how many square inches that cage must be. The engineering standard is the enforceable one, and so I carry a tape measure on my rounds, right with my copy of the regulations. Is there internal consistency of outcomes between these side-by-side standards? Not much.

The USDA revised its performance criteria in 1991 by adding "walking in a normal manner" to the other required freedoms (stand, sit, turn about freely). But can a dog walk in a normal manner in a cage that is only 6 inches longer than that dog's body? Not if "walking" includes taking one or more full strides. Few dog cages are perfect squares, though: perhaps a longer rectangular cage that met the same floor area would allow for a step or two? But as the length increases in a constant-area cage, width decreases, to the point that the cage is too narrow to meet the "turn about freely" performance standard. Likewise, dog cages that are 6 inches taller than the dog (regardless of her erect or drooping ears) allow her to stand in a "normal position" so long as that *only* means standing on all four legs; a dog who would sometimes prefer to stand on her hind legs is out of luck in such a cage.

The same mismatch holds true for resting positions, and with the *Guide*'s addition of "normal postural adjustments" to its long-standing "freedom of movement" criterion, it took on a similar performance/design mismatch to what the USDA had established. The Animal Welfare Institute's *Comfortable Quarters* (1979) contains line drawings of animals in resting postures that the cage-size charts of the current *Guide* and Animal Welfare Act prohibit. In particular, dogs, cats or rabbits who might rest with hind and forelegs extended will not be able to do this in cages that just meet the minimum stipulated dimensions, as many commercially available cages do.

I cannot say that the USDA or Association for Assessment and Accreditation of Laboratory Animal Care would never privilege the performance standard over the design standard, criticizing a facility whose cages met the rule books without providing freedom of movement, normal lying postures, or the ability to take a step or two "in a normal manner" (figures 5.1 and 5.2). I know I have never seen a site visitor overtly try to make such a determination for species which figured on the cage-size charts.

Beyond leg room: Alternative performance standards

Animal protectionists have never embraced performance standards, but mistrust of self-regulation and performance-based standards is only part of the picture. It

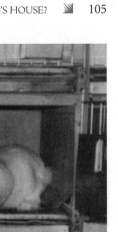

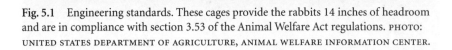

Fig. 5.1   Engineering standards. These cages provide the rabbits 14 inches of headroom and are in compliance with section 3.53 of the Animal Welfare Act regulations. PHOTO: UNITED STATES DEPARTMENT OF AGRICULTURE, ANIMAL WELFARE INFORMATION CENTER.

reflects protectionists' mistrust of scientists but should not obscure the fact that protectionists and research advocates want substantively different standards, however phrased or enforced. For decades, protectionists have called for big cages that cost big money, take up precious laboratory space, and require costly added labor.

In all aspects of laboratory animal care and use—animal housing, use of painkillers in experiments, provision of veterinary care—protectionists and research advocates have insisted there is no conflict between good science and good animal care. Protectionists claim their demands will not increase the cost of doing science, that the best scientists are already in line with protectionist ideals, or that even if costs do actually increase, better scientific data will be one happy outcome of improved animal care. Researchers insist the same: that their quality research has always depended on healthy, well-cared-for animal subjects for whom they have always provided well, except for the few "bad apples" of the occasional exposé. The 1963 *Guide* states "Rarely are the requirements of research incompatible with physical comfort" (Animal Care Panel 1963 p. 17). The Animal Welfare Institute (a private animal protection organization) publishes its own guidebook to "assist institutions in providing the most comfortable and practical housing for their animals, thus increasing the likelihood of sound scientific results" (Animal Welfare Institute, 1979, p. 1). With both groups sharing the same two goals of good

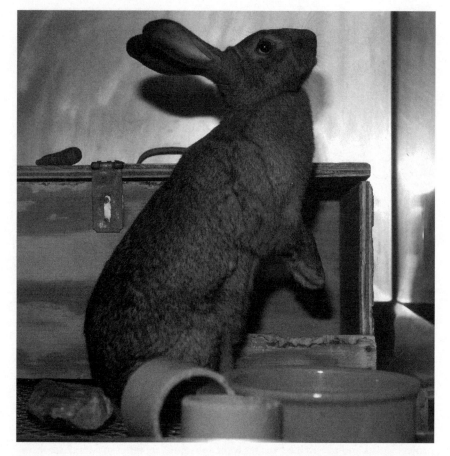

Fig. 5.2 Performance standards. This cage allows the rabbit to make "postural adjustments with adequate freedom of movement," in compliance with section 3.53 of the Animal Welfare Act regulations. Rabbits cannot stand up like this in the 14-inch tall cages in figure 5.1.

science and good animal care, their standards should be indistinguishable, but they are not.

The Animal Welfare Act is a compromise document, influenced by protectionists and by research advocates and forced upon scientists from without. The NIH *Guide* is the laboratory animal profession's vision of how animal care should be standardized—cognizant of protectionist demands and public sensibilities, but still the research community's exclusive domain. The Animal Welfare Institute's *Comfortable Quarters* fills this niche somewhat for the animal protectionist community, and its standards are worth looking at.

First published in 1955 and inspired by a British guidebook for animal care (Worden 1947), *Comfortable Quarters* predates the *Guide* by eight years and the Animal Welfare Act by eleven (Animal Welfare Institute 1955).[2] It bypasses most of the issues covered by the act and the *Guide*—sanitation, animal acquisition, re-search surgery, divisions of professional jurisdiction in the laboratory—for an ex-clusive focus on animal housing. For all its length (more than 100 pages in later editions), it finds no room for cage-size charts and tables: it is full of photos and drawings as part of a book-length argument in favor of its own set of (perhaps surprising) performance standards, summarized at the end of the book in the "An-imal Welfare Institute Policy on the use of Vertebrate Animals for Experimenta-tion and Testing."

In addition to the stand, sit, lie, and walk standards of the Animal Welfare Act and the freedom of movement and normal postural adjustments of the *Guide,* the Animal Welfare Institute's standards add some other activities: "Enclosures or cages must be sufficiently large and well constructed to permit burrowing, climbing, perching, swinging, walking, stretching, rolling, or other normal actions ordinar-ily seen in the species when not confined"(Animal Welfare Institute 1979, p. 108).

Rabbits cannot burrow in the steel-floored cages standard in most laboratories. Baboons cannot climb in the 36-inch high cage recommended by the 1985 *Guide* or required under the 1991 Animal Welfare Act standards. No dog or cat or rabbit can stretch in a cage just a few inches longer or taller than her torso. This is not just a different approach to enforcing or encouraging standards, but a different set of standards. Line drawings of the animals in these poses, and photos of cages that meet the Animal Welfare Institute's standards illustrate the pages of *Comfortable Quarters.* They do not resemble the 4-square-foot solitary caging cats or rabbits get in the other sets of standards.

The Animal Welfare Institute's standards would need more precision were they to become enforceable regulations. How much walking, for instance, would meet their minimum requirement? A step? Several steps? Nor were their standards as expansive as they might have been: running, jumping, and flying, for example, might be subsumed under "other normal actions," but given how many animal species run as part of their day, if the Animal Welfare Institute thought running was important, they should have itemized it along with walking and climbing and the others. But just as the *Guide's* authors hope to maintain its credibility with people outside of the scientific community, offering the *Guide* as "symbolic of the scientific community's ethical commitment" to animal care (Animal Care Panel 1963, p. 1), so too has the Animal Welfare Insitute sought acceptance of its *Com-fortable Quarters* with laboratory animal professionals. *Comfortable Quarters* has always included articles by well-known senior laboratory animal professionals, and in turn, *Comfortable Quarters* has appeared in the bibliography of every edi-tion of the *Guide.* Setting some bounds on the space offered to animals maintains the status of *Comfortable Quarters* as a reasonable document.

The Animal Welfare Institute is not alone in proffering alternative standards to those of the act and the *Guide.* I have found no evidence of standards that are less spacious than the act and the *Guide's* specifications for cages slightly smaller than their outstretched animal occupant, but suggestions for larger cages are numer-ous. As official policy, the European Union and the Canadian Council on Animal

Care have both employed performance criteria that differ little from the USDA and NIH criteria, but in the United Kingdom, in particular, that standard is then translated into design specifications for cage sizes three to five times larger than their American counterpart, depending on the species (Royal Society and the Universities Federation for Animal Welfare 1987).[3]

Expertise and animal cages

Mismatch between the Animal Welfare Act or the *Guide*'s stated performance standards and their specific cage-size recommendations are only a part of the concern in how to house research animals. If the *Guide* were rewritten tomorrow with cage size tables that really did allow rabbits and cats to express all their "normal postural adjustments," or if the act's cage-size formulae really did allow dogs and cats to "walk in a normal manner," we would hardly have closed the chapter on how large a cage to give an animal. Does a single step in any one direction constitute walking in a normal manner? Why must they be allowed to walk at all, as long as they can rest comfortably? Where would they go if they could take a second or third step in their cages? On the other hand, why stop at requiring space to walk? Should cages be large enough to allow dogs and cats to run if they choose? Or jump? What makes the University of Chicago animal behaviorists specify *six* full pace-lengths as a minimum cage length, rather than three, twelve, or twenty-seven? Where do these standards come from? What really are we trying to do?

Laboratory primates are at most a few generations removed from their wild-caught progenitors. Even today, many primates currently in laboratories began their lives in the jungles of Asia or the savannas of Africa: They are wild animals. Dogs and cats and hoofstock have been familiar domestics for centuries. How do we condense these animals' normal lives in the wild or in human society into the laboratory? What features must be retained and which excluded? Throughout most of their histories, the act and the *Guide* distilled the question down to one of cage size. Social considerations, for example, were cordoned off in early editions of the *Guide* as matters for in-house rule and professional judgment, not for national guidelines. Other aspects of caging were largely ignored, except for sanitizability, and absence of sharp edges or sites for injury. What about denning areas? A space to dig, or climb, or lie in the sun? A place to defecate that is more than 6 inches from where an animal lays her head?

Until the 1990s, neither the *Guide* nor the act often said where they got their standards. The *Guide*, for instance, made no effort to directly link recommendations within its text to the extensive bibliography in its Appendix. Information in the appended references only made it into the *Guide*'s text through the filter of its authoring committees, its anonymous reviewers, and their "knowledgeable experience and opinion" (ILAR 1965, p. 1). The USDA made even less effort to tie its Animal Welfare Act regulations to a publicly accessible base of knowledge.

The USDA's particular trump card was its experience in enforcing the Animal Welfare Act, something it alone had ever done. Since 1967, the USDA had been sending its veterinarian-inspectors into research animal facilities throughout the nation. In the process, they collectively saw just about every possible variant of housing conditions. Thus they could write in 1990, "based on our inspections of research facilities," that 2.5 square feet would not "provide cats with the space we believe is necessary," and they increased cage size to 4 square feet for large adult cats (Animal and Plant Health Inspection Service 1990a, p. 33464). They further agreed with unnamed commenters that stretching the front and back legs was "part of a cat's normal behavior," which must be accommodated in larger cages, but only in a horizontal direction (p. 33464). Cats who might prefer to stretch upwards, dreaming perhaps of stereo speakers and shreddable couches, were of lesser concern to the USDA, and the need for cages exceeding the minimum 2 feet were "subject to the judgment of the attending veterinarian" (p. 33464). As with cats, the USDA could not justify cages tall enough to allow dogs to stand up on their hind legs, or to hold their tails aloft: "We do not consider a dog's standing on its hind legs to be a frequent enough postural adjustment to require its inclusion as a minimal standard" (Animal and Plant Health Inspection Service 1991, p. 6444).

Just as the USDA's special database was its own enforcement experience, so the ultimate justification for its regulations was not what was best for animals or best for science, but what Congress intended in passing the act. Without congressional mandate, the USDA had no authority. Thus it retreated from initial proposals to address animals' comfort, recognizing it had overstepped its authority: "With regard to the word 'comfort' we agree [with commenters] that it is inappropriate for use in the proposed regulations. Although we encourage an environment that will promote the dogs' and cats' comfort, the intent of the regulations is to provide minimum standards for the health and well-being of the animals" (Animal and Plant Health Inspection Service, 1990a, p. 33458). The USDA did not interpret Congress's Improved Standards for Laboratory Animals as including comfort in the definition of well-being, and so removed it from its regulations as out of its jurisdiction.

Both the USDA and the *Guide*'s authors bemoaned the lack of scientific data on which to base cage-size recommendations, though still feeling the need to set some standard. Little effort went into filling this knowledge gap. The USDA convened "an expert committee of nationally recognized zoo curators, directors, and veterinarians" to set space requirements for those warm-blooded animals (such as zoo species) not initially covered by the act; the committee's consensus was that there were inadequate data (Animal and Plant Health Service 1971, p. 919). Despite the USDA's intention of requesting public data, views, and arguments on the subject, they never have specified standards for these other species. Likewise, the self-regulating scientific and laboratory animal professionals were better at pointing out the holes in the database than at working to fill them.

In 1976, the National Academy of Sciences' Institute of Laboratory Animal Resources (ILAR; publishers of the NIH *Guide*) convened a symposium on laboratory animal housing, a follow-up to a 1963 symposium on the topic. Though four editions of ILAR's *Guide* had by that time called their own cage-size recommendations arbitrary, the two-day symposium never addressed cage-size needs, focusing instead on topics like construction materials and air handling systems. One talk on "integrating psychosocial objectives" into animal facility design covered social behavior of people during their work day in the labs, not the animals who lived there round the clock. The two talks that did discuss the animals in their cages ignored cage size as a relevant topic and spoke instead of the animals' social environments, their responses to isolation and to crowding (Committee on Laboratory Animal Housing 1976). Despite the data presented on the stresses of isolation and crowding, the 1978 *Guide* continued to mention overcrowding only briefly in relation to physical comfort and to ignore social isolation, either as a research variable or a welfare concern, entirely.

In the late 1980s, the scientific and laboratory animal professionals called for standards based on science, and the USDA began citing a handful of research papers as justification for its proposed rules. Of those research reports covering species other than dogs, the most important was White, Balk, and Lang's (1989) study of cage space use among guinea pigs (see also White 1990). Submitted to the USDA in a prepublication form by the National Association for Biomedical research, the USDA cited these papers in its decision to scale back the space requirements it had proposed for breeding groups of guinea pigs (Animal and Plant Health Inspection Service).

The authors were three laboratory animal veterinarians associated with the Hershey Medical Center in Pennsylvania and with Charles River Laboratories, a major commercial breeder of guinea pigs and other rodents for research. They sited their work squarely in its political context, noting the expense of animal housing. They reminded the reader that neither the *Guide* (on whose 1972 and 1978 authoring committees Lang had served) nor the Animal Welfare Act regulations gave the source of the data used in their cage-size recommendations, and they compared their study cage to the USDA's space requirements.

In the study, harem breeding groups of one male and either three or six females were videotaped to examine their use of cage space. The males were vasectomized so that sexual behavior would continue, without the group sizes constantly shifting as litters were born. The cages were large enough (718 square inches) to slightly exceed USDA's requirements for seven adult, nonbreeding guinea pigs, but would only have met standards for three breeders. The black plastic cages were kept free of litter to improve the videotape quality, and the pigs were filmed day and night.

The authors reasoned that as population went up, guinea pigs seeking to avoid unwanted interactions would spread out over the entire cage, making full use of the available space. But if herding and grouping were more important to them, they would not spread out. The results: they found no difference in cage space utilization whether four or seven guinea pigs were living together. Moreover, their guinea pigs tended to sit along the cage periphery in a group, their rumps to the wall, avoiding the bare center of the cage (figure 5.3). Having situated their study in its political context, so, too, did the authors translate their findings into their

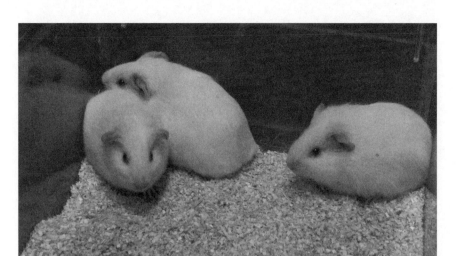

Fig. 5.3 Guinea pigs often cluster together or hug the cage walls, leaving most of the cage space unoccupied for much of the day.

political implications: "groups of guinea pigs use very little of the space available to them . . . 4636 cm^2 of floor area provides adequate space for a breeding group of 7 guineapigs, even though this is 40% less than current USDA guidelines" (White et al. 1989, p. 213).

It worked. For twenty years, the USDA had required double the cage space for breeding guinea pigs. Citing this study, the USDA proclaimed that henceforth, guinea pigs would have the same cage size regardless of whether they were breeding, pregnant, raising a litter.

With this move, the USDA set a precedent, for the first time directly linking one of its rules to a published study. For this one ruling, at least, it could not be accused of hiding behind the veil of its enforcement experience, the consensus of vaguely identified experts, or its divinations of congressional intent. Here were hard, objective facts, gleaned with a "computer-coupled video tracking system." Fact led neatly to regulation, virtually untouched by human hands, just as the scientific community had been calling for.

The trouble with tying regulations so tightly to universally accessible data, however, is that any individual study is open to alternative interpretation. The USDA had already "carefully reviewed and analyzed the material" (nearly two years before its peer review and publication) and proclaimed the data sound (Animal and Plant Health Inspection Service 1989b, p. 10910). And though the USDA's was ultimately the deciding voice, it was not the only one.

In 1989, the Animal Legal Defense Fund challenged the USDA's use of these guinea pig studies in its correspondence to the USDA. ALDF claimed that these studies neglected to take into account guinea pigs' "natural preference for the periphery of a cage for leaning against, resting, etc." ALDF wrote: "Merely because guinea pigs prefer the periphery of a cage doesn't lead logically to the conclusion that the unoccupied space in the middle of the cage can be taken away without any effect. The space equal to the area in the middle of the cage is still necessary for exercise, stretching of limbs and for space that is taken up by feeding bowls or water bowls" (Regulatory Analysis and Development 1989).

The USDA, like the NIH *Guide*'s authors, has never elaborated any theory of cage-size determination into which to plug new data. Why did it secure larger cages for breeding groups in the first place? Did it simply assume that there would always be young stock scurrying about? Neither the Animal Welfare Act regulations nor the NIH *Guide* count unweaned young, no matter how active, in calculating space per animal, and so a seven-adult harem with ten suckling young still only counts as seven animals. Perhaps it thought pregnant females had different space needs or preferred to get away from each other or from amorous males more often. Having no guiding principles on which to base cage-size regulations, it was susceptible to any claim to scientific data that could give it some firm basis for its rules. But what did the guinea pig studies really show?

The political context, intent, and timing of the guinea pig study were obvious: Even though published in a European journal, the comparison to American regulations was stressed. The authors stopped short of calling for a change in regulations, but they were clear in their conclusion that "the current guidelines for guinea pig housing based on area allocation per guineapig, cannot be supported by the behavioural characteristics of these animals or careful quantitation of their patterns of cage use" (White et al. 1989, p. 213). They had specifically avoided any attempt to assess or define stress in the animals as "subjective at best," but failed to see or acknowledge the limits to the objectivity of their own work.[4]

Look again at how guinea pigs used their available space. They spent 75–88% of their time in about 47% of their cage, mostly along the wall. Or, as the authors state, the pigs may spend up to 25% of their time in other parts of the cage. Exploring? Exercising? Getting some social distance from each other? We don't know, as this is a study of the objective movements of animals, not the subjective assessment of their motives. But it is a subjective interpretation, though phrased in impersonal language, that up to 25% of time spent moving around the larger space represents using little of the cage space available. An alternative interpretation, equally in tune with the data presented, is that spending 25% of one's time someplace (six hours a day) is quite a significant use of that space. But as the USDA was concurrently ruling (even without computerized video data) that dogs do not stand on their hind legs often enough to protect that postural privilege in law, why would it challenge the laboratory animal professionals at Charles River Laboratories?

The National Association for Biomedical Research submitted the White et al. report as evidence that large, open spaces in guinea pig cages should not be mandated. But as surely as the study showed that floor area was not important to the pigs, it revealed two things that pigs want: a wall to stand against and a group to huddle with. Either of these provisions could have been mandated in the new Animal Welfare Act regulations, but NABR did not ask and the USDA did not move to shift how it thought about cage space. You will not find, for instance, any design standard that each guinea pig receive x inches of wall space or a performance standard that cage complexity be maximized with plenty of opportunity to avoid open spaces and huddle in corners or along walls. The USDA's regulations likewise remain silent about whether guinea pigs should be housed in groups when possible, despite what the computerized video tracking system shows to be their strong preference.

The USDA listened to what the guinea pigs said they did not want (large, open spaces) rather than what they said they did want (sheltered, wall-side spaces; social grouping). These guinea pig studies also made it into the 1996 *Guide for the Care and Use of Laboratory Animals,* but by then their meaning had been reshaped: "Whenever it is appropriate, social animals should be housed in pairs or groups, rather than individually, . . . some rodents or swine housed in compatible groups seek each other out and share cage space by huddling together along walls, lying on each other during periods of rest, or gathering in areas of retreat" (ILAR 1996, p. 26).

These studies were also cited indirectly in the *Guide* (as citations within the cited references) for the claim that "some species benefit more from wall space (e.g., thigmotactic rodents) . . . than from simple increases in floor space" (ILAR 1996, p. 25). White et al.'s study had rediscovered the concept of thigmotaxis, the orientation of some animals to tactile stimuli, in their wall-hugging, contact-seeking guinea pigs. Concepts cross disciplines only with difficulty, and so while thigmotaxis may be a familiar concept to animal behaviorists, the three laboratory animal veterinarians studying guinea pig cage use may not have been familiar with it. Their work was situated in the applied and political arena of laboratory animal science, with little reference to concepts from the academic study of animal behavior. It took the work of animal behaviorists to put the guinea pig studies in that context and to rewrite their meaning, from the "space is wasted" to the "huddling along walls is beneficial" policy lesson (Anzaldo et al. 1994; Stricklin 1995). Thus, while one policy conclusion of guinea pig studies was regulatory relief from excessively spacious (and expensive) cages, the same research findings can be a tool to argue for increased complexity of caging and to strengthen the presumption in favor of social housing.

Change comes slowly. The 1996 *Guide* brought new emphasis to how animals use space and how social interaction may affect their lives, but this is not reflected in that document's cage-size charts. Rather, the new concerns are written in the new language of performance standards—complex, subtle, flexible, general principles rather than specific rules. They are embedded in lengthy text, rather than set out and apart as tables. How these new standards will affect the actual animals will depend on how laboratory animal professionals transition to the new regulatory approach, finding a language that goes beyond compliance and violations, learning that "flexible" does not mean "optional." My professional experience has shown me that that transition is only just beginning. I have seen rats, for instance, housed in variably sized groups or in solitude, even within a single research project, despite the *Guide*'s standard that "social animals should be housed in physical contact with conspecifics" and the likelihood of increased research variability with such a difference in animal treatment. Armed with nothing but a *Guide* that repeatedly emphasizes its flexibility, I have found lackluster support within institutions in addressing social isolation, especially for rodents.

Conclusion

The NIH *Guide* and the USDA have retained their charts and tables of animal cage-size recommendations, continuing a thirty-plus year tradition of design standards and an overly simplistic assumption that floor space is the important variable in animal housing. As people add on other concerns (cage complexity, social grouping, vertical space, escape from aggressors, nesting and resting materials), the concept of charts and rigid rules becomes unwieldy and irrelevant, and generally worded performance standards look more attractive. The flexibility of self-regulating performance standards, however, makes them suspect in the eyes of animal protectionists, who fought long and hard to impose more control over animal researchers.

In a political climate in which animal protectionists and research advocates distrust each other, concern about the enforceability and the flexibility of standards runs high. But enforceability was really only part of the animal protectionists' agenda in pushing for changes to Animal Welfare Act standards in the 1980s. Debate over performance versus design standards complicates the picture but does not remove the basic fact that data only enter the political arena through the lens of human interpretation. Both regulatory approaches rest on making some sort of assessment of what makes for good animal welfare. Both also require value judgments, balancing animal welfare against cost, research considerations, and staffing capabilities. How strongly must animals choose certain conditions, how often must they assume various postures or execute particular movements for those behavioral opportunities to be protected by regulation? Scientific studies may help with the assessment of animal welfare, but they do not make the value judgments.

Neither the government veterinarians writing Animal Welfare Act regulations nor the scientists and veterinarians writing the *Guide for the Care and Use of Laboratory Animals* have made explicit through the years how they translate knowledge into animal care recommendations. The anonymous review processes and expert authorship of the *Guide* perform the same political work as the USDA's claims of experience through enforcement: They restrict the relevant database to something they alone have full access to. In the 1980s, both the USDA and the *Guide* authors began to open up that process, explicitly identifying some of the scientific studies in which they find prescriptions for animal welfare policy. Opening up the process is a two-edged sword, however: It gives credibility to the people writing the regulations, but it allows greater access to people who would write the regulations differently.

The guinea pig studies I have described were but one instance of using data to generate policy, significant for how explicitly the USDA acknowledged them, but otherwise completely ordinary. The *Guide* and the act contain hundreds of recommendations and regulations on animal care and use, which must be applied to a wide range of animal species. Just as the guinea pig studies were vulnerable on methodological and interpretive grounds, so too is virtually any other study that is employed in the regulatory context. In this context, a study may be criticized on methodological grounds and faulted for producing erroneous data. But often, that is a superficial challenge: Most controversies leave the data pretty well intact with the real disagreement over interpretation of what the data mean. Witness how everyone can agree that the vasectomized guinea pig harems huddled together along the wall in large cages with bare central spaces and still profoundly disagree over what that tells us about how to house breeding groups of guinea pigs.

Similar controversies are possible with every other species. Scott Line, a veterinarian and animal behaviorist, cited some 1963 studies of chimpanzees as evidence that cage size had no effect on the development of abnormal, stereotyped behaviors (Animal and Plant Health Inspection Service 1990b). But in the hands of chimpanzee behaviorist Roger Fouts (1998), the studies are meaningless. All of the cage sizes studied in the 1963 studies were too small, in Fouts's opinion, and so small incremental increases were meaningless to the animals. Only when the larger enclosures are island-sized habitats providing a range of behavioral and social opportunities would he expect to reveal the correlation between enclosure size and psychopathology.

Nor is the problem restricted to cage-size determinations. Any time the interpretation of experimental data results in policy decisions, the stakes can be high enough to sustain an ongoing series of critiques, dismissals, and deconstructions. The competition is on to be the one to speak for animals and what they want. Science is one tool in that competition. In the coming chapters on euthanasia methods, dog exercise, and primate psychological well-being, I show the limits (not the uselessness, but the clearly limited usefulness) of science's potential to deliver us from the need to make value judgments about the lives of animals.

6

Centaurs and science: The professionalization

of laboratory animal care and use

MANY OF THE LABORATORY ANIMAL VETERINARIANS I KNOW HAVE A MISSIONARY streak: They do the work they do because they think they can make the lives of research animals better. When I first started working with laboratory animals in 1981, I encountered a curious division of labor that blunted veterinarians' potential. Veterinarians (and their Animal Welfare Act inspectors) focused in the minutest detail on how animals were housed and cleaned and fed, but they had little voice in how animal experiments were conducted. Moreover, in their zeal for health and hygiene, wood, blankets, and anything soft but not readily sterilized were banished, and animals lived singly in stainless-steel cages. But perhaps most incongruously, veterinarians as a group were far more active than the scientists who experiment on animals in battling pressures from the animal protectionists to change things.

I would not have designed laboratory animal care this way; I want veterinarians to be unequivocally effective champions of laboratory animal welfare. But there are reasons that things were the way they were. In this chapter, I explain the history of how these curious divisions of labor arose, and why I am glad they are breaking down. We'll start at the beginning.

Before he was immortalized as the constellation Sagittarius, Cheiron was a centaur on earth. Half human and half horse, he practiced the healing arts, both for humans and for other centaurs. He taught his medicine to a human, Aesculapius, whose staff, animated by two serpents, became the symbol of the medical profession.

Cheiron's personal identity and professional activities blurred the boundaries between human and animal. Throughout history and across several cultures, people who have healed other people have also healed animals. In the nineteenth century, however, as physicians established their formal and learned profession, a gulf arose between human and animal healing. Still, Aesculapius's snake entwined the healing staff, the animal symbol intimately connected with medicine. Charles Darwin further challenged human–animal dichotomies, emphasizing the continuities of the human and the animal condition, differences of degree, not of kind. The animal experiments of Magendie, Bernard, Pasteur, and Koch provided the scientific base that characterized modern medicine, a science dependent on human–animal similarities. But despite these intimate linkages of human and animal in symbol and in science, medical practitioners distanced themselves more and more from what the sociologist Everett Hughes (1958) might label the "dirty work" of veterinary medicine.

The gulf exists not because humans and animals differ so markedly in their diseases and their cures but because of matters of profession, policy, and economics. Physicians have replaced the clergy as the premier professionals trafficking in matters of life and death; who could expect them to sully their hands with colicky horses or dyspeptic swine? To many people, veterinary medicine is much closer to agriculture and to dog shows than to human medicine. It is *animal* medicine, not animal *medicine*.

Veterinarians, though, have maintained awareness of the connections between human and animal medicine, and, indeed, several veterinary training programs in this country have included class time spent with future physicians. To veterinarians, accustomed to extrapolating knowledge across species lines—from dogs to horses to chickens and whatnot—the overlaps with human medicine are obvious. Many veterinarians have X-rayed their own injuries, sutured their own wounds, treated their own infections; I certainly have. A broken toe is a broken toe, after all, whether sheathed with nail, claw, or hoof.

Medical doctors are often far less aware of what veterinary medicine comprises. Medical doctors treat human patients; veterinarians treat all other species. Their professional domains are clear and rarely overlap. But nowhere, since centaurs roamed the plains of Greece, are species boundaries blurred more than in animal research laboratories. There, the biological and medical continuities across human and animal taxa are emphasized, often in departments of comparative medicine. There, animals have long served as models of the human condition. Blurring species boundaries even further, some transgenic animals now actually carry human DNA in their genes.

The expertise of laboratory animal veterinarians is in the biological and medical continuities across human and animal taxa. They have seen themselves as central to the judicious care and use of laboratory animals. And yet, they have faced an uphill struggle trying to establish their professional niche in animal research. Even when medical doctors embark on research that uses animals, they may fail to see much worth in having veterinarians tagging along on their quest for new cures and new knowledge. Laboratory animal veterinarians have worked to overcome such prejudices of physicians and scientists since the early days of their professional specialty.

From my standpoint as a laboratory animal veterinarian, I see veterinarians as key actors in establishing the daily practices that determine animals' lives. Like the centaur Cheiron, their healing spans the human and animal realms. As long as animals populate laboratories as models of the human condition, veterinarians will be there as their doctors. Veterinarians manage animal facilities, sit on animal care and use committees, write the *Guide for the Care and Use of Laboratory Animals* and the Animal Welfare Act regulations, conduct USDA inspections and accreditation site visits, perform research on animal diseases, anesthesia, and husbandry, teach students, supervise technicians, and treat the research animals when they are ill or injured.

In this chapter, I look closely at the development of the profession of laboratory animal veterinary medicine. Veterinarians have enormous potential to be the strongest voices for animal welfare, and yet this had been blunted at times by the work they have had to do to even have a place in the laboratory. One of the curious effects of this struggle has been a professional division between animal *care* (and housing and management before the experiment begins) and animal *use* (what happens to animals once the experiment has begun). This division delayed serious and consistent oversight of animal use. Moreover, the place of veterinarians in the laboratory was secured not just because of their value in maintaining animal health but by their utility in combating antivivisectionists who were calling for tight restrictions on animal research.

It is impossible to fully understand the lives and welfare of laboratory animals without examining the role of veterinarians, which calls for a look back at how the profession of laboratory animal medicine developed.

Laboratory animal practice as a profession

The ability and interest of laboratory animal veterinarians in working for animal welfare is profoundly shaped by professionalization issues such as their legal, practical, and moral authority over other professionals' (research scientists) practices. This authority is not an automatic or natural fact of animal research, but it was shaped, fought for, and contested. In this chapter, I describe how ongoing competition among scientists, laboratory animal veterinarians, and animal protectionists to speak for animals shapes the profession, its goals, and its effectiveness.

I follow Andrew Abbott (1988) in choosing an ecological or systems model to chart the development of the profession. Two key features of this contextual model are (1) it makes best sense to look at professions in relation to the other professions around them, and (2) interprofessional relations may profitably be studied as competition for a limited resource: professional jurisdiction over one or more tasks. Professions may be born or die as a new professional task is created or an established one goes away: think about the new profession of airline pilots and the extinction of stagecoach drivers as transportation technologies evolved. Or professional groups may vie for ongoing jurisdictions, as when the young profession of psychiatry convinced people in the nineteenth century that madness was a medical, not a criminal, condition and more properly the province of specialized physicians than of legal authorities.

Types of work may differ in their prestige, the amount of preparation required for mastery, the social and economic status of the clientele served, and the need for large capital expenditures and centralized factory/hospital/office settings. The work that laboratory animal veterinarians do differs in important ways from what general veterinary practitioners do: Its connection to human medicine elevates its status and moves the work from private offices to institutional laboratory and medical-center settings. However, its differences from the standard pet-and-farm focus of standard veterinary curricula potentially render veterinarians ill-prepared for this role, and so invite competition from nonveterinarians. Its scrutiny by animal protectionists has led to government involvement in establishing jurisdictional divisions between the scientists who experiment on animals and the veterinarians overseeing the animals' care.

We will see how a jurisdictional split between animal care and animal use left scientists' experimental treatment of animals largely unregulated for decades despite passage of the 1966 Laboratory Animal Welfare Act. The priorities of laboratory animal practice have also shifted over the years, from an early focus on infection control and physical disease to greater emphasis on animal pain and distress in research to questions of how to recognize and promote happiness and emotional well-being among animals. All of this has profound effects on the welfare of the animals living in the laboratories.

Readers can find a handful of histories of the development of laboratory animal medicine—the founding fathers, the associations they formed, the training programs and certification procedures, the codes of practice, and the scholarly journals (Brewer 1980; Cohen and Loew 1984; Quimby 1994). To find lessons in these histories about the potential of veterinarians to promote animal welfare, we need to consider the professional issues that empower or emasculate veterinarians in this role. Why did the profession arise when it did? What issues did it prioritize? What autonomy and authority have veterinarians had in the laboratory? What tasks have veterinarians performed, and who would control these tasks if veterinarians did not? How exclusive is veterinarians' hold on their knowledge and skills?

Abbott (1988) mentions veterinarians only once in his treatise on professions, as an example of a profession, like nursing and pharmacy, content with a limited jurisdiction within the larger health field that is dominated by physicians.[1] He might just as accurately have classed veterinary medicine as the premier of the "animal fields," dominant to animal science, animal husbandry or animal behavior. In truth, it is both animal work and medical work and the profession's radically different status in these two different arenas has had profound effects on its development. Nowhere has this been more apparent than in those places (medical research establishments in particular) where human and veterinary medicine come into close contact. As medicine's "poor relation," veterinarians seeking employment in medical centers are at a disadvantage. But raise the status of laboratory animals through animal welfare regulations, and their doctors, the premier animal professionals, are similarly elevated.

Much of the sociological literature on professions assumes a private practice paradigm; Abbott's model is useful in its application to institutional workplaces as well. Whereas limited licensure for practice may be an important issue for professionals in private practice, divisions of labor, authority, and responsibility within the workplace loom large for others. For example, only veterinarians are licensed to perform animal surgery on pet animals in private practice. In contrast, surgery on research animals in institutional settings has never been limited by law or licensure to veterinarians, and policy issues center more on who should establish and monitor standards of practice for the myriad scientists, physicians, technicians, and students who perform surgeries, often far from the watchful eye of a veterinarian. Much of the controversy around the 1985 amendment to the Animal Welfare Act came down to disagreement over government-imposed divisions of labor within institutions: who should review research proposals, assess the psychological well-being of primates, or assess the credentials of experimenters to perform procedures on animals.

Laboratory animal veterinarians have defined their profession in terms of animal husbandry, animal health, and animal welfare, three somewhat separable jurisdictions throughout the brief history of this discipline. Three main groups have vied for control of these jurisdictions: Scientists strive to maintain their freedom to conduct research without constraints from antivivisectionists or from veterinarians; antivivisectionists desperately struggle for government regulations based on their conception of animal welfare; and veterinarians somehow carve a niche for themselves that accommodates the interests of both of the other groups. A new niche and a new profession: the professional management of laboratory animal care.

Three features of the ecological landscape in which laboratory animal medicine has developed are key: (1) the animals themselves, (2) veterinarians' relations with the research scientists whose animals they attend, and (3) the external threats of antivivisectionists to restrict or abolish animal research.

The landscape of laboratory animal practice

The animals

Animals present their own realities that shape both the practice of laboratory animal medicine and the potential of veterinarians to be their welfare advocates. The uses to which animals have been put in experimentation have changed over the years, but so have the animals themselves, unlikely though that may seem. As a laboratory animal veterinarian starting out in the 1980s, I faced many different challenges from my predecessors of the 1950s. Some of these reflect changed professional opportunities and the profound influence of current regulation; some simply reflect that the animals we work with now are a very different breed.

As veterinarians of the 1940s and 1950s found, animal health problems were rife in the laboratories, where whole experiments might sometimes be scrapped as an epidemic raged through an animal colony. They worked with wild-caught monkeys from the jungles of Asia, stray dogs and cats from pounds and shelters, and mice and rabbits from small-scale breeders, cleaning up their parasites and infections the best they could before offering the animals up for research. Even the available feeds were contaminated with *Salmonella* (Griffin 1952). Laboratory animal veterinarians of my generation take for granted the availability of clean and healthy research animals, balanced and wholesome diets, and established quarantine and testing protocols that minimize the spread of infections. We choose rats and mice, even dogs and monkeys, from catalogs that tell us their genetics and their health status.[2] We modern practitioners have it easy, and we have our predecessors in this profession to thank.

And yet, even this role, guardians of laboratory animal health, was not assured to veterinarians in the early days. Veterinarians and their critics both saw with equal clarity the mismatch between then-available veterinary education and the job that laboratory animal veterinarians would hold. When the New York Academy of Sciences sponsored one of the first American conferences on laboratory animal care in 1944, covering diseases, genetics, breeding, and housing, not a single veterinarian contributed a paper (Cohen 1959). In 1950, at a meeting convened by Chicago-area laboratory animal veterinarians, C. Neville Wentworth Cumming (an animal facility manager, who was not a veterinarian) spoke on the value of trained laboratory animal caretakers but questioned the usefulness of veterinarians in such training: "Veterinarians often strikingly lack in knowledge of the small animal. They can take care of cows, horses, and sheep, etc., but it is doubtful if veterinarians should be endorsed to train small animal attendants" (quoted in Flynn 1980, p. 767).

The first half of the twentieth century saw a gradual shift in veterinary practice. Though agricultural use of animals remained prominent throughout the century, assuring some rural veterinary employment vaccinating hogs and midwifing cattle, urban horse and dog work underwent radical changes. Automobiles and railroads displaced horses as the primary means of transportation in and between urban areas. Veterinarians in urban areas had to change with the times—either learn auto mechanics or develop a new patient base. Though some vets were sure the death of their profession was imminent, increasingly urban Americans and their pet dogs came to the rescue. By the 1950s, cats were finally seeing vets too, reflecting their new cachet as urban pets. Pet practitioners were learning that while their general veterinary knowledge helped them face new settings and unfamiliar species, the details and differences could still have life-and-death consequences (Jones 2003).

Laboratory animal veterinarians of the day were facing many similar challenges and learning similar lessons. Rabbits, rats, monkeys, and frogs were very different from the horses, cows, dogs, and swine that composed the bulk of veterinary education. Moreover, the setting for their care and use differed in important ways from the farm and the home. General principles and general knowledge are important first steps, but these could not carry the day alone. Species differences can be formidable in laboratory animal practice. How do you obtain enough blood from a mouse for disease diagnosis without seriously subjecting a sick animal to overwhelming blood loss? How do you restrain a sick, wild-caught monkey for examination? How do you interpret laboratory findings from a hamster, a baboon, or a leopard frog when neither normal nor abnormal standards have been defined?

The laboratory setting itself holds different clinical challenges, even when the species are those familiar to vets in pet or farm practice. In my years as a laboratory animal veterinarian, for instance, I have never seen a single flea, and I certainly never saw animals hit by cars; my patients come from "clean" sources and are almost never allowed outdoors. I have overseen mouse colony health programs for excluding viruses, some of which (the minute virus of mice comes to mind) are virtually incapable of causing disease, yet whose detection, and the fear that they might complicate interpretation of some experiments, could lead us to "depopulate" the entire colony (Committee on Infectious Diseases of Mice and Rats 1991). We watch the animals' health, genetics, and nutrition not just because we care about the animals but because good science demands the minimal extraneous variability among its research subjects.

Thus the animals themselves (the unfamiliar species, their infection-ridden sources, their role in laboratory life) shaped laboratory animal medicine as a profession. They gave veterinarians plenty to work on, and information on monkey and mouse health and disease rapidly accumulated. Veterinarians' early infection-control challenges shaped the professional standards they elaborated over the years. Sanitizable steel surfaces figure prominently in the NIH's *Guide for the Care and Use of Laboratory Animals* and in Animal Welfare Act regulations. In the face of rampant animal infections in the 1940s, 1950s or 1960s, wire-grid floors, steel and concrete surfaces, and solitary caging of animals are a blessing. The *Guide* and the act buttressed the calls of laboratory animal veterinarians to eliminate wood cages and straw and dirt floors from research animal housing, despite the high costs to the institutions using them. Sharing the laboratory animal veterinarians' focus on hygiene, USDA inspectors would sweep through facilities, citing rusted metal, cracks in concrete floors, and any hint of wood as violations of the Animal Welfare Act to provide animals with easily sanitized living quarters.

Veterinarians might be criticized by their scientist peers for the expense and the rigidity of their requirements, and indeed they were. But to the extent that freedom from infection correlates with animal health, comfort, or welfare, laboratory animal veterinarians could only be seen as champions of the animals. And the profession clung long to disease and health as the indicators of animal welfare and of the profession's success, largely failing to anticipate the emotional, psychological, and behavioral issues that would so dominate discussions in the 1980s.

Consider these statements from the American College of Laboratory Animal Medicine's 1974 reference volume on laboratory rabbits: "A loose [wooden] board should not be placed in the cage in the mistaken belief that the rabbit will be more comfortable. Wire floors are easier to keep clean and dry, a feature that makes solid floors completely unsatisfactory" (Hagen 1974, p. 36). That rabbits "like to chew on it," is actually a strike against wood, for it further detracts from wood's sanitizability, in a setting in which what rabbits want is seen as irrelevant (Hagen 1974).

In this text, and even in its second edition (Patton 1994), are found all of the elements that came to sound anachronistic in the 1980s. Veterinarians who had long fought for steel surfaces and solitary caging to limit contagion and animal fighting came to see all of that jeopardized in the name of "psychological well-being." Steel is so cold and sterile; solitude is so lonely. Veterinarians' prescriptions, forged in the days of rampant disease and infection, came to seem animal-unfriendly, incapable of recognizing what mattered to the animals. Only by appreciating the challenges laboratory animal veterinarians faced in cleaning up the animal quarters mid-century can one appreciate their resistance to change in the 1980s.

Researchers and the care/use divide

Histories of the early days of laboratory animal medicine show a veterinary profession vying for standing and respect within the prestigious halls of medical academia. Though some veterinarians were conducting their own medical research (not just veterinary medical research, but research centered on concerns for human health and illness), the first American veterinarian hired specifically for care of research animals was Simon Brimhall, in 1915, at Minnesota's Mayo Clinic (Cohen and Loew 1984). Before that time, animal care was seen almost exclusively as the individual researcher's responsibility, not the institution's, and so institution-level professional directors of animal care—veterinarians or otherwise—were unheard of. Throughout the 1940s, 1950s, and 1960s, laboratory animal veterinarians consolidated their jurisdiction as the directors of animal care, despite the occasional suspicions and resistance of the researchers. Brimhall's hiring represents an early example of centralization of animal care, shifting it from individual to institutional responsibility. Modern laws have reinforced this trend by centralizing legal liability for animal welfare violations. But institutions vary still in their degree of centralization and in the autonomy that various researchers might have in the daily care of their own research animals.[3]

Veterinarians were often overlooked in their early bid to manage animal care programs. If veterinary medicine is seen as the care of sick animals, it is unnecessary (and unnecessarily expensive) to have veterinarians overseeing research animal husbandry; it would be like hiring a physician to manage an orphanage or a day-care center. Early laboratory animal veterinarians strove to create a respectable professional niche for themselves where researchers had previously been content to hire and oversee their own, largely uneducated, animal caretakers (Brewer 1980). Yes, call in a veterinarian if the animals are sick, if you can even find one who knows about rat and mouse and monkey health, but why spend all that money to have a veterinarian on board full-time?

As some researchers and administrators began to see value in having research-oriented veterinarians overseeing animal care, resistance to their presence continued. Cohen and Loew, two laboratory animal veterinarians, describe a ten-year delay at the University of Chicago, from 1935 to 1945, in hiring Dr. Nathan Brewer as the first veterinary animal facility manager. As Cohen and Loew relate, "many investigators at the University feared that a veterinarian"—an "outsider," as Brewer relates his own history (Brewer [1980] p. 742)—"would dictate the conditions of care and use of animals, and they opposed the creation of this position" (Cohen and Loew 1984, p. 7).

Jurisdictional settlement by division of labor is a frequent, if typically unstable, result of standoffs of interprofessional competition. In animal research, an early, important division of labor was the separation of animal care from animal use.

The care/use jurisdictional division on a modern campus means that laboratory animal professionals (under the direction, typically, of a laboratory animal veterinarian) purchase research animals and house them in centralized facilities. During a holding period, the animals acclimate while the veterinary staff determines their health status, including quarantine, vaccination, deworming, and blood analysis, preparing them for the role for which they have been procured. Eventually, the animals are shifted from their holding period and placed on study, that is, they pass from the animal care to the animal use realm. Sometimes the change in jurisdictions coincides with a physical change in circumstances as well; the animals may be moved to new housing, out of the vivarium and into the research laboratory.

Even with the incursions into research contained in the 1985 Animal Welfare Act amendments and the establishment of animal care and use committees, the division between care and use persists. In one of the few memoirs written by a laboratory animal veterinarian, James Mahoney describes just this sort of shift in his agonized decisions over which chimps to place "in use" in which projects (Mahoney 1998). In my own work as a laboratory animal veterinarian, I have watched animals (mice in particular, though others as well) leave the centralized animal housing facility and the daily oversight of laboratory animal professionals and travel to a research laboratory for a several-day period of experimentation. Though technically still under the purview of the animal care committee and the institutional veterinarians, once removed from the centralized facility, in all reality they are largely out of veterinary sight and out of the veterinarian's jurisdiction.

As Cohen and Loew (1984) describe for the University of Chicago in the 1930s, research scientists may have feared that veterinarians would not be content with their limited jurisdiction. Scientists, in yielding control of animal care to another professional group, already risked a shift of resources away from their research toward beefed-up animal care and housing. How much more might they lose if veterinarians came to dictate actual research procedures?

Research scientists who valued their autonomy might well find reason for concern. The 1950s and 1960s were important times in the formal establishment of laboratory animal medicine as a formal veterinary specialty, with its own professional journals, specialty board examinations, and federally funded specialty training. Veterinarians drafted the first edition of the *Guide for Laboratory Animal Facilities and Care* in 1963. As laboratory veterinarians coalesced into a unified profession, they discussed their appropriate jurisdictional boundaries. They saw a larger role for themselves than just caring for animals (Clarkson 1961). The shifts from care to science in their organizational name and journal title, from the Animal Care Panel to the American Association for Laboratory Animal Science and from *Laboratory Animal Care* to *Laboratory Animal Science,* reflect this, as the profession matured and sought to define itself within the academic context.

Not only might veterinarians include more under the rubric of care than their scientist coworkers, they were also quick to point out the valuable role they could play within the realm of animal use. So Cohen, an early and influential laboratory animal veterinarian, wrote: "It is often necessary that these specialists [i.e., laboratory animal veterinarians] instruct other research workers and laboratory personnel in techniques of animal experimentation" (Cohen 1959, p. 163). His contemporary, Thomas Clarkson, similarly saw veterinarians telling scientists how to conduct their research, advising researchers not just on spontaneous animal diseases that might complicate experimental results, but also consulting on choice of the right animal for the job, offering "suggestions for inducing various disease states" for study and even aiding "with the interpretation of experimental data" (Clarkson 1961, p. 1329).[4] Quietly preparing animals for delivery into the scientists' hands was clearly far below the veterinarians' aspirations.

Thus, in the early days of the profession of laboratory animal medicine, professional competition between veterinarians and researchers led to a jurisdictional split in which veterinarians had little say in how animals were experimented upon, despite their eagerness to participate. Early legislation respected scientists' bid for autonomy and reinforced the informal split between animal care and animal use. Abbott (1984) claims that split jurisdictions tend to be unstable arrangements, and we shall see how external pressures for tighter regulations, the biases of the USDA veterinarians writing those regulations, and the laboratory animal veterinarians' expanding professional aspirations combined to erode scientists' secure hold over their research autonomy.

The antivivisectionists

Research animals, and the researchers experimenting upon them, very much shaped the profession of laboratory animal medicine, and without them, of course, there would be no profession. But antivivisectionists and animal protectionists have been a significant part of that landscape as well, lobbying for the restraint or abolition of animal use in research. Are they friend or foe to the veterinarian? How have their presence and pressures shaped the professionalization of laboratory animal medicine? How might they have influenced the potential of veterinarians to be forces for animal welfare?

Animal protectionists have exerted their influence largely through legislative and regulatory channels. Federal legislation, once finally passed in 1966, certainly has shaped laboratory animal care and use, but so too has the threat of legislation. Animal protectionists have also campaigned to influence public opinion, with or without legislative initiatives. They have sought direct influence on scientific practices, sometimes through engagement and dialogue, sometimes through acts of vandalism and threats of personal violence.

Modern readers, familiar with the media campaigns of People for the Ethical Treatment of Animals or the direct actions of the Animal Liberation Front may not realize the long history of antivivisectionism in America. England passed its first national law governing research animal welfare in 1876, ninety years before the United States followed suit; this hardly means that there were not efforts to introduce such legislation in the States during that time.

Antivivisectionism shaped the development of the laboratory veterinary profession long before legislation was passed. What prompted Brewer's promoters to propose his hiring as one of the nation's first laboratory animal veterinarians in 1935? What finally caused faculty scientists at the University of Chicago to accept that proposition ten years later? According to Cohen and Loew (1984), Chicago was home to the National Antivivisection Society and "a hotbed of antivivisection activity in 1945" (p. 8). Brewer's promoters believed that appointing a veterinarian to manage the animal facilities would "contribute to public confidence in the care and treatment of animals in research, and would help turn aside antivivisection activists" (Cohen and Loew 1984, pp. 7–8). Cohen and Loew describe no other anticipated benefits to the animals or to the institution beyond the political/public relations realm. The University of Chicago was not alone: "The antivivisection threat prompted a significant number of medical schools and research laboratories to employ veterinarians between 1945 and 1948," though combating antivivisectionism was not the veterinarians' only use, and "it soon became apparent that these veterinarians could also make tangible contributions to the solution of other animal colony problems" (Cohen 1959, p. 162).

Early laboratory animal veterinarians readily took up their role in turning aside antivivisectionists. As the Chicago area laboratory animal veterinarians in 1950 were initiating efforts to form a national organization (eventually, the Animal Care Panel, later renamed American Association for Laboratory Animal Science) of "supervisors of research animal quarters," they listed management of animal quarters, cages for monkeys, viral diseases of cats and dogs and "the ever present problem of countering the attacks of anti-vivisectionist groups in Chicago and elsewhere" as topics for discussion (Flynn 1980, pp. 768, 769). The threats of antivivisectionists has always been part of the laboratory animal veterinarians' ecology.

Chicago was home not just to the National Antivivisection Society and the Animal Care Panel, but to the National Society for Medical Research (NSMR) as well. The NSMR was formed in 1946 to coordinate efforts at combating the antivivisectionists' political agenda. The NSMR was an early supporter of the Animal Care Panel, donating office space and staff support in its early years. In return, the NSMR received the "objective studies of the Animal Care Panel" for use in its "campaign of truth" against antivivisectionism (p. 46).

As efforts to legislate laboratory animal use escalated in the mid-1960s, laboratory animal veterinarians were at the forefront in opposition. Their credentials were both professional and moral. For example, laboratory animal veterinarian Sigmund Rich testified before the House Committee on Agriculture as a professional with an "intensive and active concern for the health and welfare of animals" that the pet-theft bills facing Congress were "inimical to medical progress and injurious to our country's valuable livestock and pet animal population" (U.S. Congress 1966d, p. 104).

Thus laboratory animal veterinarians began their long career as the public defenders of research that uses animals, often more prominent in this role than many of the researchers whose animals they attended and whose research they defended.

Seeing the line between antivivisectionists and scientific researchers, laboratory animal veterinarians knew which side to stand on. Absent any federal legislation requiring veterinary care for experimental animals, the continued presence of veterinarians in the institution depended on staying in the good graces of administrators and scientists, not of antivivisectionists. None of their important work in controlling animal infections, writing professional guidelines for practice, or upgrading surgical and medical care of animals would have been possible if veterinarians jeopardized their positions in the medical centers and research institutes by consorting with the animal protectionists.

This, then, was the environment in which laboratory animal medicine first developed as a profession in the 1940s, 1950s, and early 1960s—the days before the Laboratory Animal Welfare Act of 1966. In house, veterinarians faced resistance from researchers who feared loss of autonomy should the vets assume too much authority. Clinically, they faced professional challenges in animals full of infections, low-quality facilities, and a lack of information and training in the common research species. Politically, they had achieved their status within the institution partly through their active engagement in stemming the activities of antivivisectionists, and partly (though supporting documentation on the part of research scientists is hard to come by) through their contributions in improving the quality of the animals as research tools (Cohen 1959).

The balance of authority during this period largely excluded antivivisectionists and government regulators. It reified a distinction between animal care (the province of the veterinarians) and animal use (the scientists' autonomous province). In their jurisdiction of the animal care arena, veterinarians embraced infection control as one of their highest priorities, and their animal facilities, with their concrete walls, steel cages, and solitary housing, increasingly resembled the efficient laboratories and sanitized hospitals of the medical centers they served. This care/use divide remained a consistent theme in more than thirty years of formal animal welfare policies and laws.

The care/use divide in formal policy

In the 1960s, standards for laboratory animal care became more formally codified, both in the 1963 *Guide for Laboratory Animal Facilities and Care* (and its successors, written primarily by practicing laboratory animal veterinarians) and in the 1966 passage of the Laboratory Animal Welfare Act. Each of these included some sort of boundary between animal care and animal use, emphasizing rules for animal care and leaving animal use to the discretion of the scientists.

After several unsuccessful years of animal protectionists' promoting federal regulation of laboratory animals, *Life* magazine's 1966 exposé of dog dealers may be what finally tipped the congressional balance. The exposé was the creation of the animal protectionists, with photographers accompanying Frank McMahon of the Humane Society of the United States on a raid of a dog dealer's premises, a "concentration camp for dogs" (Silva 1966, p. 22). A similar, earlier article in *Sports*

Illustrated magazine had likewise highlighted the horrors of the dog trade, with no more word on animal use than that Pepper, the focal dog of the article, had already been "used in scientific experiment and then cremated" by the time her family had traced her to the Montefiore Hospital (Phinizy 1965, p. 38).

Passage of the law in 1966 came with a price for the protectionists' agenda. The exposés focused exclusively on the lot of dogs headed for the laboratory. The *Sports Illustrated* story discussed impending legislation, refuting the Animal Care Panel's insistence that dog theft was not a problem and highlighting Congressman Resnick's insistence that he was not an antivivisectionist, nor his bill a restriction of animal use. Animal protectionists had chosen to secure control of dog dealing as their first step, sacrificing for the moment their urge to regulate scientists' practices. Christine Stevens of the Animal Welfare Institute pragmatically championed the Laboratory Animal Welfare Act through Congress; in 1966 she testified emphatically before the U.S. Senate Committee on Commerce: "We believe that animal experimentation does require regulation," she added, "but not in this piece of legislation before you" (U.S. Congress 1966c).

Congress passed Public Law 89–544, the Laboratory Animal Welfare Act, in August 1966. Section 13 of the law states: "The foregoing shall not be construed as authorizing the Secretary [of Agriculture] to prescribe standards for the handling, care, or treatment of animals during actual research or experimentation by a research facility as determined by such research facility." This preserved scientists'— or, at least, their employing facility's—autonomy over animal use, and even of determining the boundary of when animals are being used and when cared for (U.S. Congress 1966a).

The Laboratory Animal Welfare Act of 1966 preserved scientists' autonomy over their own research uses of animals, though without explicitly designating the complementary jurisdiction of animal care to veterinarians. The *Guide for Laboratory Animal Facilities and Care,* however, then in its second edition, strongly emphasized the role and authority of laboratory animal veterinarians and other laboratory animal professionals.

In 1963, seven laboratory animal veterinarians with the Animal Care Panel had authored the *Guide.*[5] It perfectly reflects the early 1960s landscape of laboratory animal medicine. In this *Guide,* laboratory animal veterinarians consolidated their stand on the importance of hygiene, disease management, and infection control in animal care and husbandry. But in the last two pages of this twenty-five-page *Guide,* veterinarians sought to breach the care/use division with their guidelines for experimental surgeries and for anesthetic and analgesic pain control.

One task of the *Guide,* though never explicitly stated as such, was to establish the relative roles of veterinarian, scientist, and "outsider" (whether antivivisectionist critic, or government regulator). The section on dog exercise, for instance, explains why the confusion of animal welfare groups and their calls for government intervention are mistaken, discounting outsiders' claims for a role in setting animal care standards. It defines a niche for "professionally qualified persons" to direct animal facilities, centralizing animal care under a new professional domain, rather than leaving it in the hands of individual scientists. The *Guide* lists the cre-

dentialing requirements for laboratory animal veterinarians and certified laboratory animal technicians, but it does not overplay its task of establishing laboratory
animal professionals' authority. Like the animal protectionists pushing for passage
of the Laboratory Animal Welfare Act, the veterinarians writing the *Guide* left the
scientists their autonomy in this first major foray into standards writing. Written
with the input of several nonveterinarian scientists, the *Guide*'s authors "emphasize that nothing in the *Guide* is intended to limit the investigator's freedom and
obligation to plan and conduct animal experiments in accord with accepted practice" (Animal Care Panel 1963).

Animal welfare groups and government inspectors are kept out. The care/use
division of authority is honored, with laboratory animal veterinarians and scientists each in charge in their own domains. The slight tinkering with the care/use
boundary in the surgery and anesthesia section, including them in the manual on
care rather than excluding them as aspects of use, foreshadowed later moves at
manipulating the care/use boundary.

The 1963 *Guide* also articulates some guiding ideologies that would continue
to influence updates of animal welfare policies. For one, while establishing the priority of research needs over animal welfare, it also asserts that such a trade-off is
rarely necessary: "Rarely are the requirements of research incompatible with physical comfort" (Animal Care Panel 1963, p. 17), and thus, rarely are the interests of
scientists, veterinarians, animal protectionists, and animals in conflict. Furthermore, physical comfort and related concerns—pain control, health, freedom from
infection—are the yardstick of animal welfare.

The early editions of the *Guide* can be read in several ways. To some extent, the
Guide is a user's instructional manual as would accompany any piece of laboratory
equipment; good research requires well-maintained instruments, quality reagents,
proper glassware, and, of course, healthy, uniform, uninfected animals. From this
perspective, animals are tools; their diseases are not significant for how they make
the animals, as subjects, *feel*, but for how they affect their usefulness in experiments. But the first *Guide*'s authors do include some provisions for animal welfare
without tying them directly to the animals' quality as research subjects. Calls for
postoperative pain relief seem to be in the *Guide* strictly for the animals' sake, as
feeling subjects and not just useful objects.

User's manual and standard of care blend imperceptibly in the *Guide* as complementary justifications for the same end result: normal, healthy animals who
feel good and function properly. Respecting the care/use divide and minimizing
their comments on use allowed the *Guide*'s veterinarian authors to avoid many of
those situations in which the two types of guidance might conflict. Comfort and
feeling good, after all, seem far more unproblematically consistent with good husbandry and housing than with induction of cancer, testing of toxic chemicals, or
other research procedures. Compliance with the *Guide* might cause researchers
some inconvenience or slight delays, and it could cost institutions a bundle in
stainless-steel caging, concrete walls, and high-tech air handling systems, but very
little in the *Guide* would derail a research project simply because of its effects on
the animals.

Read as historical text and as a reflection of the landscape of the profession at the time, the *Guide* is reactive as well as proactive, and all three major elements of the laboratory animal veterinarian's ecology are there. The animals are there: the Introduction sites the new *Guide* in a time of increased financial support for research, increased numbers of research animals, and refinements of research techniques, all of which call for "better quality animals and animal care" (Animal Care Panel 1963, p. 1). The antivivisectionists and other outsiders are there: most explicitly, they are there to be discredited in their confusion about dogs' need for exercise out of their cages, but they are also there implicitly in one of the *Guide*'s stated roles, to stand "symbolic of the scientific community's ethical commitment to provide the best possible care for animals used in the service of man and animals" (p. 1). And, of course, the third element, the scientists, are there, reassured that nothing in the *Guide* is intended to limit their freedom and obligation to conduct good animal experiments, but reminded that care and management of the animals "should be directed by professionally qualified persons" (p. 1).

Expertise and the care/use division of authority

The care/use jurisdictional boundary looks stable on paper, but it never was—not in the law, not in the *Guide,* and not in the animal laboratory. The division was weak on several fronts. Neither animal protectionists nor laboratory animal veterinarians could long be content to have their voices excluded on issues of how and when to use animals in experiments. From the early days, several issues—especially those concerning pain and anesthesia during experiments—were too close to veterinary expertise to be bounded off from veterinary input in the scientists' autonomous realm of animal use. Scientists, whose research grants bought the animals and paid for veterinarians' salaries, chafed at veterinarians' policies on running animal care programs. Later, as physical definitions of good animal care (comfort, pain management, infection control) gave way to psychological and behavioral definitions in the 1980s, control over the animal care jurisdiction required claims to behavioral, no longer just medical, expertise.

The 1966 Laboratory Animal Welfare Act did little to address the overwhelming pain and suffering that protectionists claimed animals experienced during the course of experimentation. Jurisdictional settlements and regulatory policies that shielded scientific practice from any sort of animal welfare constraints or oversight could not keep them satisfied for long. Congress amended the fledgling law in 1970.

Animal pain was the wedge by which Congress expanded authority of veterinarians and the USDA over animal use. Congress retained its assurance of researchers' autonomy, even as they began to erode it:

> Nothing in this Act shall be construed as authorizing the Secretary [of Agriculture] to promulgate rules, regulations, or orders with regard to design, outlines, guidelines, or performance of actual research or experimentation by a

research facility as determined by such research facility: *Provided . . .* that professionally acceptable standards governing the care, treatment, and use of animals, including appropriate use of anesthetic, analgesic, and tranquilizing drugs, during experimentation are being followed by the research facility *during actual research or experimentation.* (U.S. Congress 1970a; emphasis added)

Use of anesthetics was the first aspect of experimental design to be transferred to the USDA's authority. The USDA immediately categorized anesthetic use during experimentation as an aspect of "adequate veterinary care," subject to the "opinion of the attending veterinarian at the research facility" (Animal and Plant Health Service 1971, p. 935). Pain is the issue that more than any other undermined the care/use dichotomy and gradually empowered veterinarians and the government to enter the laboratories.[6]

Veterinarians watched research in progress and knew that they had much to offer. They would not stay long content supervising the animal facilities and staying out of the laboratories. Laboratory animal veterinarians found the fruits of their strong allegiance to the research enterprise, as tenured faculty with academic recognition and federal research grants alongside their MD and PhD peers. But the involvement of veterinarians can slow research (such as when they impose quarantine and holding periods on newly purchased animals before experiments begin), add costs (for the stainless-steel cages their focus on hygiene requires), add time (such as when they insist researchers come in through the night to administer painkillers to their animals), and even derail experiments (if they insist an animal is too sick to stay in the experiment).

The government veterinarians writing new Animal Welfare Act regulations in the late 1980s saw the increased status of veterinarians in the laboratories and proposed an even greater expansion of their role. This met resistance, however, though more from individual scientists than from research advocacy organizations. The language of the resistance was the dispute over veterinary expertise.

Correspondence to the USDA from the major professional associations glossed over in-house disputes between veterinarians and scientists, the National Association for Biomedical Research, for instance, treated empowerment of veterinarians more or less synonymously with flexibility and self-regulation for institutions. But other professional associations and several individual scientists disagreed. Professional competence and knowledge were often the language in which they resisted the ascendancy of veterinarians.

The American Pharmaceutical Manufacturers, for instance, worried that the USDA's proposed rules had expanded veterinarians into "the attending veterinary," with "excessive administrative and decision-making powers" not consistent with the Animal Welfare Act, or an "animal welfare Czar," as one disgruntled psychology professor wrote (Regulatory Analysis and Development 1987). Research psychologists were among the most outspoken critics of empowering laboratory animal veterinarians. The American Psychological Association told the USDA in 1987 that the powers the USDA proposed for laboratory animal veterinarians should go instead to the IACUC, "which offers a multidisciplinary perspective" (Regulatory Analysis and Development 1987).

Scientists' skepticism of veterinary expertise filled the USDA's mailboxes, with animal protectionists and animal dealers joining in. The catalog of veterinary ignorance was impressive. Veterinarians were unfit to rule on questions of animal use, given their ignorance of research study design, including surgical techniques, anesthesia, and drug use. Their expertise in animal care was similarly challenged and their knowledge gaps enumerated: kennel management, animal husbandry, animal nutrition, housing, ventilation, administration, care of agricultural animals, primate dentistry, and animal psychological well-being.

Many scientists wanted the veterinarian's role restricted to a narrowly construed jurisdiction of animal medical care; some thought even that was beyond veterinarians' competence. One scientist who used rabbits as his research subjects wrote that otherwise competent veterinarians were useless when confronted with rabbits as patients; better to consult rabbit breeders, other scientists, or the library. Laboratory animal veterinarians were seldom "pertinent" as rabbit doctors, this scientist wrote, and "the expertise of an attending veterinarian seldom, if ever, matches that of an experienced principal investigator" (Regulatory Analysis and Development 1987).

Against this skepticism, many others (veterinarians in particular) applauded recognition of veterinarians' knowledge and authority in the USDA's proposal. The American Veterinary Medical Association (AVMA) wrote that laboratory animal veterinarians are not adversaries of science or scientists. Rather, "the researcher must be encouraged to regard the veterinarian as a scientific expert and to actively enlist his or her cooperation" (Regulatory Analysis and Development 1989).

Expertise in this dueling correspondence is framed largely as a question of who has the most and the best facts. For any particular topic, the specialist will invariably, by definition, have the most information within her specialty. In the USDA correspondence, veterinarians come off as jack-of-all-trades generalists against the more specialized scientists over whom they sought jurisdiction. How could my two semesters of animal nutrition during veterinary college hold up against someone who studies nothing but? How could my training in canine abdominal or orthopedic surgery compete with the specialized knowledge of brain anatomy and surgery possessed by many experimental psychologists or neurosurgeons? Many of the researchers with whom I have worked as a laboratory animal veterinarian had specialized in their animal species—meadow voles, naked mole rats, rhesus monkeys, falcons—for years before I even went to vet school; what could I possibly tell them about their animal care and use? Veterinarians will almost always lose the expertise competition with specialized researchers, if they allow it to be framed as who knows the most about any one specific topic.

Defenders of veterinary authority in the laboratory were looking for a different sense and base for this authority than simply a large database of knowledge. They groped for a concept of expertise that would allow veterinarians to stand proudly as peers and equals with the specialized scientists with whom they worked. What they found was that veterinarians could claim expertise in the generalized knowledge they possessed, precisely because it was generalized. Veterinary expertise lies in its emphasis on integration and application of knowledge from multiple disciplines. That integration is the specialized skill of the laboratory animal veterinarian. This expertise lay in the smattering of subjects on which they knew something, but in any one of which they lacked expertise.

Alternatively, veterinarians also could (and often did) claim a specialized expertise in the clinical relationship between a veterinarian and individual animal patients, a point that both the National Association for Biomedical Research and the AVMA made in pushing for a performance based approach to limiting the number of surgeries on individual animals. Rather than arbitrarily limiting researchers to one major survival surgery per animal, they would place that decision in the hands of the animal's attending veterinarian. In such a formulation of veterinary practice, the formal knowledge of specialists and scientists might be subservient to what individual clinicians know about individual patients. However, a veterinarian who spends her day intimately involved with her individual patients risks being limited to that task, rather than the broader, policy-setting jurisdiction the USDA regulators were offering.

Ultimately, the USDA shifted many of the responsibilities it had proposed for laboratory animal veterinarians to the IACUC, and it has fallen to research facilities to determine the relative authority and autonomy of committee, researcher, and veterinarian in most of the areas that were so controversial in the late 1980s: judging who is qualified to conduct surgery and other research techniques, determining who should review and approve or disapprove research protocols, and deciding when and whether veterinarians might enter scientists' labs and risk disrupting experiments in progress.

Happiness, behavior, and psychological well-being: The final frontier?

Veterinarians, animal care and use committees, and USDA inspectors made incursions into scientists' freedom of animal use with the 1980s provisions for research protocol review. Concurrently, veterinarians faced loss of their jurisdictional control of animal care to a new group of professionals: the animal behaviorists.

Before the 1980s, veterinarians had consolidated their control of animal care through their success at controlling illness, infection, and injury among laboratory animals. Laboratory animal veterinarians described their progress in scientific or clinical terms, emphasizing the improvements in diagnosis, epidemiology, treatment, and isolation of animals. Laboratory animal veterinarians developed several technologies for eliminating infections among laboratory animals. For example, they developed Caesarean-derived rodent colonies, in which near-term baby animals, surgically removed from their mothers' uterus, could be hand-reared far from others of their species. Infections that might be passed in mother's milk, in daily contact with mother, or through life in an infected colony could be stopped through this technique; only those rare infectious agents capable of transmission through the uterus and placenta could circumvent this strategy. Laminar flow of microfiltered air, acidification of drinking water, sterilization of feeds and bedding, and an assortment of isolation cages augmented Caesarean derivation, erecting microbiological barriers behind which the new generations of laboratory rodents could stay clean and uninfected (Committee on Laboratory Animal Housing 1976; Committee on Rodents 1996; Foster 1980).

For larger animals, such as dogs, cats, and monkeys, a significant component of infection control—whether purpose-bred for research, captured in the jungles, or trucked in from animal pounds—was the limited contact allowed between animals and the choice of sanitizable and sterilizable caging materials. Dogs and monkeys housed alone in stainless-steel cages passed fewer infections and never injured or fought each other (Kelley and Hall 1995; National Research Council 1973; Zinn 1968).

This progressive decontamination of laboratory animal colonies was not just a medical success for laboratory animal veterinarians, but a political success as well. Despite the costs of their programs, laboratory animal veterinarians successfully convinced regulators and many administrators and researchers of the correctness of their approach to producing healthier animals and better science. Throughout the 1980s, however, "healthier" became uncoupled from "happier." Animal protectionists did not deny that laboratory animals were healthier than in the 1950s, but they and many laboratory animal professionals increasingly considered health but one component of happiness. And animal happiness was what they sought in the 1985 Improved Standards for Laboratory Animals.

You will not find the word "happiness" in the 1985 Animal Welfare Act, or in recent editions of the *Guide for the Care and Use of Laboratory Animals.* Look instead for "welfare," "psychological well-being," "enrichment," and even "exercise" as stand-ins. "Psychological well-being" (for primates) and "exercise" (for dogs) were the terms that senators Dole and Melcher successfully introduced into the 1985 legislation. They sensed that protection against infection, physical disease, and aggression did not encompass the full agenda that the new amendment was aiming to promote: the psychological and emotional dimensions of welfare, of happiness.

Laboratory animal veterinarians had consolidated their jurisdiction of animal care through their success in eliminating infection and trauma, but concern for animal happiness shifted that jurisdiction, or threatened to establish a new jurisdiction. The measure of that new jurisdiction was behavior, not physical health. Laboratory animal veterinarians were ill prepared for leadership in this new, or, more precisely, for neither the terms nor the ideas were truly novel in the 1980s, newly legitimated, approach to animal welfare. Veterinary curricula traditionally included precious little on animal behavior; as a veterinary student in the mid-1980s, I had a single animal behavior course available to me, the emphasis of which was treating behavior problems (barking, biting, urinating on carpets) rather than recognizing and promoting animal happiness. And most formal laboratory animal medicine publications and training programs emphasized pathology, infection, and disease rather than behavior.

Not only were laboratory animal veterinarians ill-prepared for leadership in the "animal happiness" jurisdiction that the Dole–Melcher amendments created; if anything, the new direction that the animal happiness advocates promoted ran counter to what veterinarians had so long struggled to create. Animal protectionists fought against the one-animal–one-stainless-steel-cage standard of husbandry that veterinarians had long championed. Happy animals would live harmoniously in groups in enriched environments. They would sleep on blankets, in straw, in warm wooden nest boxes. They would enjoy their human and animal friends, play with a rich array of toys, and select from a varied and interesting assortment of foods.

Many laboratory animal veterinarians and scientists saw disaster in this—a return to the days of animal fighting, rampant infections, and nutritional imbalances. One senior laboratory animal veterinarian wrote a series of letters to the USDA in the 1980s, decrying the whole project of psychological well-being, social interaction, or any other "unhealthy" approaches to animal happiness. In such letters, we see the challenge of getting researchers to comply with the laboratory animal veterinarian's prescriptions, along with the dangers of social grouping, varied animal diets, and even dog walking:

> These proposed rules are for the most part a step back in terms of animal welfare. To now allow tree limbs, dirt, gravel, etc. in indoor research facilities precludes proper sanitization, proper disease control, and will assure large populations of roaches. . . . Animal welfare will not be enhanced by these proposed rules. It will in fact frequently be jeopardized. . . . This is the most amazing proposed change and would only make sense for pet owners or some behaviorist . . . Some primate behaviorists and psychologists resist all efforts to have a clean, rodent and roach free environment. . . . Group housing is much more likely to lead to injury and psychological distress to some. . . . Aberrant behavior is the best indicator of psychological distress . . . I have not seen evidence of psychological stress in primates. Obviously, no vets (who have to deal with traumas, diarrheas, vermin control etc.) were chosen on the panel of 10 experts consulted. . . . There is not a shred of scientific evidence that the same commercial diet every day is not totally acceptable. Most primates thrive on such diets and eagerly eat them each day. (Regulatory Analysis and Development 1989)[7]

Other scientists had listened to their veterinarians over the years and shared their "medicalization" of animal welfare. For example, a psychology professor who studied squirrel monkeys wrote to the USDA in 1990, hoping to stop proposals for mandated group housing for primates. He related his experience group-housing males, many of whom were not able to obtain sufficient food, or were "stressed through constant aggressive harassment" in the group setting:

> About 18 years ago, on the strong advice of the USDA inspecting veterinarian and the University of Georgia's Laboratory Animal Care Coordinator (a veterinarian), we eliminated all group caging. . . . I believe we have been highly

successful using the criteria of the monkeys' physical condition and longevity; most of the monkeys in my care have lived 20 years or more . . . the monkeys are healthy, robust, and devoid of stereotypical behaviors. (Regulatory Analysis and Development 1990)

These two writers, one a veterinarian and the other not, indicate their long familiarity with primate care in a specific context—not a zoo or wild animal park, but a laboratory in which the animals' function supersedes their well-being (for the humans in their lives, at any rate). They are comfortable with a physical–medical assessment of animal welfare: longevity and freedom from infection and injury. Neither can escape the language of behavior (stereotypical behaviors, aberrant behaviors) in making his case for the healthy benefits of the status quo, nor could either stem the new trend of privileging the behavioral and the subjective over the physical in describing animal welfare.

The new focus in the 1980s was on behavior as the window into animals' mental states: their happiness, contentment, and psychological well-being. Anyone who would claim the jurisdiction of animal welfare specialist must either defend a different way of measuring well-being, or defend her own special expertise in reading animal behavior. Both have been tried, as the new discipline, animal welfare science, has grown and matured since the early 1980s.

Over the past two decades, both laboratory animal and farm animal specialists explicitly have grappled with how to define, recognize, and quantify animal welfare. Marilyn Stamp Dawkins summarized the field to date in her 1980 book *Animal Suffering* and brought cohesion to subsequent discussions, if not closure.

Several veterinarians, animal behaviorists, philosophers, and others have promoted their own theories of animal welfare. Some stress the more physical aspects of welfare; others focus more on psychology and its outward manifestation, behavior. Some work to integrate the two, while others emphasize how much the laboratory or the farmed animal differs from or approximates the "natural" state, either emotionally or in other ways.

Physical measures of animal welfare include productivity, especially of farm animals: how well a hen is laying, a cow milking, or a pig fattening. They can include measures of stress, or, more specifically, of so-called stress hormones, such as cortisol and corticosterone, epinephrine, adrenaline, or of brain chemistry, endorphins, and the like. Physical measures of welfare may include population data on disease incidence or recognition of pathology and disease in individual animals. Measures of immune status may be used, such as antibody production or white blood cell counts.

Physical measures of animal welfare need not ignore how animals feel (whether or not they are happy), but their proponents emphasize the physical manifestation of animals' feelings. They disagree with animal behaviorists not over whether the feelings of animals are real and important, but over the best method for knowing the feelings of the animals.[8] Many of the proponents of such nonbehavioral measures of welfare have been agricultural animal scientists, physiologists, and veterinarians (Fraser et al. 1997; McGlone 1993; Moberg 1985).

The animal behaviorists, for their part, have a range of methodologies as well. The laboratory animal veterinarian and the squirrel monkey psychologist quoted above reveal the tendency to focus on unhealthy behavior. Good welfare is presumed when bad behavior is not in evidence: the animals are not pacing or circling in purposeless stereotypy; they are not self-mutilating, banging their heads on cage walls, cannibalizing their young. They exhibit no overt psychopathology. Many of the laboratory animal veterinarians who wrote to the USDA in the 1980s used a psychopathology model of animal welfare as they argued for or against animal welfare regulations. And why shouldn't they? Animal health and disease, physical and perhaps mental, are the language of veterinary medicine.

Not all behavior specialists speak in terms of pathology. Some focus instead on welfare issues far below the threshold of inducing psychosis in the animals. Animal preference and choice are frequent objects of study. What sort of bedding do mice choose to lie in? How much do monkeys choose to play with the toys in their cage? Do guinea pigs choose to rest together or apart? Behaviorists may take this to another level of sophistication by asking how much animals will work or what pleasures they will forgo to get these preferences.

Policy debates in the 1980s carried the potential to open a new jurisdictional niche for assessors of animal welfare. For a professional group such as animal behaviorists to fill this niche (which they made no strong or organized attempt at the time to do), they would have had to demonstrate their superior ability to perform the requisite work (assessing animal welfare). That would require defining the work as a behavioral, rather than as a physiological or medical, task.

A crucial difference between behavioral and physiological measures of welfare is access to the technology. Anyone can observe and report animal behavior. Not everyone can draw blood samples, measure cortisol levels, and diagnose animal tumors or ulcers or immunodeficiencies. For all the sophisticated theory and analysis behaviorists may bring to their work, their methods are deceptively simple. They require animals and an observer, possibly some video equipment, and a stopwatch. No need to set up the laboratory equipment for radioimmunoassays of cortisol concentrations; just set up the animals and the cameras and go to work. Watch the animals; report your findings.

The apparent ease of observing behavior explains, in part, the failure of behaviorists to dominate the discussions of animal welfare policy in the 1980s, even though behavioral claims were central to policy formation. The handful of studies that the USDA cited in setting its animal welfare regulations in the late 1980s were indeed behavioral studies—of guinea pigs' use of cage space, of the distance dogs travel in small cages—but they were performed not by behaviorists or psychologists, but by veterinarians, and they were published not in animal behavior journals, but in laboratory animal journals (Hughes et al. 1989; White et al. 1989).

Though animal behavior specialists showed little effort to carve out a professional niche for themselves, others nominated them for that position. A primatologist, for example, suggested that the USDA compare the input of applied animal behaviorists (whom he analogized to human psychologists) and veterinarians (the physicians' analog) as an indicator of how the two professions approach the psychological well-being of animals differently. "Historically," he wrote, "the care of nonhuman primates *has* been the domain of veterinarians. Yet, the nature of this care, especially as it pertains to psychological well-being, has been widely perceived by the public as inadequate to some degree." Making no claim that his own behavioral research and training were appropriate to the task, he pointed out the Animal Behaviour Society, with its "entire certification program devoted to Applied Animal Behavior," which should be consulted in writing welfare regulations (Regulatory Analysis and Development 1990). However, no one certified through this program wrote to the USDA speaking on their own behalf, suggesting for example, a role on IACUCs for credentialed behaviorists. The closest anyone came to that was the American Psychological Association's insistence that some of the authority proposed for laboratory animal veterinarians be invested instead in the multidisciplinary IACUC (Regulatory Analysis and Development 1987).

It was a jurisdictional turf war that never really happened. As jurisdictions were redefined in laboratory animal policy, neither Congress, the USDA, nor the authors of the *Guide for the Care and Use of Laboratory Animals* recognized or mandated a role for behavior specialists in laboratory animal welfare. The USDA veterinarians writing the Animal Welfare Act regulations explained in 1990, in response to comments that animal psychologists should rule on primate psychological well-being, "We believe that most attending [laboratory animal] veterinarians are familiar and knowledgeable in the behavioral patterns of the nonhuman primates" and "are well-versed in what is necessary for the animals' health and well-being. We are confident in such veterinarians' capabilities to make sound professional decisions with regard to the regulations" (Animal and Plant Health Inspection Service 1990a, pp. 33492, 33498). Other than the IACUC's annual review of the animal care program, laboratory animal veterinarians retained their statutory authority over animal care.

Conclusion

Abbott proposed a sociological system in which professions compete for jurisdiction over specific tasks. His theory of professions explains much of the development of animal welfare policy in the late twentieth century. Laboratory animal veterinarians secured a role for themselves in scientific institutions dominated by researchers with MD and PhD degrees. Ironically, part of veterinarians' ability to secure a place in the laboratory rested on their willingness to be prominent opponents of the animal protectionists' agenda. It also rested on their willingness to accept limited jurisdiction over animal *care,* leaving animal *use* the private domain of the researchers doing the experiments.

By separating animal care and animal use into separate professional domains and by establishing their expertise in animal care, laboratory animal veterinarians gradually gained authority over the professionals with whom they worked. They buttressed their authority in publishing their own *Guide for Laboratory Animal Facilities and Care,* while USDA veterinarians and congressional mandate guaranteed this authority in the Animal Welfare Act.

The care/use division of professional jurisdiction has remained unstable. Animal protectionists, government regulators, and laboratory animal veterinarians all sought increased veterinary jurisdiction over animal *use,* particularly in the wake of early 1980s exposés of primate use in two research laboratories. Incursions into scientists' long-defended autonomy in their use of animals took two forms: (1) an ongoing effort on the part of veterinarians and others to define some aspects of animal use (especially pain management and surgical procedures) as a component of the veterinarians' jurisdiction over animal care and (2) increasing requirements for committee review of scientific protocols, with committees made up of laboratory animal veterinarians, laypeople, and scientists. Both approaches further eroded the autonomy of the scientists.

Shifting priorities in animal care throughout the 1980s, however, threatened to undermine veterinarians' hard-won authority. Veterinarians had defined animal care and comfort largely in physical and medical terms, such as freedom from infection, illness, or injury. They attributed their progress in taming colony-wide epidemics to their programs of isolation caging, rigorous animal quarantines, and exclusive use of hard, sanitizable caging materials. Their gold standard, a research animal housed alone in a stainless-steel cage, became anachronistic as the language of happiness, social needs, psychological well-being, and behavior gained currency. Behavioral expertise became the new route to authority over animal care, but during the five-year period in which the USDA rewrote its animal welfare regulations in the late 1980s, veterinarians retained their authority. Neither the USDA nor the 1996 edition of the *Guide for the Care and Use of Laboratory Animals* has recognized an explicit niche for behavior experts. This may yet happen, as applied behaviorists continue their own path to professionalization.

The important issue is, how might this affect the animals? That question is difficult to answer because so much of the discussion of the Animal Welfare Act was in the language of professional authority rather than specific proposals. Many laboratory animal veterinarians explicitly worried that a rush to social housing and exercise programs would undermine their disease-control interests, while many animal protectionists pushed explicitly for those very changes. Animal behavior experts were largely silent in this period. Several researchers warned (as did several animal protectionists) against placing too much authority in the hands of veterinarians, but they rarely said just what they feared would happen. Nor did they show unanimity: Some seemed to fear that veterinarians' emphasis on infection-control would put a damper on efforts to enrich their animals' lives. Others seemed to fear that veterinarians would place more and more restrictions on the freedom of scientists to conduct experiments as they thought best, just as they felt veterinarians had been doing in other aspects of animal management.

Veterinarians, animal behaviorists, and animal protectionists have often spoken in terms of pathology, disease, and deprivation—first of a physical nature, later of a psychological nature. The shift in language from physical to emotional health seems to have expanded the range of possibilities for animals. Whereas previously there were two options—normal and diseased—the language of behavior led to a third possibility, on the other side of "normal" from diseased, a state of thriving, enriched, happy animals. Speaking for animals has progressed from statements of what animals need to claims of what they want; we are moving to a time when what animals have a right to expect, to hope for, will be the language of animal welfare discussions.

7

The problem of pain

PAIN IS GOOD. WE CANNOT LIVE WITHOUT IT. WE MAY LEARN MOST THINGS BEST through positive reinforcements, rewards, and pleasures, but for some lessons, nothing is so good a teacher as pain. Pain tells us when we've pushed our bodies too far, when we've come too close to danger. Pain helps us protect injured body parts—shifting our weight from a sprained ankle, for instance—while they heal. Pain reminds us of the things we need to know to keep on living: stay away from hot stoves, don't climb too high in trees, avoid fights with those who are bigger than us. Pain has survival value.

People unable to feel pain, whether congenitally or through injury, are subject to all sorts of injuries (Bar-On et al. 2002; Levitt 1985). Eve and Adam felt no pain until their expulsion from the garden; I have no idea how they kept from injury in those halcyon days. Theologians have pondered why other animals, innocent of sin, should be afflicted with pain (Rachels 1990). But pain is good for other animals, too; it teaches the same lessons, gives the same warnings.

The "Silver Spring Monkeys," whose plight catalyzed passage of the 1985 Animal Welfare Act amendment, had been surgically rendered pain-free in one arm (Taub et al. 1994).Without the valuable information pain could have given them, they let their deafferentated arms hang limp, in harm's way.[1] The monkeys chewed on their useless arms, unaware of the damage they were inflicting upon themselves. Ultimately, the damage sustained by their pain-free limbs could have killed them, through blood loss or infection (Rowan 1998).

What makes pain so good is that it feels so bad. In a creature unable to move, pain would be sheer, inescapable torture; I certainly hope that trees, or the grass underfoot, are incapable of feeling pain. But for creatures capable of responding, avoiding, escaping it, pain is invaluable, both in the moment, and, for those animals capable of learning from it, in the future as well. (Committee on Pain and Distress in Laboratory Animals 1992; Iadarola and Caudle 1997; Nesse 1991). Pain demands attention: You *will* drop that hot frying pan *now*, and you will not repeat such a move any too quickly.

Pain is useful, in part, because it can be reduced. Move away from the heat, keep weight off the sprained ankle, run away from predators and aggressors—acts to reduce pain are typically acts of survival. The recurring image of research animals' lives in nineteenth-century etchings and in twentieth-century posters is the restrained animal in the hands of the vivisectionists, unable to escape the scalpel blade or whatever other pain is in store. Acute, inescapable pain, surgery without anesthesia, the torture of vivisection constitute useless pain, at least for the animal enduring it; it does nothing to help that animal survive.

Political history of pain

While the ability to feel pain is essential for survival, actually feeling it (or inflicting it) at any particular moment is a very bad thing. Animal pain in the laboratory has been a recurring theme of animal protectionists for well over a century. Animal pain has been the strongest argument not only for total abolition of animal experimentation, but also for reform and for government oversight. As the new-born Victoria Street Society for the Protection of Animals from Vivisection pushed for partial abolition of animal research in Britain's landmark Cruelty to Animals Act of 1876, it also pushed for reform: that all surgical experiments would be conducted under anesthesia and the animals painlessly euthanized when the surgery ended (Hume 1957; Vyvyan 1969). Pain has kept the animal care/use division unstable. Pain management has been the prime component of animal experimentation that undermined scientists' exclusive jurisdiction in the laboratory. Pain's dual nature—physical and psychological—and its ubiquitous occurrence among animals and humans makes it the leading edge for expanded concern for animals' psychological and emotional well-being.[2]

Attention to animal pain was not new to the 1985 Animal Welfare Act. For nearly twenty years, regulators had been attempting to regulate animal pain management, either by prescribing particular practices or by proscribing certain painful procedures, but mostly by manipulating the jurisdictional boundaries between scientists and veterinarians.

As did the first edition of the *Guide for the Care and Use of Laboratory Animals* three years earlier, the first version of the Laboratory Animal Welfare Act in 1966 explicitly excluded research practices from its purview. Pain management was also excluded, being more a feature of animal use than of animal care. Congressional sponsors took great pains to clarify their intent to separate care and use. Senator Warren Magnuson opened hearings on his proposed bill, saying, "I would like to emphasize that the issue before us today is not the merits or demerits of animal research. We are interested in curbing petnapping, catnapping, dognapping. . . . We are not considering curbing medical research" (U.S. Congress 1966c). His concerns were to protect pet owners and to assure humane care of animals while in the hands of dealers. His bill codified the animal care/animal use divide in laboratory settings through the "establishment of regulations for handling of animals while in the research institution, except during actual research or experimentation" (U.S. Congress 1966c).

The 1966 Laboratory Animal Welfare Act called on the USDA to develop standards for "adequate veterinary care" for animals at the dealers and at research facilities, though the USDA was not to prescribe such standards during "actual research or experimentation" (U.S. Congress 1966a). As emphasized by the conference committee that crafted the final version of the bill, "the important determination of when an animal is in actual research so as to be exempt from regulations under the bill is left to the research facility itself" (U.S. Congress 1966b).

The standards for adequate veterinary care articulated by the USDA were fairly minimal, more like what would later be called "performance standards" than like the rigid prescriptions that the USDA elaborated for the size of a dog tag to use, the size of a rabbit cage, and the temperature of a vehicle used to transport animals. The USDA articulated a jurisdictional standard, sketching out the responsibilities of the veterinarian and the animal caretaker, and the limitations thereto: "Programs of disease control and prevention, euthanasia, and adequate veterinary care shall be established and maintained under the supervision and assistance of a doctor of veterinary medicine" (Agriculture Research Service 1966, p. 16114). It stipulated daily observation of dogs, cats, and nonhuman primates by their caretakers, with sick, diseased, injured, lame, or blind animals to be "provided with veterinary care or humanely disposed of unless," importantly, "such action would be inconsistent with the research purposes" (Irving 1967, p. 3275). In contrast to the detail on the size and shape of dog tags, animal pain was not a regulatory concern.

Neither the NIH's *Guide* nor the Animal Welfare Act could continue this hands-off exclusion of research practices from its purview and simultaneously address animal pain. And neither did. The veterinary authors of even the very first 1963 edition of the *Guide* began to encroach on animal use in their call for postoperative pain management. The legislators of the Animal Welfare Act and the animal protectionists who relied upon them waited for the act's first update, four years after its initial passage, to make this encroachment. That update, the 1970 amendment, identified pain in laboratory animals as an important regulatory concern and in the process began to erode the autonomy of scientists in their laboratories.

The original 1966 law had mandated adequate veterinary care for laboratory animals. The 1970 amendment expanded the definition of veterinary care to include treatment of pain, and that meant treatment of pain during research procedures. Representative Thomas Foley sponsored it in the House as a bill that "imposes an ethic of adequate veterinary care, including the appropriate use of pain-relieving drugs" (U.S. Congress 1970b). Congress clarified its intent that these pain-relieving drugs were to be used even during experiments and that laboratory animal veterinarians were the in-house authority to dictate their use. Congress and the USDA would not dictate the prescriptions for pain management in any detail, and they recognized that veterinarians may choose to withhold such drugs when experimental needs might take precedence over the animals' feelings:

> The intent of the [agriculture] committee is the decision with respect to appropriate use of anesthetic, analgesic, or tranquilizing drugs would rest exclusively with the attending veterinarian of such research facility, and that any standards promulgated by the Department of Agriculture could be dis-

regarded by the facility if in its opinion these guidelines were not proper under existing circumstances and research requirements. Further, that the research facility veterinarian would not be required by the Secretary [of agriculture] to justify or defend his decision to not employ these agents if inconsistent with or contrary to standards recommended by the Secretary. (U.S. Congress 1970b, p. 40159)

Congress passed this amendment with confidence that it was still keeping its meddling hands out of scientists' practice. As Congressman Foley put it: "Decisions [to treat animals for pain] are exclusively in the hands of the research institutions, and their decisions are final" (U.S. Congress 1970, p. 40155). No conflict should arise between the mandate for pain-control drugs and the free conduct of good science: "Under this bill, the research scientist still holds the key to the laboratory door. However, the Agriculture Committee and the Congress expect that the work that is done behind the laboratory door will be done with compassion and with care" (U.S. Congress 1970b, p. 40158).

Dog theft and dog dealers were not forgotten in 1970, but the Animal Welfare Act and its supporters had clearly broadened their horizons, knocking loudly at the laboratory door. Concern for animal pain was the tool by which they did this, as well as their motivating concern, and laboratory animal veterinarians were their agents.

Congress and the USDA balanced their desire to promote humane experimentation and their desire to let research proceed unencumbered by expanding the definition of "adequate veterinary care" to include use of painkilling drugs during potentially painful experiments. They defined this more fully in their regulations, published about a year after passage of the 1970 amendment (Animal and Plant Health Service 1971). Adequate veterinary care was to include the "appropriate use of anesthetic, analgesic, or tranquilizing drugs when such use would be proper in the opinion of the attending veterinarian of the research facility." Veterinarians were not empowered to be loose cannons or iconoclasts, however, for their prescriptions should be "in accordance with the currently accepted veterinary medical practice as cited in appropriate professional journals or reference guides." And a performance standard of sorts was articulated, by which veterinarians and scientists would know they were complying with the regulations: the various anesthetics "shall produce in the animals a high level of tranquilization, anesthesia, or analgesia consistent with the design of the experiment [and] . . . the use of these three classes of drugs shall effectively minimize the pain and discomfort of the animals while under experimentation" (Animal and Plant Health Service 1971, p. 335).

This, then, was the regulatory mandate, calculated to satisfy the animal protectionists who had long worried that scientists disregard animal welfare in their experiments, as well as the laboratory animal veterinarians who had long wanted more of a voice in how animal studies would be conducted. It elaborated a standard of care to meet the animals' needs, while continuing to respect the fact that some experiments could be ruined by use of such drugs, which can have far-reaching effects throughout the body, and to exempt those experiments from disruptive regulation. This was the standard, but how could it be enforced?

Enforcement came in the form of annual reports by animal facilities on their animal use. Each facility submits a report of the numbers of each regulated species used, broken into categories, showing that "professionally acceptable standards" of care were followed, including pain relief during experimentation. This report was to include the number of experiments in which animals might experience pain but in which painkillers were withheld, with a brief explanation stating the reasons for withholding drugs.[3] No system was installed to verify the accuracy of these reports, though the USDA theorized that having top officials at institutions sign these reports may actually encourage facilities to minimize the number of potentially painful studies they perform without painkillers (American Veterinary Medical Association 1980).

The *Guide for Laboratory Animal Facilities and Care* followed a parallel course. Remember that this *Guide,* though largely funded by the NIH and requisite for receipt of many federal grants, is written by the research community itself, especially laboratory animal veterinarians. The 1963, 1965, and 1968 editions all called for use of postoperative analgesics "whenever indicated." Responsibility for deciding on the use of such painkillers was not assigned to anyone's jurisdiction in these early editions, but in later editions, they approximate the Animal Welfare Act: "the choice and use of the most appropriate drug(s) are matters for the professional judgment of the attending veterinarian. Research personnel must be provided with guidelines and consultation" (ILAR 1978, p. 13).

This is where the regulations and guidelines stood relevant to animal pain control in experimentation in the 1970s: A regulatory presumption in favor of pain management was in place, with veterinarians increasingly seen as both the source of information and the arbiter of anesthetic use. This mandated attention to the issue and empowerment of veterinarians certainly brought the rules closer to the ideal of the animal protectionists, the Congress, the USDA's staff of veterinarians, and the laboratory animal veterinarians employed in the various research institutions. As one USDA veterinarian wrote in 1970 for a veterinary readership: "When the administration of laboratory animal welfare legislation was assigned to a group in which veterinarians have long played a leadership role [i.e., the Animal Health Division of the USDA], it was, I believe, a significant stimulus to the placement of veterinarians in other areas of laboratory animal care" (Saulmon 1970, p. 1964).

Pain and the Improved Standards for Laboratory Animals

The Improved Standards for Laboratory Animals was the 1985 amendment to the Animal Welfare Act. As in the 1960s, its passage followed several years of multiple bill proposals in the Congress. But whereas the 1966 bill was passed after tales of dog theft were exposed, the catalyst for the 1985 passage was a pair of exposés of monkey experiments. Charges (complete with videotapes stolen from the University of Pennsylvania) of researchers abusing monkeys during the course of their experiments strained the long-stated desire of Congress to keep its hands out of dictating the conduct of research. Something had to be done, and much of that involved increased attention to pain in laboratory animals.

The 1985 amendment had a few major provisions. It mandated the formation of institutional animal committees both to oversee animal care and to review scientists' efforts to minimize animal pain in their animal use proposals. Each committee was to review, as part of its semiannual animal facility inspections, "(A) practices involving pain to animals, and (B) the condition of animals, to ensure compliance with the provisions of this Act to minimize pain and distress to animals" [(U.S.C. 7, section 13 (b)(3)]. In addition, any planned exceptions to the pain control provisions were to be filed with the committee.

Another new requirement was that scientists must now search for alternatives to any painful procedures in their experiments and report on that search to the committee. The 1970 rule that adequate veterinary care included prescription of painkilling medications became a requirement for the scientist to consult with the veterinarian on use of anesthetics. As with the mandated committee reviews and inspections, Congress was continuing what it started in 1970, to recognize a professional jurisdiction of pain management and to move it out of the autonomous domain of the researchers.

All of these issues required further elaboration in the standards and regulations that the USDA would craft over the next six years. The USDA began this process in 1986. Charged by Congress to update its regulations, it sought public input first, rather than posting proposed regulations for comment. Specifically, it wanted comments in four areas:

1. Exercise for dogs
2. Psychological well-being of nonhuman primates
3. A list of painful procedures that should require the use of anesthetics, analgesics, or tranquilizers in research animals
4. A list of major operative experiments from which an animal is allowed to recover, which should prohibit the same animal being used in another similar major operative experiment(Animal and Plant Health Inspection Service 1986)

The third and fourth points, of course, are entirely concerned with animal pain and strongly imply the USDA's willingness (congressional assurances to the contrary notwithstanding) to march through the laboratory door and start dictating scientific practices.[4] The USDA's first feint at updating management of animal pain was both proscriptive and prescriptive. It would all but outlaw some painful research practices and dictate terms for pain management for the remainder.

The Animal Legal Defense Fund (ALDF) was one of the few to respond on the USDA's stated terms (Regulatory Analysis and Development 1986). Whereas most scientists, veterinarians, and protectionists went for generalities, often claiming the impossibility (and rapid obsolescence) of developing any such list, the

ALDF submitted a detailed and lengthy list of painful procedures. The ALDF, self-described in 1986 as an organization of some 200 lawyers and 30,000 other supporters, reported on an 18-month study that it had been conducting with United Action for Animals. It had compared published research papers with USDA enforcement reports at the facilities where the studies were done and claimed that animal pain was consistently undercounted in annual reports to the USDA. It was certain that this information would encourage the USDA to develop a better self-reporting program that would allow better scrutiny of research institute reports.

The ALDF apparently saw little need for veterinarians or anyone else to diagnose pain in individual animals. Instead, it submitted nearly 200 scientific articles exemplifying the procedures that could be presumed to be painful and which would therefore call for anesthetics. Bowing to the standard that scientific necessity could preempt animal welfare, it proposed that "When the conscious response of the animal is unnecessary or merely incidental to the purposes of the experiment, a general anesthetic shall be used" for a list specifying (but not limited to) some two dozen procedures, including brain injury, eye and skin toxicity, drowning, testing of biological and chemical weapons for physiological effects, distressful methods of euthanasia, and bone fracture. The burden of proof would be on the experimenter to establish that withholding drugs was scientifically necessary. It argued as well that congressional intent only allowed animal pain in studies of the most pressing sort, aimed at curing "dread disease," as one member of Congress had phrased it[5] (Regulatory Analysis and Development 1986).

The ALDF called for regulations so explicit that little would be left for individual interpretation in the research facilities. It had already explained its skepticism about self-reporting; self-policing would not impress it much more. The ALDF wanted a strong animal care committee that would review all protocol proposals, but it did not seem to envision much need for individual diagnosis of animals in pain or worry much about who would prescribe the requisite painkillers and anesthetics.

Neither scientists nor veterinarians submitted a similar list, calling instead to leave matters to local control, in the hands of the animal committee and/or the attending veterinarian. The consensus among veterinarians and researchers was that any list would quickly become obsolete, as new experimental procedures come into use. People might wrongly assume that procedures not on the list were not painful, resulting in greater harm to animals. Some would accept a categorization scheme such as the Scientists Center for Animal Welfare had proposed: cataloging procedures into five groups, based on the severity of the intervention, and having the animal committee focus most efforts on the highest pain categories.[6] No scientist or veterinarian suggested anything like the ALDF's list of procedures that would never be allowed, or that only studies of dread disease could warrant unalleviated animal pain.

The USDA received only about 350 comments in response to its first call for information in 1986; in the subsequent 3 years it would count some 35,000. During this first round of correspondence, scientists and veterinarians were united in their call for flexibility and self-regulation, and jurisdictional differences between these two groups were little apparent. They emphasized either the judgment of the attending veterinarian or the role of the institutional animal committee in reviewing any proposals to withhold painkillers. They suggested a standard of care such as "currently accepted practices," "current professional practice of laboratory animal medicine," or "the evolving general standards of the animal research community," rather than whatever detailed mandates the USDA might come up with. The correspondence of that period contains no evidence of conflict between proposals that highlight the role of the veterinarians versus those that spotlight committees. No one was suggesting that standards might vary between and within institutions or that veterinarians, animal care committees, and research scientists might disagree within an institution on the standards and practices of pain management.

Scientists and laboratory animal veterinarians joined forces in their desire to keep government from intruding into the conduct of research, striving for the maximum self-determination for research institutions. But institutions do not make pain management decisions; individuals within institutions do. And the more autonomy could be secured for research institutions to regulate themselves, the more the importance of being the person empowered within the institution grew. For example, a laboratory animal veterinarian wrote to the USDA that the important rule would be to require the presence of a veterinarian on the team if surgery would be performed: "By creating standards that ensure proper postoperative care, e.g., that every survival surgery in non-rodent species must have a veterinarian on the research team, the need to list operative procedures [requiring pain relief] could be avoided" (Regulatory Analysis and Development 1986). This veterinarian foreshadowed the turf war that was about to ensue, though it had been brewing for decades.

In publishing proposed regulations in 1987, the USDA sought a compromise between the demands of the animal protectionists for strong and specific pain-management rules and the unified call of veterinarians and scientists for flexibility and self-regulation. The USDA proposed four categories of animal use in research and teaching with pain and distress the defining criteria, but it left the determination of when or whether to use painkillers for local review. As prompted by many of their correspondents, USDA adopted the standard that procedures painful to people should be considered painful to animals (Animal and Plant Health Inspection Service 1987).

In leaving determinations of pain management to self-regulation, the USDA did not shy from specifying how committees would review protocols nor from mandating specific jurisdictional divisions of authority within institutions. Committees were to focus heavily on the investigator's efforts to reduce animal pain and distress. Much of the committee's role during protocol review, however, was to safeguard the attending veterinarian's jurisdiction over use of anesthetics and analgesics. The committee was to require that the principal investigator consult with the attending veterinarian for category 3 and 4 procedures (those with the greatest potential for animal pain) and use painkillers "in accordance with the attending veterinarian's recommendations and established or accepted veterinary practices" (Animal and Plant Health Inspection Service 1987, p. 10302). The veterinarian would instruct laboratory workers in pre- and postsurgical care and evaluate animal surgery facilities and qualifications of researchers who perform animal surgery. Veterinarians would even develop the daily record-keeping systems that researchers were to use to assure proper drug use and surgical care.

Research scientists were left with little of their old autonomy under the USDA's 1987 proposed rules. Scientists might find some indirect autonomy in their representation on the animal care committee, but not because Congress or the USDA had preserved this for them. Congress required a committee of at least three members, including the attending veterinarian and one person otherwise unaffiliated with the institution. Presumably, most other committee members would be research scientists, though Congress did not worry about reserving such a slot for them.

Who says animals are in pain?

Two core beliefs fuel the drive of animal protectionists for stricter regulation: that animals suffer pain in laboratories and that scientists do not do enough on their own to prevent or treat this pain. To read the history of animal pain in the Animal Welfare Act, you would think that everyone agrees that animal pain is quite straightforward to recognize and treat and that scientists are simply bad actors who refuse to do their duty by their animals.

In the 1980s, the USDA sought a middle course between the demands of animal protectionists and the demands of scientists. A middle course on animal pain management implies a starting consensus on how much pain animal research currently entailed. That consensus was not there.

Are animals actually capable of experiencing pain? René Descartes is widely credited (or reviled) for articulating a mind/body dualism that included the claim that animals, lacking human rationality (as evidenced by their lack of human speech), did not really experience pain as we know it. They were body only, automata or machines; no mind, and certainly no soul. In a much-quoted letter, he claimed that his "opinion is not so much cruel to animals as indulgent to men . . . since it absolves them from the suspicion of crime when they eat or kill animals" (Descartes 1649). And at least some of his followers did find great license in his words. Nicholas Fontaine related an anecdote of experimenters at a seminary in France in the late seventeenth century: "They administered beatings to dogs with perfect indifference, and made fun of those who pitied the creatures as if they felt pain. They said the animals were clocks; that the cries they emitted when struck were only the noise of a little spring that had been touched, but that the whole body was without feeling" (Fontaine 1738, p. 201). If that dismissal of apparent animal pain could work 300 years ago, perhaps it could work today as well: scientists today could head off much controversy and restrictive regulation if they believed, and could convince the rest of us, that animals were truly incapable of feeling pain.

Bernard Rollin, a philosopher who has spent much of his time interacting with scientists and veterinarians, has encountered frequent denials that animals perceive pain in any way comparable to the way we humans do. He quotes the associate dean of a veterinary college, for instance, as claiming that "anesthesia and analgesia have nothing to do with [animal] pain; they are methods of chemical restraint" (Rollin 1989, pp. 117–118). Rollin reports that in the 1960s, at least one major veterinary teaching hospital did not stock narcotic analgesics for animal pain control, or even bother to obtain a license to do so. "Increasingly, I found myself in the position of being forced to 'prove' [to scientists of all varieties] that animals were conscious, and to provide good, 'scientifically acceptable' grounds even for claiming that animals feel pain" (Rollin 1989, p. xii).[7]

I have found a less absolutist stance in my conversations with scientists and in reading their correspondence to the USDA. Amid the hundreds of scientists' letters decrying the Animal Welfare Act regulations, none claimed that animals cannot experience pain. Rollin and others may be the reason that in the late 1980s no one would willingly commit to such a belief in writing, so much a minority opinion as it would be. It is equally possible that scientists writing to the USDA knew that the law had already been passed, and with it the mandate to do something about animal pain. Categorically denying animal pain perception would be irrelevant in that context. Still, I have never had a scientist where I worked try to tell me that animals do not feel pain as a general rule, despite the myriad times I have heard, in essence that "*this* particular animal undergoing *this* procedure is not in pain." This can happen even when we stand together watching an animal's response to a scalpel or needle.

Radical theories that fly in the face of common sense, whether ancient or modern denials of animal consciousness (Carruthers 1992)—Watson, Skinner, or other behaviorists' dismissal of the mental lives of animals, or anyone's denial that animals in general feel pain—find little place in the policy arena. The action is in determining when (not whether) animals might feel pain, and who is qualified to make that determination.

Scientists may well believe that animals can feel pain and still resist giving a particular animal a painkiller. They have a wide range of reasons to resist government prescription of pain medicines for their animals, regardless of how deep or shallow their concern for animal welfare. Anesthetics and analgesics can be expensive. Many are controlled narcotics that require extensive administrative efforts (record keeping, Drug Enforcement Agency licensing and inspections). Their proper use may require round-the-clock attendance on the animals to redose every few hours. Even the most modern analgesics have undesirable side effects (respiratory depression, intestinal upsets, decreased blood clotting) that may impact animal health or create research variables. Few have been extensively evaluated for proper dose and administration in laboratory animal species.

There are many studies in which treating animal pain would result in bad science. These are the studies that institutions report as "category E" in their annual reports to the USDA. For example, if I am assessing whether a new painkiller could help arthritis, I could induce arthritis in rats by injecting an immune stimulator, or adjuvant. While some of the rats may find relief with the new painkiller, I will probably need an untreated control group to truly assess the value of my new therapy. Without a control group, I would not know if pain-free rats receiving the new medicine are pain-free because the new medicine is so effective or because my method of inducing disease did not work in this particular instance (Houri and O'Sullivan 1995; Wilder 1996; Williams 1998)

In addition to the costs and inconvenience of treating animal pain, I've suspected a psychological reaction among the scientists I've known. Many of the scientists I work with have come of age since Singer published *Animal Liberation* in 1975; they have received their training in the era of expanded government regulation of animal use. They believe that animals are sensitive creatures and that harming them is wrong. They very much want to go home at the end of the day satisfied that they are among the ranks of the better scientists whose experiments may kill, but do not hurt, their animals. Protecting their self-identification as someone who would not hurt animals could lead these people, ironically, to refuse to see that their animals might indeed be in pain, despite their good character and their best intentions. To diagnose pain would be to diagnose themselves as people who inflict pain. If my observations are true, this desire to avoid identifying as a person who could hurt animals can result in underdiagnosis, and more important, undertreatment of animal pain.

In the political arena, no scientist is likely to say she has no concern for her animals' welfare. Rather, it is all about knowing what animals want—whether and how much pain they feel in particular circumstances. Scientists, animal protectionists, and veterinarians each have their own ways of knowing when animals in general, or any particular animal, are in pain and in need of treatment.

Know pain, know gain

Let's agree that animals do not want to be in pain and that we are going to do what we can to honor that. The ease with which science's defenders and critics discuss animal pain glosses over the deep epistemological questions of when, whether, and how animals experience pain and who is able to recognize it. The easy consensus that animal pain must be minimized breaks down in the face of specific cases, such as determining what procedures do or don't cause pain or which individual animals are or are not experiencing pain. Scientists, veterinarians, and animal protectionists tend to rely on different conceptions of animal pain, and even more so, of the ability to know if an animal is in pain, as they compete for the right to speak for animals and to determine animal welfare policy.

Read through the congressional testimony on the Animal Welfare Act and it seems straightforward: Animals often suffer pain during experiments; the ethical-cum-legal imperative is to do the best to obliterate that pain without undermining the scientific objectives of the study. Animal protectionists know this. It is abundantly evident to legislators.

Read through the pro-research materials that seek to minimize the intrusion of costly and detailed regulations into scientific practice, and the opposite is just as clear: Scientists are fully cognizant of the potential for animal suffering and committed to minimizing it. "The biologist yields to no one in his reverence for living things," wrote Lester Dragstedt, a physician, in the *Journal of Medical Education* in 1960 (p. 2). "It is evidence of the scientist's reverence for life that he avoids all unnecessary suffering in his work" (p. 2). The American Medical Association repeated this position thirty years later in its white paper on animals in research: "Most experiments today do not involve pain, most animals used in experiments do not suffer pain, and the degree of pain that is inflicted during some experiments has been greatly reduced through the establishment of rules for the humane conduct of experiments" (American Medical Association 1992, p. 17).

The point is made in the many public information materials put out by numerous research advocacy groups, including the National Academy of Sciences: "Most animals experience only minimal pain or brief discomfort when they are used in research. . . . Animal activists are wrong when they accuse researchers of inflicting needless pain on experimental animals" (Committee on the Use of Animals in Research 1991, p. 23).

Laboratory animals do not speak human languages and can only enter the welfare policy dialogue through their human interpreters. A host of human interpreters compete to speak for animals, often with little agreement among competing factions. Why should legislators believe the animal protectionists' claims about what pains the animals suffer? The protectionists are not in the labs to see it. But then, why should they trust the scientists' assurances that animals are not in pain? Their interest in avoiding restrictions will surely lead to bias. Knowing this, both the protectionists and the scientists have claimed the veterinarians as their witnesses, implicitly affirming the veterinarian's competence and integrity.

Much of the work of bringing the private experiences of animals into a public forum has required the "scientization" of pain. Discussions of pain among scientists and veterinarians are often dominated by conceptions of pain as a physical and quantifiable phenomenon, not the subjective and emotional jumble of feelings that a common-sense or empathic reading (a layperson's reading) might produce. But pain resists this reduction and can resist easy diagnosis, even for experts. There is no blood test, for instance, to measure pain levels, only indirect and equivocal behaviors and signs: depression or agitation, vocalization or silence. Even the most obvious signs—limping, for instance—can have alternative readings. A dog or a human with a short leg, for instance, will limp without pain simply because of the anatomic asymmetry.

Look at the monkey in figure 7.1. Is this animal in pain? How would you know? Unless the observer is very familiar to the animal, most of what you'd see in the animal's behavior is the reaction to a stranger, not the subtler signs of pain. He

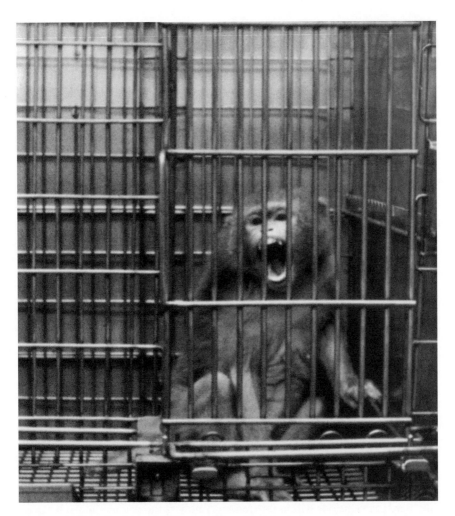

Fig. 7.1 Is this animal in pain? How would you know? COURTESY OF VIKTOR REINHARDT.

is not likely to allow a close examination, except under sedation, which will also mask the evidence of pain.

This scientization is the professional way of objectifying pain into something that people can see or hear or feel and discuss. Animal protectionists also must objectify the inner experiences of animals to make them visible and tangible for their audience. Most of us have seen photos of the faces of laboratory animals intended to depict pain: typically these are monkeys, not because they experience more pain necessarily or because people in general care more about them than about dogs or cats or horses or because they are used in more painful experiments. These things may be true, but more, monkeys' faces look so expressive and so human, and animal protectionists choose these images wisely. They choose their words carefully as well, describing animals' experiences in graphic terms—being thrown into a dog-dealer's truck, sitting in excrement, injected with toxins—and inviting the audience (legislator, public sympathizer) to empathize and analogize: How would *you* feel in this situation?

In contrast, when scientists describe animals behavior in more neutral language, they invite the audience to set aside emotion and anthropomorphism. Saying "x was aversive at all concentrations" instead of "the animals acted as though they were in pain no matter how low the dose" is not just word economy. Better (i.e., more scientific) is the translation of subjective experience into objective laboratory data: brain waves, blood cortisol levels, vocalizations, seconds elapsed before flicking the tail from a noxious stimulus.

Scientists, veterinarians, and protectionists are not competing just to convince an audience that animals are or are not in pain in any particular set of circumstances. They are vying to establish their credentials as the group best poised to identify and manage animal pain in general.

It became clear throughout the late 1980s that the USDA was not going to ban specific procedures or to mandate specific painkillers. The National Association for Biomedical Research (NABR) had urged its membership to promote self-regulation, and veterinarians and animal committees loomed large as the most credible defense against excessive government intrusion. NABR and other professional scientific and veterinary organizations downplayed any potential for conflict within institutions in their portrait of veterinarians, animal committees, and scientists working together harmoniously to advance good science and good animal care. NABR and laboratory animal veterinarians shared an agenda: flexible self-regulation for scientific institutions that would not equate with laissez-faire business-as-usual for individual scientists in their laboratories. This approach posed problems, however.

Whereas scientists and laboratory animal veterinarians stood easily together in their 1986 bid to maximize institutional home rule, the USDA's 1987 proposal to place home rule primarily in the hands of veterinarians and animal committees uncovered the tensions within institutions. Pain was the major concern breaking down the traditional divide between animal care and animal use and therefore was the issue over which scientists most faced loss of autonomy in the conduct of their experiments. The USDA chose committee review of animal use protocols before the start of an experiment as the primary tool for minimizing animal pain and for spreading authority among scientists, veterinarians, and committees. For this reason, decisions about which protocols to review, what to include in a review, and who would review them became so important to anyone hoping to shape the regulations.

Scientists and veterinarians had stood together to subvert what seemed like common sense, to convincingly argue that neither what looked painful to animals nor what felt painful to people might necessarily feel painful to animals. Knowing animal pain is a job for experts—not government officials, and certainly not animal protectionists. Once pain recognition became the province of the experts, however, the competing expertise of veterinarians and research scientists became the issue of importance.

It is mostly in the USDA correspondence from individual scientists and their professional associations that the cozy collegiality between scientists and veterinarians breaks down. Many scientists found veterinarians ill-equipped to be their peers, much less their overseers. They saw laboratory animal veterinarians as simply the USDA's agents, with review of animal protocols the tool by which USDA officials (veterinarians themselves, and with what appeared to be a sympathetic ear for the animal protectionists) would erode scientific freedom and tie up animal experimentation in a bundle of costly red tape. In reality, the USDA was proposing in 1987 what it had started in 1970: empowerment of veterinarians to manage animal pain during experiments. The only new twist was that the committee would assure that veterinarians were playing this role.

Jurisdiction on paper had not necessarily resulted in jurisdiction in the workplace, despite the actions of Congress and the USDA in 1970. Several scientists wrote in 1987 as though the veterinarian's involvement in prescribing pain control were completely new to them, as telling a reflection on the limited force of the 1970 law as any. For example, one scientist (the vice-chair of his campus's Institutional Animal Care and Use Committee) worried that "requiring the use of anesthetics etc. in accordance with the veterinarian gives the veterinarian control of scientific protocols" in excess of congressional mandate (Regulatory Analysis and Development 1987). His concern came seventeen years after Congress first mandated such veterinary involvement, which was evidently not much in force on that particular campus during that interval. Years before that scientist's 1987 letter about veterinarians' "new authority," the American Veterinary Medical Association had reported on Animal Welfare Act regulations for its members in 1975, stressing the laboratory animal veterinarian's responsibility for the appropriate use of anesthetics to control pain at all times, throughout entire studies. But the AVMA noted, apparently in response to concerns of laboratory animal veterinarians, that if the institution does not give the veterinarian the necessary authority to fulfill these responsibilities, "the attending veterinarian may wish to attach a statement to the annual report form, listing such lack of authority or any restriction of limitation placed upon him by the responsible officials of the registered facility" (American Veterinary Medical Association 1975, p. 260).

Some veterinarians moved to consolidate the role that the Animal Welfare Act had assigned them some seventeen years earlier. USDA had proposed a definition of painful procedures to include those that cause pain in people. But that would mean that anyone could pronounce an animal procedure painful. One laboratory animal veterinarian, working in a medical school, "found that veterinarians are more knowledgeable concerning the detection of pain in animals than most investigators. After all, that is our job" (Regulatory Analysis and Development 1987). Another worried that a human standard of pain might imply that a physician-researcher with a medical degree would be the one to decide what was painful to animals: "Could this be reworded such that the decision will remain in the hands of the attending veterinarian?" (Regulatory Analysis and Development 1989). For another, veterinarians were the "breath of fresh air" who could get scientists to re-evaluate the procedures they'd been doing year after year, and any language that gave the animal committee greater authority than the veterinarian should be struck (Regulatory Analysis and Development 1987).

While some animal protectionists were content to empower laboratory animal veterinarians to rule on animal pain, rarely would they grant them absolute authority. Most called for a strong role for the animal committee (no doubt assuming that the nonaffiliated community representative would bring a pro-animal flavor to committee deliberations), including review of all animal protocols, not just the most painful category 3 and 4 protocols. They called for enhanced and highly detailed annual reports, describing all painful procedures, explicitly discussing the alternatives that were considered (and rejected) and the rationale for withholding painkillers—all accessible to the protectionists through Freedom of Information Act requests. And they still hoped for national rather than local standards and policies, suggesting, for instance, that all of an institution's written animal care policies be reviewed by a higher authority, perhaps a panel of NIH scientists.

Protectionists had limited faith in veterinarians partly because the vets worked for the research institutions, their loyalties divided between the animals and their employers. But they also challenged the competence and professional standards of veterinarians as well. Some applauded the USDA's proposal that use of anesthetics and painkillers be "in accordance with . . . the accepted or common veterinary use of such drugs," and that pre- and postsurgical care be "in accordance with established veterinary medical and nursing procedures" (Animal and Plant Health Inspection Service, USDA 1987, p. 10314); others were unimpressed. As one animal welfare organization wrote about "common veterinary usage" of painkilling drugs: "Most veterinarians in private practice does [sic] not prescribe analgesics. This could be used as a basis for greatly limiting the use of pain-relieving drugs, which would be in violation of the Act" (Regulatory Analysis and Development 1987).

Scientists, too, examined the state-of-the-art of pain management among veterinarians and found it lacking. Like some protectionists, they too argued for a more powerful animal committee, of which the veterinarian would be but a single member (though, unlike the protectionists, they surely counted on a committee more heavily weighted with research scientists than with community representatives). A physician, chair of his medical college's animal committee, wrote that a veterinarian would be "clearly redundant" on an animal project if an MD surgeon and MD anesthesiologists were working together (Regulatory Analysis and Development 1987). Another scientist noted that veterinarians have "no generally agreed-upon standards" on postsurgical painkillers, or even on intraoperative anesthesia for minor surgeries. Clearly, many scientists were unimpressed with their veterinarians' credentials as animal pain experts.

Further working against veterinarians' jurisdictional consolidation, scientists pointed out that there was little accepted or established use of veterinary drugs for laboratory animal uses. Most animal drugs are tested for the common domestic species in common clinical situations; farm animals and pet animals are the major market for veterinary pharmaceuticals. It is illegal to label drugs for indications or species for which they have not been specifically tested. You cannot buy analgesics marketed and labeled for pain control (or any other use) in mice, nor are there drugs tested and approved for placement of brain electrodes in even the most common of domestic species. Therefore, most use of drugs in laboratory animals are extra-label uses: They are prescribed for species and situations for which they have not been tested, labeled, and marketed. Without this market-driven database, on what could a veterinarian base her prescription of drugs for animal subjects?

Surprisingly, two veterinary associations, the American College of Laboratory Medicine and the American Veterinary Medical Association, corresponded with the USDA in 1987 on several topics related to the authority, responsibilities, and credentials of laboratory animal veterinarians, but neither group claimed any special expertise about animal pain. Only after many scientists spurned the proposals to empower veterinarians did the AVMA advance such a claim. In 1989, as the USDA worked to finalize its regulations, the AVMA wrote: "The attending veterinarian is the scientist who is trained to make precisely these judgements [about pain management during experimentation] and his or her expertise should be utilized to the fullest extent possible. This has not always been the case in the past . . . the researcher must be encouraged to regard the veterinarian as a scientific expert and to actively enlist his or her cooperation" (Regulatory Analysis and Development 1987).

Having once taken up the role of defining veterinarians as animal pain scientists, the AVMA went further. Agreeing that most drug use in laboratory animal practice was untested and extra-label, it found authority for veterinarians where scientists had anticipated quackery. It is precisely because there is no database for research animal uses that the individual attending veterinarian must be empowered to make the "final professional judgment for the animals in his or her care" (Regulatory Analysis and Development 1987). Takacs (1996) has described an "argument from ignorance" in his study of biologists as expert-advocates for biodiversity. Expertise can confer power, but so can ignorance, as long as *everyone* is ignorant (about the effects of deforestation on biodiversity, about subjective experiences of pain in animals), and you are best poised to shine the light in that ignorance (Takacs 1996, p. 83). The AVMA put forth for pain control what has frequently been the argument for performance standards in animal welfare policy: If we don't know enough collectively to write rules that enhance animal welfare, then welfare will best be enhanced by leaving it in the hands of separate animal care committees and scientists, but above all, laboratory animal veterinarians.

What the AVMA did not make explicit, and neither did anyone else arguing for a strong role for veterinarians, was how the veterinarian would base her professional judgment. Would she find a database that she alone, not the scientists whose animals she tended, would have access to, or would be competent to interpret? Might her authority rest in a close clinical relationship with the individual animals in her care? Or did she perhaps have some sort of experiential or craft knowledge of pain management that eluded scientists, knowledge that allowed her to prescribe pain medications early in a project's planing stages, even before animals had been purchased or examined?

A primer on animal pain, circa 1985

At the time of the Animal Welfare Act amendments of 1985, I had left my work as a laboratory animal veterinary technician and was in my third year of veterinary school. As correspondence flooded Washington in response to USDA's 1987 proposed regulations, I was graduating from veterinary college, beginning my career as a laboratory animal veterinarian. I had just completed four years at one of the finest veterinary colleges in the world, my brain saturated with state-of-the-art veterinary medicine. And I confess that I had not learned nearly enough about recognizing or treating animal pain.

My veterinary professors were not quite the Cartesian dualists that Rollin describes; they did not deny that animals could experience pain. In truth, such a denial would have been a much more consistent reckoning with pain than what I encountered. During my veterinary training, animal pain appeared and disappeared like the Cheshire cat, its significance, and the attention we should pay to it, constantly shifting.

Veterinarians cannot deny animal pain because it is much too important a diagnostic tool. My orthopedics professors were the most invested in pain-as-diagnostic. They taught us to press and palpate, to flex and extend joints, to localize the painful part of a limping dog's leg. A swollen and painful joint might be arthritis; pain along the long limb bones might indicate cancer in an older dog, inflammation of the bones (panosteitis) in a growing pup. Accurately localized pain would sharpen our focus for the next diagnostic step: the X-ray. A nonpainful lameness would point us in other diagnostic directions.

My bovine medicine professor scorned modern laboratory tests and told us to "ask the cow where she hurts." He showed us how to push up under a cow's chest with a broom handle, imitating the grunt she would make if she had an infection in the pericardium surrounding her heart. Pain helped distinguish the swelling of an abscess (painful) from the swelling of a tumor (often painless). We learned to look for pain where our "lay" clients might not: the painful tooth that explains why an animal stops eating, the painfully inflamed bladder of a cat who has suddenly lost her toilet manners. And we learned to respect pain for the way it could inspire a horse to kick, a dog to bite, a cat to lash out, all with painful consequences for the veterinarian.

At other times, however, pain seemed to disappear. Our teachers seemed unable to agree on whether gouging out a calf's budding (and unanesthetized) horns was significantly painful. Though general anesthesia was the standard of practice for castrating a dog, young pigs got no such pain control. Time and again we were told that an animal was just "resisting restraint," or was just "uncomfortable," not really in pain. Many animals *do* resist restraint. What I lacked was training in how to reliably recognize whether pain was also present along with the restraint and the discomfort.

Only occasionally during my education was pain considered an unpleasant experience worthy of treatment in its own right. Typically, the best we would do by pain was to treat the underlying cause and let the gradual cessation of pain (if it successfully ceased) reveal the progress of our cure. We would treat an infection with antibiotics, and though it might take hours or days for the infection to subside enough to lessen the pain, only rarely might we add painkillers as part of our therapeutic regimen. A dog with bad teeth got an appointment for dentistry, but no pain treatment while she waited. Imagine telling a human patient not to bother with aspirin now, because a pain-causing infection would subside in a few days or because the dentist was available within the week. Pain itself can be treated even as the underlying cause of pain is under treatment, but you would never know that from reading either my veterinary class notes or my own clinical records.

Pain was most relevant to surgery, where it was the province of the veterinary anesthesiologists. They taught us anesthesia was not an either/or, all-or-nothing proposition. Different parts of a surgery stimulate pain sensation to differing degrees, so careful monitoring and adjustment throughout the procedure are necessary. Too little anesthetic, and your patient may feel the operation; too much, and you risk an anesthetic death. With gas anesthetics, we can adjust the flow minute by minute to tailor the anesthetic to the individual animal and that moment's manipulations. With injected anesthetics, the kind so often used in research surgeries on rodents, a one-dose-for-all injection typically risks that some individuals will be somewhat underanesthetized, some dangerously overanesthetized, and some, at least for some stages of the operation, just right. I wince when I review animal protocols with this impersonal one-dose approach to anesthesia and wince again for my realization that the researcher got the dose from books that veterinarians wrote.

Curiously, though we learned about surgical anesthetics in exquisite detail, postsurgical pain management got short shrift in our veterinary educations in the mid-1980s (and even less attention in earlier generations). I remember far too vividly an incident from my surgery class as a third-year veterinary student. My surgery beagle howled (mournfully?) while recovering from the practice ophthalmic surgery that we students had performed, but we were talked out of giving her an analgesic. After all, her howling could be just some residual excitation from the preanesthetic, oxymorphone, that we had administered. But back in 1986 no one tried to teach me (nor do I recall asking) how to tell whether she might also be in pain as well as in excitation. Nor did anyone give her pain the benefit of the doubt and administer a painkiller in the face of uncertainty.

While scientists had been denying or discounting the pain of their research animals over many years, veterinarians (clinical veterinarians on farms and in pet practices, not just laboratory animal veterinarians) had simultaneously been downplaying their animal patients' pain. To do otherwise could have had unpleasant and inconvenient implications for their practice. Serious attention to pain could raise the cost of veterinary medicine, especially in the days before synthetic opioids and potent analgesics with long durations of action. It could mean long hours attending to animals overnight after surgery, rather than leaving them quietly unattended. Analgesic drugs cost extra money, require extra record keeping (many are controlled narcotics) and can have side effects that require additional monitoring. Their use in farm animals may render the meat or milk unusable for human consumption, as very few drugs may legally be used in the last few days preceding slaughter, in the attempt to keep drug residues out of the meat that people eat. Often in farm practice the decision is whether to treat an animal, or to send her to slaughter untreated, her meat and milk, and her pain, untouched by drugs. Veterinary surgeons long relied on the idea that postoperative pain is a good thing, best left untreated, if it keeps animals from putting weight on a recently pinned fracture or from straining a surgical incision. It was rare that a dog in the 1980s or earlier received postoperative painkillers.

A veterinarian genuinely concerned about postsurgical pain in laboratory animals had few tools and little guidance available in those days. For example, in the American College of Laboratory Animal Medicine's texts on rabbits and mice, postsurgical care is covered with absolutely no whisper of postsurgical pain management, no matter how invasive the surgery (Bivin and Timmons 1974; Cunliffe-Beamer 1983). Veterinarians who searched for information in veterinary texts would find meperidine (trade name Demerol) and pentazocine (trade name Talwin) as two of the only opioid drugs for postsurgical pain. With effective duration of actions of only two to four hours, serious attention to pain management would become a round-the-clock pastime (Holmes 1984; Jenkins 1987).

Ironically, in my early years of practice in laboratory animal medicine, in the late 1980s and early 1990s, laboratory dogs were receiving postoperative pain medication more routinely than your pet dog would. By then, both the Animal Welfare Act regulations and the NIH *Guide* defined abdominal procedures (such as spaying) as "major surgery," and presumed postoperative pain medication unless there were a scientific justification to withhold. By then, longer-acting painkillers such as butorphanol and buprenorphine were becoming available. The standard of practice was shifting. What was once a standard (at its best) of treating animal pain only when unequivocally diagnosed was becoming a standard of withholding treatment only when certain that it would cause problems. Swapping tales with other newly graduated veterinarians, most of them in private pet-animal practices, I realized how little pain relief pet animals—spayed dogs, declawed cats, and others—were receiving, and I sanctimoniously lectured them on all the newest painkillers available for their animal patients.

After fifteen years of practice, I still find animal pain diagnosis incredibly challenging. Pain (especially deep and chronic pain) can manifest in contradictory ways: agitation or depression, increased or decreased appetite, vocalization or quiet. Worse, almost all these signs can have other explanations. A monkey may pick at her sutures after surgery because the incision hurts or because she's feeling fine and it's something to do in an impoverished environment. Different species and different individuals may show pain differently. Rabbits get still and quiet, but a dog in a lot of pain may yet wag his tail and lick your face and wait until he's alone to curl up and whimper. Even response to therapy can be equivocal. If I give a painkiller and the animal's behavior does not change, does that mean the behavior was not indicative of pain, or that the drug at that dose cannot control that particular pain? If behavior does change, I may still be uncertain why. For example, our favorite rat analgesic can cause abnormal appetite (pica) at higher doses whether or not the rat was in pain before its administration (Roughan and Flecknell 2002).

Abbott (1988) writes that the nature of professional practice is to take the general, theoretical, formal knowledge of a field and apply it to specific situations. The challenge for veterinarians was to show that they had the best professional body of knowledge and were the most competent professionals to apply it to individual cases. In making this move in the late 1980s, they were playing a game of catch up. And they were playing this game in the face of the ubiquity of pain as something we have all experienced, something people may only reluctantly recognize as a province for specialized experts. Veterinarians' prior inconsistent attention to animal pain, both in the clinic and in the research laboratory, left both their commitment and their competence in question as the USDA worked to assign jurisdictions in the 1980s.

The 1980s saw a groundswell in veterinary and scientific interest in animal pain. Though most scientists see animal pain as an unwanted by-product of their experiments, there are those who formally study animal pain. Animals have served as a model of human pain for decades, as scientists have worked to understand the basis of pain perception and to develop newer and better painkillers for human use. The interest in studies of animal pain is not so much *whether* animals feel pain, but *how much*. A metrology of animal pain has grown, embedded first in studying animals as models in the development of analgesics for human use, but now trickling down for application to animals themselves. Analgesiometry, the quantitative assessment of the efficacy of a painkiller, depends on quantifying the amount of pain being experienced or relieved. Pain researchers may apply stimuli that the animal can terminate on his or her own (moving a tail away from a source of heat, for instance) or stimuli that cannot be easily terminated (such as injecting irritating materials into the abdomen or forepaw) (Dubner 1987; International Association for the Study of Pain 1983). Either way, the basis of analgesiometry involves measuring behavioral responses to standardized stimuli. Behavioral assessments may be as simple as timing how long a rat will keep a foot on a hot plate before terminating the contact or as complex as studying whether animals learn to avoid a chamber in which they have experienced a painful stimulus.

Throughout the 1980s and into the 1990s, formal attention to animal pain and animal pain control boomed, with scientists and veterinarians working together. Much of that work began well before passage of the 1985 laws, reflecting, I hope, changing concerns within institutions and not just fear of impending regulation.

The AVMA sponsored a symposium on animal pain at the 1982 meeting of the Federation of the American Societies for Experimental Biology (Kitchell 1983). In 1987, the AVMA Council on Biologic and Therapeutic Agents hosted a Collo- quium on Recognition and Alleviation of Animal Pain and Distress. With funding from the USDA, NIH, and several industry sponsors, it brought together aca- demic veterinarians and other scientists (including some physicians) and philoso- phers to set the stage for an era of increased ethical concern about animals, to initiate a program of study on animal pain and its alleviation, and to show the vet- erinary profession's willingness to take up the challenge of addressing animal pain and distress. Publication included a panel report on future directions for research and policy (Panel on the Recognition and Alleviation of Animal Pain and Distress 1987). A year later, the National Academy's Institute of Laboratory Animal Re- sources convened a similar panel (with some overlap), publishing its report in 1992 (Committee on Pain and Distress in Laboratory Animals 1992).

These publications tended toward the theoretical, the scientific, the physical. All three acknowledged the ethical climate in which they were written, a time of increased public concern for animals, particularly research animals. They were also quite clear, especially in their overviews, prefaces, and introductory notes, that there is an emotional and cognitive reality to pain in animals. They distinguished the experiential character of pain from nociception, the neurophysiological input that pain-sensory nerve fibers deliver to the brain.

But though recognizing ethical, cognitive, and emotional dimensions to ani- mal pain, these groundbreaking texts were highly technical and scientific. The 1982 conference focused heavily on nociception—what Rollin (1992, p. 61) calls the "plumbing of pain"—as opposed to how pain feels. The emphasis is on the ob- jective and the standardizable. In one paper, human verbal reports of pain are questioned as sometimes misleading; better to develop measures of "pain reactiv- ity" that can be used in humans and other species (Vierck et al. 1983). It is not sim- ply that the experience of pain can be reduced to the neurophysiology of nocicep- tion, but that human self-reports of how pain feels are less relevant, in the scientific context, than what the body reveals to the objective scientist. This scien- tization of pain may reinforce boundaries around pain expertise, excluding "lay" outsiders, even as it works to create a new professional discipline of animal pain studies. So much for the USDA's belief that human pain would be a good guide to animal pain: It's not even a trustworthy guide to human pain!

Still, this highly technical volume on animal pain contained several important policy elements, including some that animal protectionists might applaud. It was the first workshop to focus on animal pain as significant in its own right, not just as a model of human pain. While surprisingly few of the papers contained even a cursory statement that animal pain must be minimized, that commitment is im- plied throughout. Significantly, the editors emphasized (alongside their caveats about overindulgence in anthropomorphism) that the uncertainty of knowing pain in animals does not imply that they don't feel it.

Laboratory animal veterinarians practicing in animal facilities have limited need for the science and standardization of pain research. What we want are some sure-fire ways of diagnosing pain and comprehensive formulary of which pain-killers to use at what dose in which species for any given application. And we are getting there. Through texts and e-mail discussion lists, with anecdote balanced against controlled studies of pain and pain-relief, laboratory animal veterinarians are developing a database of animal pain management practices (Flecknell 1996; Flecknell and Waterman-Pearson 2000; Kohn et al. 1997). These professional dialogues blend formally published peer-reviewed information with the experiential craft knowledge of veterinarians who prescribe the drugs.

Assurance that these developments in pain management actually make for happier and more comfortable animals remains a challenge. Mary Phillips's (1993) ethnographic study of laboratory practices revealed a widespread tendency in the laboratory not to take pain seriously, to define it away with the flimsiest of excuses. But that was a decade ago, and a very busy decade it has been; similar studies would help to document current laboratory practice. Social scientists can document their observations of laboratory workers' behaviors toward the animals. Indeed, in my own practice and observation, I find a wide range of behaviors toward animal pain management. Some scientists think it's amusing to worry about mouse pain, but comply with campus standards nonetheless. They will argue that if their mice simply survive a procedure, then all is well. Plenty of others recognize that there is plenty of room for animal pain and morbidity short of outright mortality and eagerly work with training staff to update their anesthetic and analgesic protocols.

Conclusion

The profession of laboratory animal medicine first developed through veterinarians' efforts to control disease and infection and supply healthy animals for experiment. Veterinarians nurtured a professional jurisdiction over laboratory animal care that left scientists free to conduct experiments as they saw fit. Concern for pain in laboratory animals has been the important tool in breaking down the care/use divide that has long separated the professional jurisdictions of veterinarians and scientists. Congress and the USDA progressively eroded scientists' autonomy and scientific freedoms in the Animal Welfare Act, not so much through detailed rules for experimental design, but through the creation of Institutional Animal Care and Use Committees and the expanded empowerment of laboratory animal veterinarians.

Pain has dominated animal welfare policy debates of the past three decades, overshadowing other forms of poor welfare (psychological distress, boredom, anxiety, unhappiness) and even casting killing and death into the background as minor concerns. Many of the provisions of the 1985 Animal Welfare Act amendment are built on the concern for animal pain.

Though laboratory animal veterinarians were well acquainted with anesthetics and pain control for surgery, they were ill-prepared to take over an expanded pain management jurisdiction in the 1980s for the many types of pain (and distress) that animals might suffer outside of surgery. Often, veterinarians and scientists claim that while animals in general can and do experience pain, a particular animal in a particular setting does not. Pain control is a labor-intensive activity requiring animal examination and monitoring, sometimes on a round-the-clock schedule. Drugs are expensive and entail complicated paperwork (as they are controlled narcotics). Pain control efforts undermine the public assurance that most research procedures (or clinical practices) are not inherently painful in the first place.

The USDA chose a flexible performance standards approach in which animal care committees oversee researchers' efforts to minimize animal pain and distress, including their search for alternatives to painful procedures and a mandatory consultation with a veterinarian. Performance-standards approaches to pain regulation allow flexibility, but taken seriously they are enormously demanding of time and resources. As well, we need better social ethical tools for how to make decisions about animal welfare in the face of what I expect to be the irreducible residual uncertainty—that there are limits to our ability to know and speak for animal minds—and that we need better decision-making strategies that factor in this uncertainty.

Scientists and veterinarians have shifted their conception of pain over the years, from the purely physical nociceptive model that best fits reductionist and objectivist ideals of the biological researcher, to something that recognizes the essentially subjective, experiential, and emotional aspects of animal pain. Veterinarians who claimed pain as their expertise by reducing it to a purely physical phenomenon limited their effectiveness to speak on broader matters of welfare, happiness, and other subjective and valuational matters.

I next move on to examine some cases in which the tension between physical and experiential aspects of animal welfare continues. In one instance, pain diagnosis takes a turn for the purely physical, as I examine the controversy over how to tell whether decapitated rats still feel pain in their disembodied heads. Later, we look the other way, at provisions for exercise and psychological well-being that were made possible only after pain had opened the door to serious discussion of animals' inner experiences. As always, the competition to speak authoritatively for the animals shapes the policy work. Before we get to these divergent cases, chapter 8 emphasizes that expertise has not been the only platform on which people have based their authority to speak for animals. Expertise exists alongside advocacy, the moral authority people have claimed to say what animals want.

8

The animal advocates

Dear Dr. Crawford:

If you are really a Dr. of Veterinary Services and a true humanitarian you will please support the Enforcement of the Improved Standards for Laboratory Animal amendments and the proposed animal welfare regulations under the Animal Welfare Acts.

Sincerely,

A true animal lover.
—Regulatory Analysis and Development 1987

THE USDA PUBLISHED PROPOSED ANIMAL WELFARE REGULATIONS IN THE *FEDERAL Register* on March 31, 1987, inviting public comments to be addressed to staff veterinarian Richard Crawford (Animal and Plant Health Inspection Service 1987). Poor Dr. Crawford: the USDA counted some 7857 comments submitted for his review (Animal and Plant Health Inspection Service 1989a). The majority of these letters to the USDA were impersonal; others, like the handwritten note quoted above, did indeed presume to know the good Dr. Crawford. He was a veterinarian, after all, and that meant two things: He possessed knowledge, and he had dedicated his life to animals. One writer reminded him, "Because of your position and your pledge as a Veterinarian, to limit and eliminate animal suffering, you are in a unique position" (Regulatory Analysis and Development 1987). Yet another called on Crawford to stand up with her against the bullying of the National Association for Biomedical Research: "The NABR would have everyone believe that these horrible conditions do not exist but I know and you as a Veterinary, know that they do and it is up to us to see that these situations are cleaned up. This is our chance to show the NABR that we mean business. Don't let the animals down, they are depending on you" (Regulatory Analysis and Development 1987).

For these letter writers, the veterinarian's knowledge and commitment to animals went hand in hand. For others, the commitment of veterinarians to animals was more complex. Just as the presumption of veterinarians' complete knowledge of animal welfare, pain management, and care was challenged by both scientists and animal protectionists in the 1980s, so too was their eligibility for the emerging role of animal advocate.

Both animal protectionists and research scientists challenged veterinarians' expertise on several fronts. Protectionists often thought common sense and extrapolation from the human condition were sufficient to determine what mattered to animals and how they ought to be treated; in this regard, veterinarians had no special expertise to offer. Scientists, on the other hand, often denigrated veterinarians' generalized and applied knowledge, which was shallow when compared point-by-point with the specialized knowledge of researchers. Often, however, veterinarians' knowledge and competence were taken as given, and at issue were their accountability (by virtue of the jobs, licensures, and accreditation they held) and their commitment to animal welfare (whether sworn in a professional oath or demonstrated in their performance).

As they had done in prior decades, animal protectionists tried in the 1980s to enlist veterinarians, in laboratories, in the government, and in the protectionist organizations themselves, as allies in reining in the freedoms of scientists to use animals as they saw fit. The relationship between protectionists and laboratory animal veterinarians had never been an uncomplicated alliance, however. For that reason, the animal protectionists also sought their own standing within the laboratories by pushing for inclusion of their own as animal advocates on the newly mandated IACUCs.

In this chapter, we look at the interplay of expertise and advocacy in animal welfare policy-making: Does expertise lead automatically to advocacy? Does advocacy require expertise? Should there be a special advocacy or accountability role for veterinarians that goes beyond doctoring the animals? As veterinarians, protectionists, and research advocates debated these questions with the USDA regulations writers, the animals themselves and controversial questions of who knew what was best for them, were often lost in the cross fire over who cared most about what was best for them.

Veterinary accountability and authority

Congress made two separate decisions to empower veterinarians in the early days of the Animal Welfare Act: first in 1966, when it chose the USDA (with its staff of veterinarians) over the scientists and medical doctors at the NIH to administer the new law, and then again in 1970, when it expanded the definition of "adequate veterinary care" for laboratory animals. Both reflect assumptions of where the competencies and commitments of veterinarians, as well as Congress's evolving ideas of what should be regulated in the laboratory. Neither move guaranteed that when the law underwent its upheaval in the 1980s veterinarians would emerge as the champions of laboratory animals.

Both the NIH and the USDA were candidates to administer laboratory animal welfare regulations when Congress passed the law in 1966. The USDA had a long history of law enforcement and inspection responsibilities (such as enforcing quarantine requirements for infected herds of cattle or performing carcass inspection at slaughterhouses). It already had a cadre of veterinarians working as field inspectors who could be enlisted to go into the laboratories and the premises of dog dealers for animal welfare inspections. However, their efforts had been entirely directed to agriculture and farm animals, and they had little training to evaluate the laboratory practices of medical schools or drug companies.

The NIH, in contrast, had much more experience in animal research, both in its own intramural research programs and in funding research around the country. But this was rarely a regulatory role: It funded and promoted research, with minimal restrictions for responsible use of either animal or human subjects, and even less ability for enforcement. In theory, the NIH could withhold funds from institutions not abiding by its guidelines, but its limited ability to detect noncompliance contributed to the rarity with which such funding restrictions occurred.

Ultimately, Congress awarded enforcement of the Animal Welfare Act to the USDA—a task the USDA was not necessarily eager to receive. Some fifty bills had been proposed throughout the 1960s before the Laboratory Animal Welfare Act of 1966 was finally passed. The NIH had opposed many of these regulatory proposals as far too stringent, losing whatever credibility its leaders ever had with the animal protectionists. Once the animal protectionists got their exposé of dog theft published in *Life* magazine and their legislative efforts found success, handing over enforcement to the NIH seemed too much like "sending the canary home by the cat" (Stevens 1968, p. 52). Protectionists saw the NIH's publication of the *Guide for Laboratory Animal Facilities and Care* and its own proposed laboratory animal legislation not as good faith efforts to improve animal welfare, but as the combined efforts of scientists and the NIH to forestall meaningful regulation (Nace 1994; Stevens 1990). The NIH, in short, was not to be trusted with the fledgling law and the animals it protected.

Who better to protect the laboratory animals than the dedicated veterinary staff of the USDA? "Welfare of animals should be the responsibility of the body that is primarily interested in them," testified faculty surgeon Nicholas Gimbel of Wayne State University, noting that he somehow knew that if he were a dog, he would want the USDA administering the law (quoted in Stevens 1966, p. 76). The NIH had no expertise in commercial dealings of animal acquisition, and the USDA's expertise on medical research was limited. But given that the 1966 Laboratory Animal Welfare Act was basically a pet-theft bill, the decision to empower the USDA's veterinary staff went well with the congressional decision to restrict coverage to animal acquisition, transport, and care outside of experimentation—the care/use divide that I have described. As the care/use divide steadily crumbled through subsequent amendments of the Animal Welfare Act, the USDA's historical focus on regulatory enforcement and its primarily veterinary staffing combined to flavor the direction the law and its enforcement would take, moving laboratory animal veterinarians to center stage in issues of animal care and use.

During the first two decades of the Animal Welfare Act, the veterinarians in the facilities and their veterinary inspectors in the USDA learned together how to exercise their new powers. Despite the inherent antagonism in the inspector–inspected dynamic, they came from similar backgrounds and shared a professional language and some common goals. In many facilities, although there is no legal requirement for this, it is the facility's laboratory animal veterinarian who accompanies the USDA inspector on his or her rounds. The two veterinarians may interact repeatedly over the course of several years. As a fledgling laboratory animal veterinarian in the 1980s, I learned (as I believe most laboratory animal veterinarians quickly learn) to sidestep inspectors' questions and to steer them gently from problems we would not want in an inspection report, but I also learned to shape inspection reports to my advantage. Laboratory animal veterinarians know to call items to their inspector's attention to get government sanction of their own priorities, with statements like "We're trying to get these dog runs upgraded as soon as we can find the funding," or "We've been working with this research team to improve their record keeping." At the end of the day, the laboratory animal veterinarian would have the USDA's written inspection report in hand, with thirty or sixty days to upgrade dog runs or improve record keeping. The rapport of the laboratory animal veterinarian with the USDA inspector thus could result in administrative funds to upgrade dog housing or in the IACUC's insistence that a principal investigator and her graduate students adopt the veterinarian's conception of acceptable record keeping. This informal, behind-the-scenes collegiality held well enough over 20 years for the USDA to attempt in 1987 to enlist laboratory animal veterinarians in the regulatory effort in a more formal way.

The USDA and other state and federal agencies have had a long history of enlisting veterinarians in private practice in their regulatory efforts, where human health or animal agriculture could be affected by animal infections. Private veterinarians may be accredited by the USDA to perform tuberculosis tests in cattle, for instance, and their rabies vaccination and health certificates are legally recognized documents. The USDA sought to import veterinarians' legal accountability from other areas it regulated into animal welfare regulation. When Congress established an annual reporting system in 1970, for example, the USDA wanted the facility veterinarian to sign it, certifying that pain control drugs had been used as appropriate (Schwindaman et al. 1973).

The USDA found little agreement from laboratory animal veterinarians on their proposal. The USDA's model of accreditation is all about knowing regulatory requirements and does nothing to recognize the specialized training that laboratory animal veterinarians acquire. Anybody can be trained to competently administer a rabies vaccine to an animal, for instance, but only a veterinarian can legally certify that it was performed. What animals want and need is tangential to who signs what forms. Laboratory animal veterinarians feared an untenable hybrid role, simultaneously employed by institutions to run their animal care programs and deputized by the USDA to report on the shortcomings of the institutions.

The USDA reworked its proposals, following the NIH's lead and assigning most responsibility to the institution, rather than to any particular individual, and it quickly dropped any talk of formal accreditation of laboratory animal veterinarians. But dropping talk of formal regulatory roles for veterinarians did not resolve questions of how much oversight scientists would be under, and who would be overseeing them. It did not resolve questions of who was looking out for the animals.

Veterinary credibility

The USDA's rules writers, mostly veterinarians, wanted research facilities run by veterinarians with knowledge and authority. Laboratory animal veterinarians had credibility with the USDA regulators, but they wanted public and in-house credibility as well. That credibility includes presumptions about what veterinarians know, but it mostly centers around what veterinarians do—the jobs they hold, the things they see.

The credibility of veterinarians was a hot political resource, and not just for the veterinarians. Both animal protectionists and scientists claimed to speak for the reality of the lives of research animals: which animals felt pain and distress under what circumstances. Each side enlisted its own resources in arguing for greater or lesser restriction of animal experimentation. Protectionists had photos and videos, along with scientific journal articles describing unspeakable tortures. Scientists faced a trickier challenge. To be sure, scientists emphasized the lifesaving value of their medical research, but they also wanted to assure the public and the government that the cost to animals of this medical progress was not nearly so high as the protectionists were claiming. They could point to the NIH *Guide*, their twenty-year exercise in self-regulation. They could point to the animal beneficiaries of animal research, pet puppies whose lives depended on the vaccines for which laboratory dogs had given their lives. But frankly, they needed a credible ally, and laboratory animal veterinarians were the obvious candidates.

In 1950, T. J. Blakely of the National Society for Medical Research (NSMR) had called on the newly organizing laboratory animal veterinarians of the Animal Care Panel to add their "objective studies" to the NSMR's "campaign of truth" about animal experimentation. Over the ensuing decades, laboratory animal veterinarians took up the call and continued throughout the late 1980s period of regulation writing to offer their animal expertise, often in sharp contrast to common sense assumptions about animal welfare. Crawford and the USDA received letters from laboratory animal veterinarians claiming, for example, that not all fatal toxicity studies are painful to the animal subjects, or that dogs exercise just as much in small cages as in large exercise pens.

But Blakely and the NSMR knew that veterinarians' objective studies would not be enough: they needed advocacy. The "interest in the welfare of animals exhibited by the [Animal Care] Panel can be a decisive factor" in swaying animal lovers to be supporters of medical research (Blakely 1950, p. 47). Laboratory animal veterinarians took up this call, and over the years sent the USDA dozens of such character references supporting scientists' bid for continued self-regulation. In such letters, veterinarians' credibility is only partly based on their expert knowledge of animals. Rather, laboratory animal veterinarians can claim, "I was there; I saw; I know," as they attest to the serious concern of scientists for laboratory animal welfare.

Research advocates have not been alone in seeking veterinarians' credibility as a political resource. Animal protectionists have also readily supplemented their photos and narratives of animal suffering with veterinary testimonials, though it was the USDA veterinarians more than the laboratory animal veterinarians who were most often enlisted. The Animal Welfare Institute, for example, was not content to rest with just any allegations of laboratory excesses in its congressional testimonies or its call for its members to write letters to the USDA: it cited USDA inspection reports as its legitimate source of knowledge of the inner workings of laboratories. Its explicit mention that veterinarians conduct the inspections and document the problems stands in interesting contrast to its stand on USDA's proposals for self-regulation: In urging its membership to protest this capitulation to research interests, the Animal Welfare Institute conveniently downplayed the fact that the USDA's version of self-regulation was empowerment of facility veterinarians. It is one thing to exercise concerned citizens that facilities will make their own rules on painful experiments or dog exercise programs and quite another to convincingly argue that even the facility's veterinarians should not be so empowered. Clearly, not all veterinarians are equal in the eyes of protectionists. But it is their position, rather than their training, that separates the credible watchdogs at the USDA from the laboratory animal veterinarians in the facilities. Though laboratory animal veterinarians typically are much more highly trained than the USDA's vet-inspectors, protectionists see them as mired in conflicts of interest.

People trust veterinarians. They (not the activists with strongly shaped opinions, but the individual who more or less believes in research, wants the animals not to suffer, and mostly does not want to think about it) do seem comforted to know that there are vets in the facility watching out for the animals. It should surprise no one, then, that animal protectionists and defenders of research would each add their own veterinary testimonials to the other rhetorical tools in their political armamentaria.

While opposing factions have been quick to hitch their political agendas onto the public credibility of veterinarians, they have often remained quite ambivalent about the actual individuals occupying the role. This became increasingly obvious as the USDA moved to empower IACUCs, rather than individual laboratory animal veterinarians, in its attempts to keep the regulation in self-regulation.

Animal advocates and animal committees

What better way to conduct the business of animal welfare than through that ubiquitous creature of the late twentieth century: the committee. Committees are the centerpiece of research self-regulation, both for human experimental subjects and for animal subjects. The current requirement for animal committees followed their introduction as an optional component of animal care: in the 1972 NIH *Guide* (in which a committee is suggested as "one effective way to develop and monitor policies to guide animal care"; ILAR 1972, p. 19); in the USDA's 1971 Animal Welfare Act regulations (in which a committee is an acceptable alternative to the attending veterinarian for certifying appropriate use of anesthetics and painkillers in the institution's annual report); and in 1971 requirements for recipients of Public Health Service/NIH funds (in which in-house oversight by a committee is an acceptable alternative to Association for Assessment and Accreditation of Laboratory Animal Care accreditation). These proposals for animal care committees followed comparable calls for human subjects review committees in the World Medical Association's 1964 Declaration of Helsinki, and in the 1966 policy of the Public Health Service for grant recipients (Penslar and National Institutes of Health Office for Protection from Research Risks 1993; World Medical Association 1997).

The 1970s versions of animal care and use committees (not mandatory at the time) called for a minimum of three members, of which one must be a veterinarian; the other two slots were up for grabs (scientists? animal caregivers? administrators?). That the veterinarian was the only member whose presence is stipulated is no great surprise, considering that it is predominantly veterinarians writing both the *Guide* and the Animal Welfare Act regulations. Over time, both the size and the role of the animal care committees grew. In 1985, Congress passed two animal laws, both requiring formation of committees: In November, the Health Research Extension Act mandated a three (or more)-person committee (including one veterinarian and one unaffiliated member, without further elaboration) and in December, the Animal Welfare Act passed with a similar committee requirement. The main difference between the two formulations of committee structure was the decision in December to elaborate that the Animal Welfare Act's unaffiliated member was to "provide representation for general community interests in the proper care and treatment of animals" (U.S. Congress 1985a). This last provision reinforced protectionists' hopes that they would have some voice in how animals are used in experiments, and the idea that an IACUC member might serve as an animal advocate gained momentum.

But do research animals really need an advocate? The very word "advocate" implies adversarial relationships between the scientists and their animals, and many scientists and veterinarians have argued that the concept does not apply. Much of the correspondence from both scientists and veterinarians to the USDA in the late 1980s reiterated the principle that unhealthy, stressed, unhappy animals do not present the standard normal population required for sound research. Unless a researcher is focused on studying poor health, stress, or unhappiness, he or she needs animal subjects that are at their best. This principle is reflected clearly in the NIH *Guide,* which best articulates laboratory animal professionals' (veterinarians primarily, but scientists as well) standards of conduct. It is reflected in the posters the NIH distributed in the 1980s to animal laboratories. A mouse sits on a

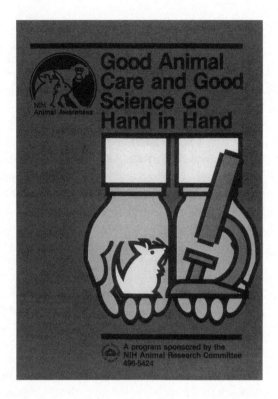

Fig. 8.1 National Institutes of Health poster. NATIONAL INSTITUTES OF HEALTH OFFICE OF ANIMAL CARE AND USE.

human hand, the other hand holds a mouse-sized microscope; the caption reads: "Good Animal Care and Good Science Go Hand in Hand." Good science (technically good, not just morally good) itself is the animals' advocate (figure 8.1).

In calling for the widest possible self-regulatory latitude, several scientists reminded the USDA of researchers' pragmatic interest in well-cared-for animals. But several went beyond this, insisting that most scientists were people of good character, who could be counted on to treat their animals well, regardless of pragmatic self-interest.

The paradigm examples of professional self-regulation in America are physicians and lawyers. Their highly specialized professional knowledge has historically combined with their professional ethic of public service to legitimate a system of peer review, limited entry (through elite educational requirements and state-operated licensure), and relative freedom from government regulation. Their relative autonomy has rested not just in the presumption that doctors (or lawyers) alone know enough to review each other's practices, but that members of these and other elite professions take an oath to public service that has seemed credible in light of their professional prestige. To be sure, doctors and lawyers have lost some of their prestige over recent decades, and the benign paternalism they offered has not always held up well in an era of informed consumers, patients' rights, and malpractice lawsuits.

Research scientists enjoyed even greater autonomy in the early part of the twentieth century than did doctors and lawyers. Entry to their ranks was not regulated by law, and no state licensure was required; as long as they had funding, they faced few restrictions. Like physicians, scientists lost stature during the 1960s. As dog theft exposés of the 1960s and monkey research exposés of the 1980s threatened their autonomy, scientists faced an uphill battle in trying to replace laissez-faire so late in the twentieth century with the state-endorsed self-regulation physicians and lawyers operated under.

Scientists have long struggled against public suspicion of their laboratory practices: read Marlowe's *Doctor Faustus* or Shelley's *Frankenstein* for portrayals of how poorly scientists have been thought to regulate their professional practices. Susan Lederer has described the early twentieth-century fears that unrestricted animal experimentation would encourage physicians to next turn their human patients into laboratory animals (see also Lederer 1995). What could scientists offer to vouchsafe their call for autonomy in their use of animals? Where is their Hippocratic oath? Their benign paternalism? Indeed, in their correspondence to the USDA, some scientists elaborated on how they inconvenienced themselves and their staffs to give animal welfare its full due. Several laboratory animal veterinarians added their testimony on the character and caring of scientists as well.

If good science demands good animal care, then good (technically good, not just morally good) scientists will also demand good animal care. Why, then, do we need regulations, guidelines, and oversight? I see two reasons. One is humanity: There are bad apples. The other is that there are plenty of situations in which the simple aphorism does not hold: Good science does *not* always require good animal care.

Much of the Animal Welfare Act amendment focused on making bad scientists better by catching villains and knaves through increased in-house oversight and inspections. But simply weeding out a minority of inhumane scientists would not have met the demands of protectionists. The 1985 amendment reflected the protectionists' assumptions about scientists. It pushed both the good and the bad to do a better job: having veterinarians prescribe the painkillers, requiring database searches for alternatives to painful procedures, and instituting dog and monkey care that makes these animals healthier, more normal, better research subjects. The law reflected a presumption that while bad apples are rare, most scientists are lazy, cheap, uninformed, or unconcerned enough to need a push toward better hand-in-hand animal care and science.

Like scientists and veterinarians, many animal protectionists (reformers, not the abolitionists and antivivisectionists) worked with the NIH's hand-in-hand maxim. They had to; it was their best defense against charges that their animal welfare demands were too costly. If the two truly go hand in hand, then any increased costs to improve animal welfare would also be justified by the improved science that results.

As I have witnessed, the hand-in-hand aphorism breaks down more than we'd like to admit. Sometimes "good" science hurts animals, or good animal care compromises science. Rarely did protectionists or scientists admit that there could be inherent conflict between the needs of animals and the needs of the research. In the protectionists' view, if research hurts the animal, then someone (a bad scientist, no doubt) must be doing something wrong: The scientist hasn't done a thorough enough literature search, hasn't used the right analgesics, hasn't listened to the veterinarian, or hasn't spent enough grant money on the animals.

Sometimes, after all of the efforts at reduction and refinement and replacement to minimize the suffering of sentient animals, the best a scientist can come up with is a project that still harms and kills animals. Even an experiment thoroughly refined by a careful researcher and a conscientious IACUC may entail significant animal suffering, despite the happy promise of the "good animal care, good science" slogan. As described in chapter 2, the USDA recognizes that some studies (in USDA's category E) would be invalidated by use of painkillers. An example are the untreated control animals in pain and analgesia studies, who may be left untreated as the comparison group against which animals receiving some experimental pain medication are judged. For these animals, there may be some refinement that will improve their lives (such as soft bedding and easier access to food and water for rats on arthritis studies who would have trouble walking around), and this may even make them better subjects somehow. But they're still in untreated pain—is this what the NIH's poster is promoting?

The more serious reality is that, often, good science and good animal care do track independently. As an example, return to the monkey described in chapter 2, the one who receives head implants under surgical anesthesia. Her tour as a laboratory animal generating data for the scientist really will not begin until after a few weeks of postsurgical convalescence. During that period, the scientist may or may not give the animal analgesics. The quality of her care will greatly depend on this pain management, but chances are good she'll recover well enough for her role in research regardless of the degree of pain she experienced during her first few days of convalescence. The quality of the science will probably be just about as good, independent of how well the animal's pain has been managed. In the convalescent period, limitations on the pain relief this animal receives might relate more to issues of cost and convenience: Will the scientists come in through the night to administer expensive but short-duration analgesics? If the quality of the science unequivocally rested on the scientists camping out through the night to administer to the animal, they would do it. Would they still do it if the only benefit were to the animals?

Several individual scientists recognized these limitations as they wrote to the USDA. They sensed that IACUCs would be making value judgments, weighing costs to animals versus benefits to science, not just policing for derelict scientists, and they wanted to be sure the deck was not stacked against them. They had no illusions that animal research could be done without costs to the animals, and they did not pretend otherwise. Unsure of the loyalty of laboratory animal veterinarians to science if animal welfare was at stake, they called for assurance that scientists would be well-represented on committees.

However, it was the animal protectionists who feared most how the IACUC deck would be stacked. Their bid to reserve the unaffiliated seat on the IACUC for one of their own reflects both their mistrust of scientists (hardly a surprise) but also their wariness about laboratory animal veterinarians. Some questioned how much veterinarians could truly advocate for the animals (though advocacy is not what Congress called it when establishing that IACUC seat), given their conflict of interest as employees of the institution. In voicing such a concern, veterinarians' knowledge and competence was not the issue, but the implications of their status as employees.

By the time debate was heating in the late 1980s about the unaffiliated IACUC member under USDA regulations, many institutions were acquiring experience with how the committees could work. The reason: The Health Research Extension Act of 1985, which never generated the heat that the Animal Welfare Act amendments caused, had gone into effect in early 1986. It required institutions receiving federal funding to establish committees of five members or more, complete with a veterinarian, a scientist, a nonscientist, and an unaffiliated member. The year 1986 was a period of some experimentation, trying to figure out what made a good animal committee. Some institutions took the risk of appointing outspoken animal rights activists and antivivisectionists. Others were more conservative, appointing scientists from other institutions or members of pro-research organizations. As USDA sought to define its own expectations of IACUCs over the ensuing years, protectionists protested allowing scientists, or even veterinarians, from other institutions to qualify as unaffiliated. Protectionists also wanted proportionate representation and claimed that if a three-person committee required at least one unaffiliated member, then larger committees should have proportionate numbers of unaffiliated members.

Protectionists have seen animal advocacy and IACUC membership as issues of character and commitment and have suggested various strategies for assuring that animal welfare organizations have some voice in the selection of an unaffiliated IACUC member (Levin and Stephens 1994). Implicit in their demands for representation are their philosophical commitments to what it means to speak for animals. When the USDA proposed that all IACUC members have knowledge of animal care and research, protectionists balked. Who would evaluate this person's knowledge? As the National Anti-Vivisection Society, for example, wrote to the USDA in 1987:

> We strongly disagree with the language that all committee members "shall possess sufficient ability to assess animal care, treatment, and practices in experimental research as determined by the needs of the research facility." Although this language makes sense, it does not if applied to the outside, public member. Any intelligent, humane-minded person is supposed to occupy the public member seat based upon congressional intent. However, this language can easily exclude any layperson who has no knowledge of animal care and experimental procedures. (Regulatory Analysis and Development 1987)

The American political system is not well equipped to pass laws protecting animal interests. An animal's legal status is as human property (even wild animals legally are essentially government property in most circumstances). The Animal Welfare Act is couched in terms of human interests, and the job of the unaffiliated IACUC member is phrased as representing society (and the general society's interest in animal welfare) rather than representing the animals. When animals are misused in laboratories, it is the public sensitivities and the (human) public good that suffer. The preamble to the 1985 Animal Welfare Act makes this clear: "For the purposes of this subtitle, the Congress finds that . . . the use of animals is instrumental in certain research and . . . measures which help meet the public concern for laboratory animal care and treatment are important in assuring that research will continue to progress" (U.S. Congress 1985a).

Assurance of public concern can be the role of the right public IACUC member, if she or he is believably a member of the relevant public. Animal protectionists might argue convincingly that a Harvard scientist, for example, would be unlikely to represent general society's interests on Boston University's IACUC. How closely the protectionists' own agenda mapped onto the general society's interest in animal welfare, however, remained an open question. As some scientists pointed out, a quick visit with the abandoned or abused animals at a local animal shelter quickly reveals that public concern regarding the welfare of animals is variable at best. As long as protectionists could make the case that their proposals for animal welfare were neither too costly nor too restrictive, they actually might meet the interests of the public. It was a case worth arguing, at any rate, for protectionists eagerly coveted the unaffiliated seat on the IACUC as their chance to advance their animal advocacy.

Advocacy for vulnerable subjects

Proposals for animal care committees were based on human subjects review committees, but the structural resemblances between human subjects committees and animal subjects committees can be misleading. That the NIH should be quick to adapt the human subjects review system for use with animal subjects is reasonable. In-house committee review is a low-cost regulatory approach that is highly palatable to the professionals under review. It grants researchers flexibility and autonomy and is based on a respectful presumption that research scientists can be trusted to police their own ranks (Finsen 1988). Empowerment of review committees spreads ethical responsibility out, including both the committee and the researcher (Prentice et al. 1988). The same NIH Office for the Protection from Research Risks that was overseeing human subjects reviews for campuses receiving federal funding was also overseeing animal subjects reviews up until February 2000; institutions submit assurances of compliance to the NIH, detailing how the respective committees will assure that use of animal and human subjects conforms to government-elaborated principles. Both animal and human subjects committees require scientists and nonscientists as members, along with a member who is otherwise unaffiliated with the institution. Only the animal subjects committees require a veterinarian as a member, of course, and it is interesting that human subjects reviews do not necessarily require a physician. However, the principles informing the two types of review are radically different, limiting the value of human subjects review as a model for animals.

One reason to hope that animal subjects review could be piggybacked onto the human subjects approach was the long, serious attention that human subjects have historically received. Three major documents are central to the American approach to human subjects: the Nuremberg Code of 1949, the World Medical Association's Declaration of Helsinki of 1964, and the U.S. government's Belmont Report (National Commission for the Protection of Human Subjects of Biomedical and Behavioral Research 1978). The Nuremberg Code (written in conjunction with the trials of Nazi medical experimenters after World War II) elaborated some basic principles for use of human subjects (The Nuremberg Code 1949). Experimenters should minimize potential harm to human subjects (by preceding most human experimentation with animal studies, among other safeguards)[1] and maximize the benefit by restricting experimentation to studies likely to "yield fruitful results for the good of society." The World Medical Association's Declaration of Helsinki (written in 1964 and revised in 1975 and subsequently) reiterated most of the Hippocratic provisions of the Nuremberg Code, adding the need for consideration and guidance by a human subjects review committee. The Belmont Report followed exposés in American research such as the infamous Tuskegee syphilis studies and led to national standards for human subjects research.[2] Building on the codes of Nuremberg and Helsinki, the Belmont authors added a concern for distributive justice in choice of human subjects, spreading benefits and risks out among populations and individuals in equitable ways (National Commission for the Protection of Human Subjects of Biomedical and Behavioral Research 1978).

These three documents have provided a framework and a set of principles for fine-tuning the protection of human subjects over the ensuing decades. In their unified insistence that researchers maximize societal benefits while minimizing risk to subjects, they might serve as a model for animal subjects review. Indeed, the U.S. government's *Principles for the Utilization and Care of Vertebrate Animals Used in Testing, Research, and Training* calls for a comparable balancing of benefits and harms. Principle II describes the benefit: "Procedures involving animals should be designed and performed with due consideration of their relevance to human or animal health, the advancement of knowledge, or the good of society" (p. 20864). Principles IV through VII direct attention to the harms to animals (mostly pain, including the standard that what is painful to humans should generally be considered painful to animals) and the obligation to minimize them. Principle IX calls for committee review if pain or distress is likely to be inflicted (U.S. Interagency Research Animal Committee 1985). Minimize harm to experimental subjects; maximize benefit to society. Place responsibility on the research investigator, with oversight from an appropriate committee. So far, human subjects and animal subjects reviews are similar. However, both ethically and practically, the centerpiece of protecting human subjects is not the paternalistic assessment of benefit and harm by the academics (though committee and researcher both must do that), but, rather, something that is entirely absent from animal subjects protection: respect for persons as autonomous agents (Penslar and National Institutes of Health 1993).

Respect for persons entails the general Kantian imperative that we should, to the greatest possible extent, treat people as ends, not as means. It means as well that we respect each other's autonomy. The first basic principle of the Nuremberg Code states the case: "The voluntary consent of the human subject is absolutely essential." Research ethicists since then have been elaborating the meaning of informed consent for human subjects: how to inform the subject of the best assessment of potential risks and benefits, how to assure that the potential subject has truly comprehended this information, and how to assure that consent is totally voluntary. Under American law, institutional review boards (IRBs) review the researcher's script for informing subjects and forms or methods for acquiring and documenting consent (U.S. Department of Health and Human Services 1991). As with animal subjects reviews, provisions are available for modifying some of these requirements when study design requires (though with stricter limits on what risks an individual human, informed and consenting or not, may face).[3]

Informed consent safeguards individual autonomy by restricting society (in the form of medical and research establishments) from using people solely as means to societal ends. It allows individuals to determine their own assessment of costs and benefits to themselves and to freely participate or not, including the provision that they can choose to leave the study even once it's begun. As Robert Veatch (1993) has written, it can be just as hard for experts to understand what "lay people" know about themselves as it is for the laity to understand what experts know. All of the researcher's weighing of costs and benefits is in service to the autonomous individual's free choice of how her mind and body are to be used, for as the Declaration of Helsinki states: "Concern for the interests of the subject must always prevail over the interests of science and society [and] the right of the research subject to safeguard his or her integrity must always be respected" (World Medical Association, p. 925). How might this apply to animals?

By most philosophers' and behaviorists' accounts, nonhuman animals lack the mental capacity for full autonomy and for informed consent as we know it, and I will not argue with the philosophers on autonomy. But informed consent? In one sense, I have indeed asked animals almost every day for their consent as research subjects. Their resounding "no" would quickly put me out of a job as a laboratory animal veterinarian, as so much of my work has been helping researchers to overlook the animals' dissent. Yes, I have known dogs who would willingly go in and out of their cages, and even hold out a steady paw for blood sample collection. But the rest? The rats and the monkeys and the frogs and the cats have withheld their consent; they have safeguarded their integrity, often in graphic, vocal, and violent ways. I can show you how to restrain a nonconsenting cat for a blood sample or how to trap a nonconsenting baboon in a squeeze-back cage for injection of a sedative. I've pinned snakes with sandbags to hold them still for X-rays, wrapped rabbits in towels for physical exams. An assortment of rat and mouse and rabbit and monkey restraint devices are available through mail-order catalogs for use with our nonconsenting subjects. If voluntary consent were our standard for animal research, the whole business would end—not because we cannot understand what the animals are telling us, but because we can.

If human subjects principles are to inform animal subjects practices, we would need a different concept of informed consent. And we have a candidate in the provisions for vulnerable human subjects. Informed consent breaks down when potential human subjects are either incapable of understanding the information (young children, the severely mentally handicapped) or incapable of giving free consent (the incarcerated and the institutionalized) or both (children in orphanages, hospitalized mental health patients). Recognizing that some research projects may require study of people in these populations, ethics codes and federal policies suggest ways to safeguard their well-being.[4]

Take the case of children: informed consent of their legal parent (both parents, for particularly risky studies) or guardian is required, along with the child's own assent, when age and maturity make that possible. Laboratory animals, lacking guardians and parented by animals themselves incapable of informed consent, may be more comparable to children in orphanages or who are wards of the state or other institutions. Here is the where the concept of a subject advocate comes into human research ethics. By federal law, "the IRB shall require appointment of an advocate for each child who is a ward . . . an individual who has the background and experience to act in, and agrees to act in, the best interests of the child for the duration of the child's participation in the research" (U.S. Department of Health and Human Services 1991). The advocate must be unaffiliated with the research, except in her IRB role as advocate, and with the guardian organization.

The elaboration of this role of advocate reflects the evolution of thinking on protection of human subjects, especially vulnerable subjects. Lederer (1995) has described some of the research uses of orphans in America in the early twentieth century (i.e., pre-Nuremberg, Helsinki, and Belmont). At that time, permission of the orphanage director was sufficient for access to orphans as medical research subjects. Far from being a class in need of special protection, wards of the state were seen back then as repaying their debt to society through their voluntary or involuntary, informed or uninformed, enrollment in experimentation.

Animals are the ultimate vulnerable subjects in research. They are not just wards of the institution, and they are not simply held in confinement. They are property. In many instances, their very existence stems from their usefulness for science. Add to this status their inability to truly understand, from human mouths, the costs and benefits of the research they face.

Seeing animals as vulnerable subjects would tip the balance even further toward protecting the individual than informed consent provisions for autonomous adults do. Autonomous adults may choose to participate in quite risky research; the IRB's job is to make sure they understand what they are getting into and that they are doing it of their own volition. With vulnerable subjects, a more paternalistic ethic prevails, and risky studies are generally limited to projects that target the particular vulnerable population (e.g., studies of diseases that are prevalent among prison inmates or studies of various childhood diseases) and that might help the individual subjects as well as the general population.

The animal protectionists' proposal of an animal's advocate flows from this use of advocates for vulnerable subjects. By human subjects standards, animals definitely qualify for appointment of an advocate. But who? To be sure, the protectionists coveted this role for themselves. They sought criteria by which to verify that the public member of an IACUC truly represented an animal protectionist point of view. Some scientists suggested that the entire IACUC, including the animal researchers on it, should be seen as the animals' advocate (Prentice et al. 1988). But if the IACUC is primarily composed of animal researchers, what kind of advocacy could protectionists, or animals, expect from such a group?

Laboratory animal veterinarians nominated themselves as advocates, sometimes explicitly, sometimes not. Even when they did not use that word, they saw a role for themselves that was quite independent of their expert knowledge of animals. One veterinarian wrote that it was his role to instill sensitivity to animals into the scientists. Others emphasized their relationship to their animal patients as their basis for advocacy. Perhaps the veterinarians suggested their advocacy too late, after too many decades of joining with research scientists to oppose animal welfare regulations. Protectionists rebuffed veterinarians' claims to advocacy with charges of conflict of interest. There's the obvious potential conflict just from being an insider. Tannenbaum (1995) has also noted that not only is a laboratory animal veterinarian an employee of the institution proposing to use animals, but often he or she is the director of the animal care facility (a frequent arrangement and one endorsed by the NIH *Guide*). As such, she or he has a stake in actually increasing the amount of animal use and thereby maintaining staff and budget (Tannenbaum 1995). Just as federal policy requires that the advocate of orphan children not be the director of their orphanage, so protectionists called for an outsider, rather than an animal facility director, to serve as the animals' advocate.

Virtually no one has made a strong public case that animal research technicians play the advocate role on IACUCs. I have worked with dozens of animal technicians (and was one myself, before starting veterinary college) and have found them as a group to be highly conscientious and concerned about the animals in their daily care. They are often the people who know the individual research animals best and who witness (or perform) the hands-on manipulations and research procedures (figure 8.2). Though some technicians and managers themselves have argued the value of such input on committees (Heidbrink 1987; Stephens 1987), none of the dominant voices—either protectionists, veterinarians or scientists—has advanced their cause to the USDA.

Regardless of who filled the role, imagine applying vulnerable subjects standards to animals. Unable to freely give informed consent, their role in potentially harmful studies would be limited not just to projects that targeted their animal

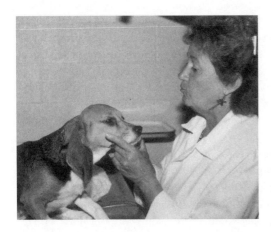

Fig. 8.2   Laboratory, husbandry, and veterinary technicians frequently have the closest relationships with the animals, but they have rarely been promoted as required members of Institutional Animal Care and Use Committees.

species, but probably to studies that might help those individual subjects as well. Research would stop even faster than if we left it to the animals' consent or dissent. We have to either jettison the vulnerable subjects model or scuttle animal research. If the vulnerable subjects model does not easily fit into research animal ethics, what could an animal advocate actually hope to do?

What animal care and use committees do

Demographic statistics on IACUCs' unaffiliated members are currently unavailable. A small handful of institutions have appointed animal activists to their IACUCs over the years, ranging from animal shelter managers to far more strident animal rights activists. Reports of the unaffiliated members' experiences are informal and anecdotal. Orlans (1993) reported on an informal telephone survey of seven "animal advocate members" of IACUCs, reflecting dissatisfaction, frustration, and isolation. Several IACUC public members wrote to the USDA in the late 1980s, hoping their experience on NIH-mandated IACUCs would shape the USDA's mandates on the same. There, too, the letters represent a spectrum of experiences and opinions. Some did report feeling isolated and wished there were another unaffiliated member or animal protectionist on the committee. Another objected to censorship from the IACUC chair and the facility veterinarian, claiming they went so far as to dictate the terms of minority opinions the member would write.

Philosopher Steve Sapontzis described his experiences in the late 1980s on a university IACUC to me. It may serve as a useful model for others. Sapontzis has argued that we should indeed use a similar ethical standard for research on animals as we do for research on other vulnerable subjects, and he would appoint a guardian for animals just as children have an advocate or guardian appointed. That guardian would watch that research was limited to projects that are innocuous to the animals, that are therapeutic for the individuals involved, or that somehow provided them adequate compensation (Sapontzis 1987, 1990).[5] In serving on an IACUC, he tried to apply this principle, knowing that he would be outvoted on the vast majority of protocols. Nonetheless, he believed that he got the IACUC to discuss issues it might otherwise have taken for granted and shifted animal care and use practices incrementally closer to his ideal. Lawrence Finsen (1988) argues that institutions appoint their members with complete freedom and may have very little to lose by appointing an animal protectionist (who would almost always be outvoted, and therefore unlikely to cripple any institution's animal research program) but who might provide insights and ideas that other IACUC members would overlook.

Animal protectionists seized on the role of the unaffiliated IACUC member to advance an agenda that went beyond the 1985 animal welfare laws. Liberationists like Sapontzis worked to maximize that position's potential for animal advocacy, though it is by no means clear that that was Congress's intent. Protectionists thought of IACUCs as ethics committees that would approve only those projects with an acceptable balance of costs and benefits, as animal ethics committees in some other countries apparently do. That is not necessarily what Congress called for.

Industry representatives, more than their university counterparts, were familiar with quality control audits, part of their compliance with the very stringent quality control required by the Food and Drug Administration under the Good Laboratory Practices Act of 1978. Writing to the USDA in the late 1980s, they emphasized the role of the IACUC in auditing for regulatory compliance, as opposed to determining how research should be conducted. They found ample evidence of congressional concurrence in the language of the 1985 act: exceptions to pain-control provisions, for example, are to be filed with the committee, not reviewed and approved (though the act also mentions concerns about deviations from "originally approved proposals" without saying who would have originally approved the proposals). The committee inspects facilities, reviews animal care programs in progress, and certifies inspection reports for submission to the USDA. Prior review and approval of animal use protocols was a modification sought by the protectionists and promoted by the USDA, but was not a provision in the congressional act.

Congress stipulated what the principal investigator must do before starting a project: consider alternatives to painful procedures, consult with a veterinarian if planning painful procedures, and detail and explain planned exceptions to Animal Welfare Act standards in a report filed with the IACUC. Apart from receiving this report for filing, all of the IACUC's mandated functions come after the fact, in their inspections and inspection reports (U.S. Congress 1985a). Congress had similarly limited the role of the IACUC earlier that year, in the Health Research Extension Act that sets animal welfare standards for recipients of NIH funds, but that had not stopped the NIH from requiring prior approval of protocols from the IACUC (Office of Protection from Research Risks 1986; U.S. Congress 1985b). If the USDA was exceeding congressional mandate in its empowerment of the IACUC, it was certainly not heading off alone in that direction.

Philosopher and bioethicist Lilly-Marlene Russow (1995) has argued that neither the IACUC as a whole, nor the veterinarian, nor the unaffiliated IACUC member could possibly serve as an advocate in the sense used in human subjects review, deciding on the animal's behalf whether participation in an experiment is in that animal's interest. Nor can IACUCs be the ethical arbiters of animal protocols if they are prohibited from considering the scientific merit of a protocol, as so many scientists and veterinarians urged upon the USDA. Keeping their hands out of dictating or even evaluating the science of a proposal, focusing solely on refinements in animal care, IACUCs are prohibited from conducting any meaningful cost–benefit analysis (Russow 1995).

Few people realize that virtually nothing is prohibited by the Animal Welfare Act, so long as it can be justified to the animal care and use committee. Nor do IACUCs, by and large, function by rejecting animal protocols when the ethical costs are too high. Unlike granting and funding agencies where money is a limited resource, IACUCs have no limit on the number of protocols they can approve. They can approve all or none, but as Russow points out, their general operating philosophy is roughly: Given that this project is going to be done, is it being carried out as humanely as possible (Russow 1998)? This is especially true if a project has been favorably peer-reviewed by a competitive granting agency such as the NIH. Given this as their starting point, how does one assess the effectiveness of IACUCs?

First, we recognize that rejection of protocols is not what IACUCs do, and so measuring their rate of rejection would be virtually meaningless. Frans Stafleu (1994) tried that, in a country in which animal committees are seen unambiguously as ethics committees (as opposed to simply auditing and inspecting committees, as some would have American IACUCs be). He gave mock animal use protocols to scientists, students, and animal technicians to evaluate and found that while the three groups might rate expected animal discomfort and human benefit differently, almost all would allow the protocols to proceed; the cost to animals must be extraordinarily high or the human benefits extremely questionable for a committee to reject one of his hypothetical protocols (Stafleu 1994; Stafleu et al. 1989) American researchers have used mock or sample protocols to analyze how American IACUCs function. Though finding considerable variability among and within IACUCs, Dresser (1989), Plous and Herzog (2001), and others have found what I have found: The IACUC's focus is much more on reworking the details of a protocol than judging its ethical acceptability or handing down a rejection.

I've worked in IACUC protocol review since its mandated inception in 1986 and have rarely seen a protocol rejected. That does not mean that the IACUC is ineffective. In fact, I believe that IACUCs have been enormously powerful in promoting animal welfare over the past fifteen years, and most people I know who have worked in this field share that assessment. But IACUC protocol rejection is rarely the route taken.

An IACUC approaches protocol review as a contract negotiation. They might send a protocol back to the research investigator with suggestions, questions, and challenges, and the more questionable the project's apparent cost–benefit balance (and not just with high-profile species of concern, to the IACUC's credit), the tougher the questions posed. And even while an IACUC would rarely reject a protocol if the scientists firmly insisted on their own plans, scientists do frequently change their research design in response to the challenge. Occasionally, the researcher does not resubmit a protocol after the IACUC's initial deferral, sometimes because funding has fallen through while the IACUC review was in process; sometimes because the IACUC has set such a high bar with its animal welfare questions that it cannot be surmounted. It is the scientist's decision how much effort to put into meeting the IACUC's challenge, and sometimes he or she will simply not try. Should we score these situations as victories for the IACUC process?

Talk among IACUC specialists and laboratory animal professionals often centers on the "three Rs" of research alternatives: replacement (of sentient animals), reduction (of animal numbers), and refinement (of potentially painful procedures). Replacement includes the search for non-animal methods of testing products for human safety, for example, but also of replacing experimental animals with tissue culture methods. Reduction, and even more so, refinement, are the prime focus of IACUCs and of laboratory animal veterinarians. They will couch this in technical language as matters of expertise and information: the assessment of animal pain, the dosage of analgesic drugs, the statistical power of sample size, the scientific justification for withholding painkillers. Quantifying how successfully they move scientists toward these alternatives is not easy.

The ethical basis of this work remains clear: Even painful animal experiments may be allowed, but only once alternatives have been thoroughly investigated and the protocol justified to the IACUC. But as long as animals are in cages and in experiments, assessing the value of this approach relies on expertly assessing the animals themselves. At bottom, however, American IACUCs are much more technical committees than ethics committees. Their work centers on reducing the costs of animals, largely regardless of any weighing of the potential benefits.

To the abolitionists, this will seem like tinkering. Animal protectionists envisioned a bigger role for IACUCs, and one that excluded rather than refined painful experiments. And they wanted a place at the IACUC table for one of their own, an animal advocate unaffiliated with the research institution, standing up to the scientists. IACUC committees have not evolved in that direction, the law has never required or encouraged it, and very few IACUCs hold a seat for a representative of an animal protection organization.

Conclusion

And so we come full circle. Animal protectionists may downplay expertise in favor of commitment, character, and accountability, but the current nature of animal protocol review, in which virtually any research procedure may be approved so long as it is justified by its scientific value, keeps bringing back questions of expertise.

How does "scientific justification" find its way onto the list of technical and empirical questions? How did it become the expert domain of scientists and veterinarians? In the next chapter, I describe the scientific justification for using physical methods (decapitation) to euthanize animals (as opposed to an overdose of anesthetic, which might affect the scientific data and samples being collected). That anesthetic drugs might interfere with data interpretation is a scientific explanation, but explanation is only synonymous with justification if we grant that all scientific "needs" trump all animal interests. To go beyond that, to perform a true ethical weighing of justification, requires not just the empirical information, but a consideration of values as well.

In animal research, we have no Belmont Report, Nuremberg Code, or Declaration of Helsinki. Neither the NIH *Guide* nor the Animal Welfare Act gives the slightest indication how to weigh competing interests and values. The "good animal care, good science" slogan suggests that the two never compete in animal research, but often they do, and just as often, they are largely independent of each other. And we certainly have no provision for individual animals to assert their autonomy, demand respect for their personhood, and opt out of "volunteering" for experimentation. Still, local oversight of animal research in the hands of IACUCs goes beyond local oversight of competency and adequacy of facilities: It becomes the closest thing we have to an ethical consensus on the justifications of animal use.

Animal protectionists seized on the idea of a community representative on IACUCs to hedge their bets against veterinarians with conflicting interests. While they hoped a veterinarian would be a moral force as well as a medical expert, protectionists have never completely trusted veterinarians. Animal protectionists sought their own seat on the IACUC, in which they could serve as advocates concerned solely for the welfare of the vulnerable animal subjects. With rare exceptions, they have not gotten what they sought, and many IACUCs would only choose an unaffiliated community representative who was willing to grant the validity of animal experimentation.

When institutions choose unaffiliated IACUC members based on their willingness to pledge allegiance to animal research, and veterinarians seek to establish their legitimacy based on their scientific knowledge, ethical consensus comes quickly, but shallowly. If IACUCs serve only to audit that minimal standards are being met, that easy consensus may be both efficient and sufficient. If we want something more, we will need veterinarians who find their authority in their relationship with their animal patients, and we will need a multitude of voices— animal caregivers and animal protectionists, physicians and nurses, scientists, and others—as we learn to listen to and speak for the animals.

I close this chapter with a quote from my September 7, 1995, interview with Dr. Joe Spinelli. When we met, he was the head laboratory animal veterinarian at the University of California-San Francisco medical center, where coincidentally I now work. He told me of a conversation he had had years earlier with a prominent cardiovascular surgeon:

> I got a phone call from a cardiovascular researcher, a real curmudgeon, and he said, "What is the most important function of your department?" I said, "To serve the needs of the faculty," and he said, "Wrong. You're here to serve the needs of the animals. Think about it. The science will get done. That's what people here know how to do. But they aren't thinking about the animal welfare. There's almost nothing you can do to stop the science; your job is to make sure that the animals are treated OK." He had the big picture; I didn't.

9

Death by decapitation: A case study

ON OCTOBER 30, 1993, DR. MARTIN FETTMAN, THE FIRST VETERINARIAN TO TRAVEL to outer space, killed six rats aboard the American space shuttle *Columbia*. These rats were not stowaways, but laboratory rats, brought into space along with 42 others, for studies of weightlessness, "space anemia," and other biological problems. Though rats had flown on other American space missions, and all had been "sacrificed" to obtain tissues for study, this was the first time in which the killing took place while on board, under conditions of micro-gravity.

The six rats were killed by decapitation in a hand-operated guillotine (figure 9.1). Modeled like a desktop paper cutter, but with a V-shaped notch for the rat's neck, the rodent guillotine, unlike its human namesake, does not require gravity for its operation. The rats received no anesthesia.

The news media chose various ways to color their coverage. *USA Today* went to press with grim humor, with headlines such as "Space to be Final Frontier for 5 Rats" (Marshall and Halvorson 1993) and "Heads They Lose—In Space" (Hoversten 1993). The *Washington Post* was more subdued, first describing the dissection without clarifying whether the rats would be alive or dead (Harwood 1993b), and in a later article detailing that the rats would be "beheaded and dissected . . . virtually disassembled, [their organs] harvested" (Harwood 1993a, p. A7). The Associated Press highlighted the grisly: "The veterinarian . . . chopped the heads off six rats . . . [in] an enclosed chamber so no body parts would float away" (Associated Press 1993, p. 11).

Coverage in veterinary and science media was both more and less detailed about the project, carefully downplaying the rats' fates. *Lab Animal*, a trade magazine for laboratory animal professionals, managed to cover the rat experimentation, including tissue sampling deep within the inner ear, of bone and of muscle, without ever mentioning that the astronauts killed the rats in the process (Nasto 1994). Fettman's (1995) description of his own work likewise mentioned collecting tissue samples without mentioning the animal sacrifice that made this possible. Meanwhile, the *Journal of the American Veterinary Medical Association* was so devoid of research information in its four full pages of coverage that the reader could almost infer that the rats were there more as companions to the flight crew than as research subjects (Spencer 1994).

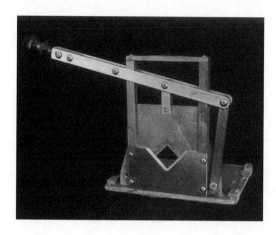

Fig. 9.1   Rodent guillotine.
PHOTO BY CHRISTOPHER READ,
USED WITH PERMISSION.

Whatever their tone, most of these articles assured the reader that this procedure was necessary for scientific progress. In response to criticisms of animal protectionists, NASA scientist and project director Frank Sulzman joined veterinarian-astronaut Fettman in explaining to the public, as they would to an Animal Care and Use Committee, how killing the rats without anesthesia was essential to keep the tissues free of chemicals. Other NASA scientists followed up with an article for laboratory animal professionals explaining how alternate euthanasia techniques would adversely affect the science in progress (O'Mara et al. 1994).

Though a rare issue in the popular press, the question of how to kill rodents for research has been quite controversial among laboratory animal professionals. Remember that no experimental procedure is forbidden in the animal research laboratory, but in the era of IACUCs, some procedures—multiple survival surgeries, use of paralytic drugs—call for stronger justification than others. The NIH *Guide for the Care and Use of Laboratory Animals* and the Animal Welfare Act require special justification for euthanasia methods that depart from recommendations of the AVMA Panel on Euthanasia. Since 1986, that panel has called for special justification for use of the rodent guillotine, whether in outer space or on terra firma.

The AVMA Panel's determination that decapitation is a potentially painful way to kill rodents is one of the most controversial issues in laboratory animal policy, though it has failed to capture the attention of the public or animal protectionists. The decapitation controversy is another case study of the use of scientific data to establish animal welfare policy. It is a case in which experts disagree and raises questions of how to set policy before closure of such a controversy. The case illustrates the interaction of theory and data in interpretation of experiments. It reflects the current primacy of pain as the concern of animal welfare policy makers and the lack of attention to death as a harm to animals. It raises questions as well about whether the scientific use of statistics in animal studies inappropriately leads veterinarians away from their traditional clinical focus on individual patients. I begin with some history, followed by an analysis of what is going on in this controversy.[1]

The rodent guillotine in public policy

In 1961, the AVMA Council on Research appointed a panel of veterinarians to study and make recommendations for techniques of killing the large numbers of unwanted small animals (i.e., dogs and cats) in animal shelters and pounds (American Veterinary Medical Association 1961). The AVMA has since convened six such panels and published updated recommendations in its journal (Andrews et al. 1993; Annis et al. 1963; Beaver et al. 2001; McDonald et al. 1978; A. W. Smith et al. 1986; C. R. Smith et al. 1972).

With each successive revision, the panel has expanded its scope: more species have been covered, more techniques have been reviewed, and more of the settings in which animals are killed have been considered. Thus, in 1972, minks, birds, and rodents were added; horses entered in 1978; reptiles, fish, and amphibians in 1986; and marine mammals in 1993. The 1972 report was the first to include mention of the laboratory setting. It was the first to consider the rodent guillotine.

The panel has also modified its stated criteria for evaluation of euthanasia methods, most notably from the first report to the second. In 1963, the panel cited literature review, observation of techniques in field conditions, and the experience of veterinarians and other professionals equally in basing its recommendations. In 1972, the panel began to scientize its report: reference to experience and observation were dropped, and "only those methods or agents for which reliable information could be obtained were included" (C. R. Smith et al. 1972, p. 761). In 1978, the panel called for further research. With each successive panel report, the number of literature citations has grown, from 14 in 1963 to 215 in 2001, and the panel has not shifted from its stated commitment to basing its evaluations on "reliable information" and to limiting its discussions to methods for which there was "currently available scientific information" (Beaver et al. 2001, p. 671). Throughout successive panel reports, animal pain has remained the overriding concern, with animal and human psychological distress, human safety, compatibility with the purpose of euthanasia, economics, and legal availability of narcotic drugs also listed as important considerations.

In 1972 and again in 1978, the AVMA Panel described decapitation as rapid and inexpensive. When properly operated, the guillotine "produces euthanasia" (C. R. Smith et al. 1972) or "instant death" (McDonald 1978) in small laboratory animals. No literature was cited or other evidence offered to support this assessment, despite then-new prefatory language that only techniques "for which reliable information could be obtained" would be considered.

A few months after publication of the 1978 panel report, a British veterinarian, A. L. Warren, wrote a letter to the AVMA, challenging the panel's assertion that decapitation produced instant death (Warren 1979). He called attention to Mikeska and Klemm's 1975 study reporting that electroencephalograph (EEG) brain wave recordings from rats' decapitated heads were activated for up to 29.5 seconds after decapitation. Warren took this study to show that rat brains remained conscious for several seconds following decapitation and that their "pain was extreme."

Mikeska and Klemm (1975) had fitted eight rats with EEG electrodes and recorded brain wave activity before and after decapitation. They collected conventional brain wave data for six of the animals. In these animals, brain waves were "activated" from the control pattern to low voltage, fast activity (LVFA) waves, for 5.6 seconds in one to 29.5 seconds in another, with an average 13.6 seconds before the brain waves went flat. In the remaining two animals, they measured "ultra-slow" brain potentials; in these animals, an "extremely large, low frequency change in potential" occurred, lasting up to 80 seconds after decapitation (p. 178). Mikeska and Klemm interpreted these two types of brain wave data, recorded after "the massive nociceptive stimulus of decapitation," as corroboration that "decapitation appears to be inhumane, [even though it] is perhaps a necessity for many neurochemical experiments" (pp. 175, 179).

The 1986 AVMA Panel took heed of Warren's letter and used Mikeska and Klemm's article as the basis for a new caution about rodent decapitation and the possibility of conscious pain perception. The panel recommended that until better information was available, animals should be sedated or lightly anesthetized before decapitation, "unless the head will be immediately frozen in liquid nitrogen subsequent to severing" (A. W. Smith et al. 1986, p. 265).

Around the time of this 1986 revision, the AVMA Panel report began to gain added regulatory weight in American animal welfare policy. Scientists in the neurological and pharmacologic sciences suddenly faced not just a new proscription against a preferred method of euthanasia, but a proscription now buttressed by law.

Pain counts, death doesn't

The controversy over death by decapitation is a controversy about pain. It is a controversy over whether the guillotine hurts the animals, not a controversy about their deaths. We will look at how scientists and veterinarians in this controversy vie to determine how much conscious perception of pain animals experience during or subsequent to this technique. But first, we should pause to ask why pain is the high-priority question in the first place when animal's lives are at stake.

Since its initial 1963 report, the AVMA Panel has consistently declined to consider questions of when, whether, or why animals should be killed, restricting itself to evaluation of *how*. "Euthanasia" or "good death" in this veterinary definition means a death free of pain and distress, even if the animal is young and healthy and apparently capable of living out a good life. This is in sharp contrast to its definition in the human medical context, where the goodness of death rests in delivering the patient from a life wracked with pain and disease, rather than the technique employed (Carbone 1998). The rodent guillotine controversy likewise differs from debates about human capital punishment in which the focus is overwhelmingly on whether the state should kill offenders, with far less discussion of how.

Hurt versus harm. Veterinarians and scientists discuss whether killing hurts animals, causes them pain. Among philosophers the livelier debate is whether death per se, even a gentle, painless death, is itself a harm to animals.[2] In public policy, pain counts for everything. Animal death is only significant in its relationship to pain. Animal euthanasia appears only twice in the 1985 amended Animal Welfare Act, both times as a prescription, along with anesthetics and analgesics, for pain relief:

> The Secretary [of Agriculture] shall promulgate standards to ensure that animal pain and distress are minimized, . . . including adequate veterinary care with the appropriate use of anesthetic, analgesic, tranquilizing drugs, or euthanasia . . . [and that] the withholding of tranquilizers, anesthesia, analgesia, or euthanasia when scientifically necessary shall continue for only the necessary period of time. (U.S. Congress 1985b)

Euthanasia is treated similarly in Public Health Service policy, where killing animals is a potent and permanent painkiller.[3] In these public policies, animal euthanasia converges on the human sense of the word: mercy killing to deliver the patient from a life wracked with pain.

However, there is no evident sense in any of these public policies that killing healthy, pain-free animals is itself to be avoided. There is no endorsement, for instance, of finding adoptive homes in which retired laboratory animals could live out their lives as pets (Carbone 1997a). Scientists often buy research animals as sources of cells or tissues, killing them upon receipt to harvest what they need. Only in language on finding alternatives that reduce the numbers of animals does one find a policy impetus to minimize animal killing. In the Animal Welfare Act, even that language on alternatives is directed only at alternatives to "procedures likely to produce pain to or distress in an experimental animal," not alternatives to killing (U.S. Congress 1985a, Sec 13(a)(3)(B)).

In my professional experience working with IACUCs and with veterinary students, I have found strong but mixed feelings about animal killing. Nothing distresses first-year veterinary students more in their early discussions of veterinary ethics than the prospect of being asked to euthanize a healthy dog or cat simply because the animal's owner has decided that she or he is too inconvenient, illbehaved, or unattractive to live in the home. In contrast, animal care and use committees often treat protocols in which animals would be killed painlessly as relatively low concern, though if the number of animals is high, they will balk and ask for further justification.

The Scientists Center for Animal Welfare is a moderate-to-conservative animal welfare organization that has long promoted a five-tier categorization scheme to better standardize animal protocol reviews. It lists painless killing of animals in its second tier "ethical concern" category of procedures "expected to cause little or no discomfort," along with blood collection and simple injections. These procedures call for lower levels of justification and scrutiny than a potentially painful surgical protocol (such as surgical removal, under anesthesia, of the reproductive organs, or spaying), after which an animal might live several years. Mild pain thus ranks higher than killing (Scientists Center for Animal Welfare 1987).

In practice, among these specialists and within the general public, thoughts about animal death and killing are complicated and contradictory; killing animals is inconsistently seen as a sad event, a convenience, an act of mercy, an inevitability, and the only way to get some of the foods that we love to eat. But really, how could it be otherwise?

The ethical principle that killing animals is justified so long as pain is excluded is intrinsic to justifying meat production and consumption. Meat is central in the diets of the majority of Americans. Tannenbaum (1995) has argued that that cultural and historical fact is itself moral evidence that meat eating is justified.[4] But can it put the pleasure of meat eating on a par with killing animals for lifesaving medical research that could not be done any other way?

Meat is central to the American diet, and it is also central to the American propaganda wars about animal welfare and animal rights. Both animal protectionists and animal-use advocates see the political significance of vegetarianism. "The symbolism of meat-eating is never neutral," writes Mary Midgley (1983). "To himself, the meat-eater seems to be eating life. To the vegetarian, he seems to be eating death" (p. 27). For budding young animal rights advocates, embracing vegetarianism is a first step in making the personal political (Adams 1990; Curtin 1991).

Vegetarianism is an important political tool for advocates of animal use as well, the dark warning to youngsters of what will follow if they chant for animal rights. Threats of enforced vegetarianism help animal-using industries (farming, research, fur-production) to work together and face the animal rights movement as a bloc. But even political debates about vegetarianism often sidestep animal killing and focus instead on pain.

Critics of meat consumption emphasize the pain that animals experience, perhaps believing that a "painless death" depiction of life on the farm would not move many people to vegetarianism. Consider this passage from the animal protection magazine *ASPCA Animal Watch*: "There was a time when the American farm was a quiet, bucolic place. Hens walked around outdoors, scratching in the dirt and interacting with one another. Cows grazed with their calves in lush green pastures, and sows lounged under shade trees, occasionally nuzzling their piglets" (Pavia 1998, p. 28).

The article goes on to encourage cutting back or eliminating animal products from your diet, not because the animals are killed, but because of the unnatural crowding, drugging, rough handling, and pain of modern animal farming. A sufficiently uninformed urban writer might limit a bucolic idyll to hens and cows, happily producing their bounty of eggs and milk and living out their lives under blue skies. He might throw in a horse or two, dreamily pulling a plow through the field. He might exclude animal death, the oxymoronic "humane slaughter," from his agricultural utopia. But sows and piglets? Their presence can only mean that killing and death are not far from sight. Could any fantasy of life on the farm include pigs as anything other than pork chops about to be realized? There are only so many truffles to be rooted out of the ground, after all. If this is the way animal farming ought to be done, then killing is obviously acceptable to that vegetarian author. As Pollan (2002) writes, "what's wrong with animal agriculture—with eating animals—is the practice, not the principle" (p. 110).

For their part, defenders of animal farming deny that animals are in pain, period. Painless death in a government-supervised slaughterhouse is a brief detour en route from farm to supermarket. Death cannot be avoided in turning animals into meat, but the significance of death can be translated and blunted by making pain the central question.

Deny the harm of animal death, and animal users become the true advocates of animal welfare. They have to be, the argument goes, because professionals who depend on animals for their livelihood have a personal stake in animal welfare. A farm animal veterinarian writes: "Since the advent of civilized society, animals have been under the stewardship of man. They have served as beasts of burden, producers of food, and as companions. Our entire civilization has been based on animal welfare," (Herrick 1990, p. 712). He goes on to list some of the ways people have used animals (transportation, food, clothing, companionship, medicine), and says, "Animals have enabled us to be here today. In fact, that is what veterinary medicine is all about—animal welfare" (p. 712). Denying killing as a harm to animals is essential to this rhetorical project of turning "animal welfare" and "animal use" into synonyms.[5]

The "animal user" bloc is not monolithic, however, as when biomedical researchers claim the highest ground over others: they are fighting for cures for dread disease, after all, while the others are trifling with human vanities (fur) or tastes (meat). In one such departure from solidarity, a research technician defended animal research in *Newsweek* magazine in 1995. Her vegetarianism and refusal to wear cosmetics, leather, or fur, though otherwise irrelevant to her work as a technician, establish her credentials as an animal lover and secure for her the moral authority to testify from the inside to the goodness of animal research (much as I've described the role of laboratory animal veterinarians in chapter 8). In her article, killing animals *is* morally significant, justifiable for medical progress but not for food or fashion, and even in research, she asserts, wisely avoiding statistics in her argument, not all laboratory animals are killed at the end of the study (Szymczyk 1995).

This juxtaposition of killing animals for food or for science is a tricky one to use in political campaigning, for or against animal research. Animal protectionists distance themselves from the appearance of radicalism when they focus on animal pain and avoid condemning animal death, whether in the lab or on the farm. Those animal protectionists who focus on reform rather than on abolition typically dress their distaste for animal killing in a vaguely phrased plea for alternatives, failing to make explicit whether they mean alternatives to pain, to death, or to both. Nor do research advocates easily or often grant moral high ground to vegetarianism the way the *Newsweek* piece does: allowing criticism of killing for food just invites the slippery-slope extension of killing for science.

The protectionists' focus on pain rather than on killing may be part of an activist's triage, not just a political strategy but an attempt at political prioritizing as well. As one animal rights advocate who had worked as a community representative on a university IACUC told me during our interview: "Well, there's a lot of intense pain and suffering. Death is almost just a relief, so when you're reading through the protocols and Oh God, great. They're just gonna take them and keep them a short time and then kill them" (anonymous interview, September 9, 1995). Another interviewee said, "They're gonna induce all this pain, so the death pales by comparison." The protectionists' conviction that overwhelming pain and misery are inescapable for the laboratory animal lend their assent to the division, and comparative ranking, of pain and death for laboratory animals (anonymous interview, September 9, 1995).

Theory, data, and the assessment of animal pain

Separating pain from killing paves the way toward the scientization of euthanasia. By scientization I mean the attempt to push an issue as far as possible from the complexity of ethics or values or politics or anything remotely subjective, or even human. The AVMA makes the attempt in its "Positions on Animal Welfare," updated by the AVMA's Executive Board in 1994. It recognized then that veterinarians have "ethical, philosophical, and moral values" to consider, but it tried to leave them in the individuals' hands (American Veterinary Medical Association 1998, p. 51). As an organization, the AVMA hoped to stay out of the moral and political fray, and still take leadership on questions of animal welfare. "These AVMA position statements deal primarily with the scientific aspects of the medical well-being of animals," even as they take the political stance that animal welfare implies prioritizing human uses of animals over claims of animals' rights (American Veterinary Medical Association 1998, p. 51).[6]

The ruling of the AVMA Panel on Euthanasia on decapitation is a case in which animal welfare is reduced even further to its strictly scientific and objective dimensions. More than any other controversy in animal welfare studies, it held the potential to eliminate human interpretation entirely from the picture, directly translating rats' subjective experiences into brain wave tracings on an EEG chart, untouched by human hands. However, its failure to eliminate the human element of interpretation from the scientific assessment of pain makes this an instructive case study.

Scientists and veterinarians use several methodologies to measure animal welfare: behavioral observations, hormonal indicators of stress, clinical indicators of disease. Mikeska and Klemm (1975) used none of these in their guillotine study. None of these is applicable to studying the effects of guillotine, but brain wave tracings remain available for study, describable in the most objective and quantitative language of frequency, duration, voltage.[7] But these apparently clean and hard data require interpretation and strong allies if they are ever to carry weight as scientific facts, especially when those facts engender policy implications that many scientists find unacceptable.

Limits on use of the rodent guillotine could profoundly affect scientific practice, though I know of no statistics on its use throughout the United States. Decapitated rats are enough a standard subject of drug metabolism and brain chemistry studies (both of which might be confounded by use of anesthetic drugs) that stakes were high for many scientists, and their laboratory animal veterinarians, to resist this restriction.

Several veterinarians and scientists criticized the AVMA Panel's adoption of the Mikeska and Klemm study, usually noting the political context of the panel's impact as they criticized the study itself. The common theme was criticism of the data; this was but a single study, never replicated; only six rats were used. The data were suspect (Allred and Berntson 1986, 1987; Holson 1992; Hughes and Warnick 1986). Despite this, though, no one really challenged the brain wave data in any detail. No one challenged the placement of the electrodes, for instance, or the confounding variables of studying chemically paralyzed rats, maintained on mechanical ventilation before decapitation. Brown (1987) noted that the crucial EEG tracing was not even included in Mikeska and Klemm's 1975 article where other experts might examine it; nevertheless, he did not suggest that other experts would read the amplitude, frequency, or duration of the brain waves any differently. No critic suggested that replication would yield anything but the same EEG tracings. Indeed, if such replication was attempted, the results never saw publication. Quite the contrary, some critics pointed out that this brain wave pattern after decapitation was already known and described (Lorden 1987).

Thus the data, while their validity was broadly questioned, were left to stand, inscriptions that all could envision though few had seen, as critics offered alternative readings of their meaning. Absolutely everyone in this controversy agreed that brain waves were detectable from decapitated rats for up to half a minute before the EEG goes flat. Despite the criticisms of Mikeska and Klemm's study, the controversy was not about data after all, but about interpretation: what do these brain waves represent?

Allred and Berntson (1986) noted the political significance of the rat guillotine in making their point in the *American Journal of Nutrition:* "Euthanasia by stunning and decapitation is far too important a tool to be banned on the basis of a highly questionable interpretation of a single report" (p. 1861). They wrote that the type of brain wave pattern described might be elicited with the presentation of food; with oxygen deprivation to the brain cells; with anesthesia; or with electrode movement artifacts. Joan Lorden (1987) claimed the pattern was a "hallmark of paradoxical (REM) sleep" (p. 148). Robert Holson (1992) agreed, noting that similar brain waves could be seen in rats decapitated under anesthesia, and that they might persist for even longer in such animals. He further asserted that the anatomy of pain sensory nerve pathways made it impossible for severe pain to result from a correctly placed cut.

Critics of Mikeska and Klemm's interpretation were generally agreed in one central assumption: that the drop in the brain's blood pressure that followed decapitation was so fast that persistent conscious pain perception was impossible. Robert Derr (1991) formalized this assessment, publishing calculations based on blood flow factors, data relating consciousness to cerebral blood oxygen saturation, and the biochemistry of hemoglobin. He concluded that consciousness in the severed rat head could not possibly exceed 2.7 seconds, a "time short enough," he concluded, "to render decapitation of rats humane" (p. 1399). Ironically, Derr reasoned that the massive stimulation of pain nerves and their repeated firing following decapitation would lead the rats' brains to consume their limited oxygen supply even more quickly and sink into unconsciousness faster; in other words, the more intense the pain of decapitation, the less time that pain is likely to persist. Equally ironically, while people were criticizing use of data based on six decapitated rats, a crucial assumption in Derr's calculations (the brain oxygen level required to sustain consciousness) came from an early 1960s study of four human volunteers (Cunningham et al. 1964; Derr 1991).

Data are interpreted within a theoretical context. For some people in this controversy, the central theoretical assumption is that decapitation—severing (and thereby stimulating) every pain-sensory pathway entering the brain from the spinal cord—must be painful. Mikeska and Klemm (1975) started with this assumption, writing in their 1975 paper that decapitation "is a massive nociceptive stimulus" and "an extremely traumatic procedure" (pp. 175, 178). They believed "the widely held thesis that discomfort, pain, and associated affective reactions would be manifested as EEG activation" (p. 175). Their adherents agree: the data only make sense to them if they start with the assumption that decapitation has got to be painful, for however briefly. Mikeska and Klemm's data simply provide a time frame for how long pain might be experienced.

In contrast, defenders of the rodent guillotine share a central assumption that decapitation, severing as it does all blood vessels supplying the brain, must be fast. The severity of the stimulus is irrelevant if the oxygen-starved brain immediately loses consciousness. Given this presumption, the long duration of rats' brain waves in Mikeska and Klemm's study are an anomaly to be accounted for, unreplicated and untrustworthy, nonspecific reflections of any of a number of nonconscious brain events, or simply, irrelevant.

A person can only interpret data in the context of his or her theoretical commitments. Thus, Holson (1992) cited research showing that similar brain waves are recorded in the severed heads of both anesthetized and unanesthetized animals. An anesthetized animal should not feel pain, and so "incontrovertibly . . . the presence of such an activated EEG can not be interpreted as evidence for conscious-ness in the severed head" (p. 254). Neither the anesthetized nor the unanesthetized animal feels pain in this fast procedure. Not so, counters Klemm. Convinced that the guillotine's blade is a powerful nociceptive stimulus, he takes such data as confirmation of his own findings. Decapitation is so powerfully painful, such a "sensory bombardment of the brain," that it can easily override the effects of anesthetics. Both the anesthetized and the unanesthetized animal feel this over-whelming pain (Klemm 1987).

The sociologist of science Harry Collins (1985) applies the term "experimenter's regress" to this sort of controversy and describes it as a problem of calibration. An illustration of this regress: we may calibrate a thermometer by making sure it reads 212°F in boiling water, and we know the water is at 212° because we measure it with our thermometer. If we find situations (say, at high altitudes) in which boiling water does not read 212° on the thermometer, we may not have a way inside the system to determine whether water boils at different temperatures at high altitudes or whether thermometers function differently.

Brain wave patterns are first calibrated by looking at behavior and seeing the accompanying EEG pattern. Thus one can catalog the brain wave patterns seen with eating, dream sleep, conventional sleep, waking, and pain. This catalog of brain wave patterns, characterized by frequency, duration, amplitude, and location, is then used to define and characterize less well understood mental states, like anesthetization, for example, or coma. Klemm writes about the paradoxical activation seen with ether anesthesia, an apparent instance of behavior–EEG dissociation, if one expects quiescent EEGs during sedation or anesthesia. It is no anomaly to him, though; having undergone ether anesthesia himself, he can attest to how noxious the experience is, at least to a human, and so finds activated brain waves hardly surprising. Other drugs, he argues (alcohol, atropine, and scopolamine are examples) may affect brain activity in ways that alter behavior and brain waves separately, making precise characterization of the observed subject's conscious state difficult. Dream sleep, or REM sleep, is another example; do the activated brain waves present indicate that EEGs are not a good reflection of mental activity, or do they evidence that this type of sleep consists of considerable mental activity (Klemm 1992)?

In these examples, the EEG is calibrated by reference to observed behavior or, in humans, to reported mental states. It is then turned back on itself to diagnose the presence of mental states. When there is an apparent discrepancy, such as activated brain waves in what should be a dead brain, there is no way within the system to resolve the discrepancy. Appeal must be made to theoretical assumptions that are essentially outside of the data-calibration system.

The decapitated head may simply have no precise correlate in ordinary experience. It is rapidly losing all blood pressure and oxygen to the brain cells. Perhaps it is receiving an unparalleled level of nociceptive input from the severed spinal cord. Neural and hormonal communication between the brain and the rest of the body have been completely cut off. If the EEG pattern in the severed head has some characteristics in common with wakefulness, pain perception, anesthesia, sleep, oxygen deprivation, and eating, how can the scientist say which of these states it most closely approximates? Theoretical statements about the unique nature of decapitation can always be marshaled to challenge any attempt at precise definition. Observation of behavior has limited value here, with such disruption of the neural pathways and such a quick passage to death. And reports of human volunteers are unavailable for comparison, of course, as, by definition, no one has undergone the procedure and lived to tell about it.

In sum, do we know that decapitation is painful because we find persistent LVFA-type brain wave activity for up to half a minute? Or do we know that the persistence of LVFA-type activity is not a useful index of consciousness or pain precisely because it can even be found in the decapitated rat's brain?

Resistance to the AVMA Panel on Euthanasia report as public policy

The USDA's Animal Welfare Act regulations and the *Guide for the Care and Use of Laboratory Animals* have both referenced the report of the AVMA Panel on Euthanasia as their standard for humane killing techniques. But what to do with scientists' and laboratory animal veterinarians' resistance to the panel's stance on decapitation?

The panel (whose membership changes almost completely with each incarnation) seemed uncomfortable with the gravity of its report. Alvin Smith, chair of the 1986 Euthanasia Panel, published a letter in the AVMA's journal in 1988 emphasizing the panel's preface that the report was written as a guide for professional judgment, not as a rigid statute.

In 1992, the fifth AVMA Panel on Euthanasia convened. Though well acquainted with the critiques of the 1986 panel's acceptance of Mikeska and Klemm's study and its conclusions, the panel found but a single new set of experimental data to consider (Andrews et al. 1993).

Vanderwolf and colleagues (1988) had reported decapitating rats with or without pretreatment with the drug atropine. The brain waves they recorded for an average of 15–20 seconds after decapitation could be largely prevented by pretreatment with atropine. In this, they more closely resembled anesthetized or conscious but immobile rats' EEGs than they did moving rats or rats in pain. Their conclusion: "the presence of atropine-sensitive forms of cerebral activation cannot be regarded as unequivocal evidence of consciousness" (p. 343).[8]

The 1993 AVMA Panel did not adjudicate competing claims of Klemm and Vanderwolf. In the face of uncertainty and competing claims, it retained its caution about the potential painfulness of conscious decapitation and asserted more explicitly the IACUC's role in reviewing the scientific justification for requiring this technique for particular projects (Andrews et al. 1993). In its 1993 report, the AVMA Panel cited both Mikeska and Klemm's 1975 study and Vanderwolf's putatively contradictory findings to ground the AVMA's conclusion that "data suggest that electrical activity in the brain persists for 13–14 seconds following decapitation" (Andrews et al. 1993, p. 241). It also cited Vanderwolf, Holson, and Derr's papers for the apparent counterclaim that decapitation "may induce rapid unconsciousness" (p. 241). The two claims are not contradictory, however: a painful experience of 13.6 seconds, followed immediately by loss of consciousness, meets both of these criteria—painful and rapid—so long, and only so long, as everyone agrees to define 13.6 seconds as "rapid."

The 1993 panel report followed the years of Animal Welfare Act regulations writing and picked up on the emphasis for flexibility and home rule. It dropped the 1986 panel's recommendations for anesthesia or for freezing the head and emphasized instead the role of the IACUC in reviewing euthanasia proposals. Unfortunately, it retained unnecessary vagueness in the report. The section specifically dealing with decapitation calls attention to Klemm's data that suggest persistent consciousness even after expertly performed decapitation. But the preceding general introduction to physical methods of euthanasia (which include gunshot and electrocution, as well as decapitation and cervical dislocation) mentions no concern about persistent consciousness and expresses reservation solely about the competence and skill of people who will be performing the procedure. Decapitation requires greater skill and precision than barbiturate injection or carbon dioxide asphyxiation, and for this reason alone the AVMA Panel classifies it a "conditionally acceptable," at least, in this earlier page of its report. The 2000 report of the AVMA Panel on Euthanasia acknowledges controversy, but moves even further from believing the potential for painfulness, with reservations primarily for skill in execution (Beaver et al. 2001). Its only new information after eight more years of controversy was a suggestion on how to restrain rats with less distress before their decapitation.

In interviews with numerous laboratory animal veterinarians and IACUC members, I have found a range of standards in use. In some institutions, where IACUC members believe that decapitation must be painful, a high threshold of justification is required. They are not content to hear that a particular euthanasia drug may affect the system under study; they want evidence that this has been studied and demonstrated and may even call for a pilot study to investigate this. At other institutions, where the IACUC and attending veterinarian are skeptical of Mikeska and Klemm's single study, the threshold of justification is far lower, the primary concern being whether the personnel involved are trained and competent.

The authors of the *Guide for the Care and Use of Laboratory Animals* opted to stay with the AVMA Panel. In 1985, they had written both that the AVMA Panel report usually should be followed (with exceptions only as approved by the attending laboratory animal veterinarian) *and* that physical methods such as decapitation were acceptable for small rodents (ILAR 1985). This was the year before the 1986 panel report challenged the humaneness of decapitation. The 1996 *Guide*, much to my surprise, dropped explicit endorsement of physical euthanasia methods and continued its endorsement of the AVMA Panel (ILAR 1996). Both the *Guide* and the AVMA Panel recognize a role for IACUCs in allowing flexibility as needed, but both have converged in shifting the burden of justification onto those scientists who want to use the rodent guillotine in their work.

The USDA has never enjoyed a reputation for flexibility in its Animal Welfare Act regulations, and so its proposal in 1987 to formally recognize the AVMA Euthanasia Panel's controversial 1986 report drew some fire (Animal and Plant Health

Inspection Service 1987). Scientists, research advocacy groups, and laboratory animal veterinarians wrote to the USDA during this period, asking that the AVMA panel *not* become the USDA standard; the AVMA's handling of decapitation was generally the reason. The American Physiological Society (1987), for instance, suggested that if the AVMA Panel must be used, the USDA should use the previous (1978) edition, rather than the current, controversial 1986 version. Though many scientific associations at the time were urging the USDA to base its regulations on scientific information, the American Physiological Society preferred the AVMA's prior acceptance of decapitation, made without reference to published studies, to the AVMA's later caution, based though it was on a published research paper (American Physiological Society 1987).[9]

Among laboratory animal professionals, the AVMA's euthanasia report has not fared well. True, their most important document, the *Guide for the Care and Use of Laboratory Animals,* endorses it, secure in the principle that an IACUC may allow departures from its recommendations when scientifically justified. But in many other guidelines, standards, and manuals, laboratory animal veterinarians have expressed their resistance. The Institute of Laboratory Animal Resources (ILAR; publishers of the *Guide*) updated its book on laboratory rodents in 1996. It describes death from cervical dislocation as "instantaneous" and states that the acceptability of the procedure is limited to the competence of the executor. It goes on to describe decapitation as controversial, but assures the reader that Robert Derr's (1991) theoretical calculations (rather than Mikeska and Klemm's data, which they do not mention) provide evidence that unconsciousness follows decapitation within 2.7 seconds. The ILAR text concludes its exoneration of the guillotine by reminding the reader that this is the route, not killing through anesthetic overdose, to artifact-free tissue collection (Committee on Rodents 1996).[10] ILAR's earlier book on pain and distress in laboratory animals similarly recommended rodent decapitation when anesthetic chemicals were to be avoided, listing aesthetics, skill, and danger to human fingers as the only reasons to avoid the guillotine (Committee on Pain and Distress in Laboratory Animals 1992). The Foundation for Biomedical Research took up the issue in its 1987 handbook for animal researchers:

> On the basis of this one report, the AVMA panel on euthanasia ruled that decapitation alone was not a humane procedure. . . . Fearing the loss of a necessary research tool, but not wishing to treat animals inhumanely, neurochemists and others in the animal research community have reexamined the interpretation of the 1975 EEG study. . . . The American Physiological Society's Committee on Animal Care and Experimentation has led to a widely shared feeling that the lone 1975 study is not persuasive . . . and have requested that the [1986 AVMA Euthanasia Panel] revision be rescinded. (Foundation for Biomedical Research 1987, p. 34)

The Canadian Council on Animal Care writes that "with the separation of the spinal cord from the brain, painful stimuli cannot be perceived" (Olfert et al. 1993, p. 242). Likewise, European authors have stated quite flatly that decapitation "causes immediate loss of consciousness," with no mention of controversial science (Flecknell 1995, p. 379). Even the one laboratory animal veterinarian on the 1993 AVMA Panel on Euthanasia ignores the brain wave data in his USDA-sponsored "primer for research personnel," asserting, in contradiction to the AVMA report he coauthored, that the potential for "operator error" is the only reason for classifying decapitation as conditionally acceptable (Bennett et al. 1994, p. 60).

The Humane Society of the United States has posted on its website its unpublished critique of carbon dioxide euthanasia of rodents. As a basis for comparison, it starts with the "assumption that any euthanasia procedure that causes distress for 13.6 seconds or more should be used, if at all, with circumspection and caution," and it concludes that decapitation is preferable to carbon dioxide inhalation (Humane Society of the United States 2002). The black box has all but closed on this controversy, now that the largest animal welfare organization has joined the researchers in its acceptance of the guillotine.

Stakeholders and controversy

The duration of the decapitation controversy is remarkable in light of the imbalance of stakeholders in the issue. Scientists whose work used the technique were, of course, most intimately affected (at least, among humans). Most euthanasia techniques induce various artifacts such as changes in regional brain chemistry (O'Mara et al. 1994), in epinephrine levels, and in liver metabolism (Allred and Berntson 1986) after anesthetic overdose, or in lung structure after carbon dioxide inhalation/asphyxiation (Danneman et al. 1994). Some scientists I have known prefer decapitation and cervical dislocation due to humane concerns, citing the excitation and distress that they have witnessed in rats or chickens placed in carbon dioxide chambers. The number of scientists using rodent guillotines, like the number of research rodents in general, is uncounted in the United States, but the concerns of these scientists were strong enough to move the American Physiological Society to speak out against the AVMA's attempt to dictate scientific practices.

This issue has not caught much attention among animal protectionists. Though some did urge the USDA to keep the panel recommendations in the Animal Welfare Act regulations, they did not refer to the decapitation issue as an example of the panel's value. I found a single letter (among the 36,000 that the USDA counted) submitting an opinion piece on decapitation from the *Chronicle of Higher Education,* but that letter's concern was for killing animals at all, deriding the very notion of doing that humanely (Mathias 1987). When animal protectionists did discuss euthanasia methods, their attention was diverted by fears that the USDA's definition of acceptable euthanasia techniques—methods in which animal pain or distress are not evident—might allow succinylcholine and other poisons that the AVMA had condemned. These drugs paralyze animal muscles, suffocating them without inducing unconsciousness, while paralyzing as well any struggling that would provide evidence of animal pain and distress. At any rate, antipathy to rodent guillotines in no way moved animal protectionists as much as a focused concern for loss of the tool moved scientists, and the animal protectionists had little role in sustaining the decapitation controversy.

Nor have veterinarians generally been important stakeholders fueling the controversy one way or the other. Rodent guillotines are far out of the realm of veterinarians in pet or farm practice and thus far from the veterinary mainstream. Most practicing veterinarians use the commercially available euthanasia solutions (or send farm animals off for slaughter) and are done with it, with no concern for the postmortem artifacts or specialized needs of killing animals for research.

Laboratory animal veterinarians and veterinary researchers are the only veterinarians whose work might be affected by a policy on decapitation, and I have found their opinions (in my interviews and in USDA correspondence) to vary greatly among individuals. None of their professional associations has weighed in on this controversy. Several wrote letters to the USDA, urging that choice of euthanasia method left in the jurisdiction of veterinarians in the Animal Welfare Act regulations. One laboratory animal veterinarian wrote, ignoring the work of the AVMA panels: "Since little can be known of the relative painlessness of each [euthanasia] method, the choice of methods should be left with the individual institution" (Regulatory Analysis and Development 1989). Even the AVMA wrote that its panel report should be superseded as necessary by IACUCs and laboratory animal veterinarians (Regulatory Analysis and Development 1987).

With no large, motivated constituency to resist this shift, the controversy is finally closing. The handful of academic veterinarians (anesthesiologists, behaviorists, neurologists) who kept open the possibility of pain in decapitation have not pursued it. This tentative and ambivalent veterinary initiative to control scientists' and laboratory animal veterinarians' use of this euthanasia practice has effectively ended.

A clinical perspective on the decapitation controversy

Before I end this chapter, let me ask what a veterinarian's clinical perspective might bring to this decapitation controversy. I do not think we veterinarians individually can contribute much new information per se. As a veterinarian, I have no idea how I could assess different techniques in any but the crudest fashion: how can I begin to guess what a disembodied head is or is not experiencing? If the meaning of rats' brain waves is determined facility by facility (as several letter writers suggested to the USDA in their rejection of the AVMA Panel's status), what can we say when the assembled body of experts is ambivalent in their interpretation? IACUCs can review the decapitator's credentials and competency and review the scientist's need to use this potentially painful procedure, but they do not determine whether decapitation per se is a painful procedure.

I have had thankfully few encounters with rodent guillotines. I have certainly seen the blood, the wide-eyed vacant stare, the rhythmic opening and closing of the animals' mouths. But as for what the animals experienced, if anything, once the blade had passed, I cannot say. I assume it hurt, because that makes sense to me, just as I assume it passed quickly. How quickly? Nothing in my veterinary training or experience has taught me to interpret these brain waves, or to read animals' minds, with precision.

I believe the data can be relevant and that clinicians offer a different framework in which to interpret them. The difference lies in the relationship of a clinician with his or her patients as individuals, versus that of a scientist (including veterinarians when they are generating laboratory data as scientists). Clinicians apply their generalized knowledge to the individual patient; scientists deduce their generalized knowledge from studying several representative individuals. Time has been a central consideration in the decapitation controversy—time to unconsciousness, time to a flat EEG—should clinicians see time differently than scientists do?

Policy discussions around decapitation are full of words like "momentary," "instantaneous," "immediate," and "rapid" and are focused on the conscious experience of the animals. The ideal of both animal protectionists and research advocates seemed to be instantaneous unconsciousness, after which time to death is less important. The USDA initially defined euthanasia in its 1987 proposed Animal Welfare Act regulations as "instantaneous unconsciousness and immediate death without evidence of pain or distress," not much of a departure from the definition already in place (Animal and Plant Health Inspection Service 1987). As scientists and laboratory animal veterinarians wrote to protest elevation of the AVMA Panel to statutory authority, some also challenged the "performance standards" of immediacy. One veterinarian wrote, suggesting deletion of the words "instantaneous" and "immediate" because "the meaning of the words cannot be complied with; there is always a passage of time and the sophistication in being able to measure this instant is continually improving." Qualitative terms such as "instantaneous" and "immediate" have no scientific definition: How many nanoseconds in an instant, or vice versa? Such words were increasingly out of place in the scientists' debates about Mikeska and Klemm's (1975) study. They remained in the policy language, however, though the USDA downgraded "instantaneous unconsciousness and immediate death" to the equally imprecise "rapid unconsciousness and subsequent death" in its final regulations (Animal and Plant Health Inspection Service 1989a).

Six of Mikeska and Klemm's eight rats contributed the controversial data of EEG activation; the other two contributed data for a different measurement—a "massive and long-lasting shift in ultra-slow activity"—that generated considerably less press and controversy, despite Mikeska and Klemm labeling it "probably the most outstanding event following decapitation" (1975, p. 178). The six rats did not respond identically, assuming their brain wave patterns can even accurately be called a response. In fact, the expectation that living creatures will not respond identically in an experiment is a major reason to use multiple animals and statistical analyses.

Mikeska and Klemm (1975) reported two sets of data, the length of time following decapitation during which they considered the EEG pattern activated, and the total length of time until the brain waves went flat and the animals were unequivocally dead. They reported the range of times, the mean (or average) and the standard error.[11] They found that the EEG was activated for anywhere from 5.6 to 29.5 seconds, with a mean duration of 13.6 seconds. The total duration of EEG activity (including the period after activation, as it was approaching the flat EEG of death) ranged from 19.0 to 46.5 seconds, with an average of 27.2 seconds. Mikeska and Klemm (1975) believed the initial period of activation "clearly indicates a conscious awareness of pain and distress" (p. 178) following the extremely traumatic (p. 178) act of decapitation.

Recall that most of Mikeska and Klemm's critics did not deny the traumatic nature of decapitation, merely the length of time during which consciousness or pain perception could be sustained in the decapitated brain. Time is of the essence. The rapidity of death is the major route by which even a painful event might be rendered humane for the AVMA Panel. Scientific assessments of rapidity are found both in brain wave data and in theoretical calculations. Minimizing the time that rats could be conscious or in pain shifts the procedure closer and closer to what Derr (1991) called "a time short enough to render decapitation of rats humane" (p. 1399). Derr was the most active in shifting this time, throwing out Mikeska and Klemm's data altogether in favor of his theoretical calculations, moving the period of possible consciousness down to a fleeting 2.7 seconds. Some critics of the AVMA picked up on Derr's calculated 2.7 seconds, but others used Mikeska and Klemm's reported average data to minimize the apparent impact on rats.

Derr presented a theoretical rat, an animal existing totally in theory and calculation, a hybrid of rat and human literature, immune to actual data. There is also a *statistical* rat in much of the decapitation literature, the rat whose average duration of brain wave activation is 13.6 seconds. Death is hastened by invoking Mikeska and Klemm's 13.6-second average, rather than the range of up to 29.5 seconds in their longest living rat. Thirteen to fourteen seconds is the commonly cited time frame in my interviews and in the literature. But notice the rhetorical function this serves of minimizing the period of possible painfulness, discounting the experiences of individual animals in favor of the "statistical rat." In pushing the time frame from 29.5 to 13.6 seconds, proponents of the guillotine approach Derr's 2.7 seconds—a time frame they, too, consider short enough to discount even the most intensely painful of procedures. By concurring with this definition, the few critics of the guillotine retained their reasonable stance, their scientific outlook, their right to remain in the dialogue, and their focus on what the brain waves might mean. But they lost the individual animals.

Animal care and use committees may want to know what the average animal experiences in a particular situation, or they may want to know the worst-case scenario for the individual most severely affected. These are two different questions, requiring different readings of the available data, and it is a question of ethics, not data, as to which question should inform IACUC policy, whether animals at the statistical extremes should get full ethical standing and consideration.

I argue that the nature of clinical practice and training should lead veterinarians in particular away from negating the individual in favor of the statistic. Indeed, the reader may have noticed my choice of the phrase "up to half a minute" throughout this chapter as my personal resistance to closing off this question of ethical standing or losing the ethical issue in the scientific language of statistics. If decapitation is indeed painful to animals, we need to worry about those individuals whose brain waves are activated for a full half minute.

Clinical veterinarians should also challenge the validity of arguments based solely on animals studied under ideal conditions. Conahan and others have found evidence that the time and restraint in positioning rats in their guillotine results in measurable increases in stress-related hormones (Conahan et al. 1985). Mikeska and Klemm's data were obtained from animals chemically paralyzed, who are easily positioned for a perfect cut. Why does this antemortem rat-and-human struggle disappear from the decapitation controversy? In one of the guillotine's rare appearances in the nonscientific literature, Maggie Smith described her graduate school experiences as the best "rat person" in her physiology laboratory: "Overconfident and careless, I failed to stick his [the rat's] head in far enough, and so cut off his nose. He started spurting blood and screaming" (Smith 1995, p. 86). Though claiming to have only done this once, laboratory culture taught her that it was "bad form" to cut off rats' noses or faces or parts, none of which would lead to painless instantaneous unconsciousness. And yet, where are the data, for all the efforts to reduce decapitation to a question of skill, on how often experienced operators get it right?

These are the animals a clinician must not overlook: the mispositioned animals mutilated rather than decapitated; the struggling, resistant and frightened animals; the animals who for whatever reason sustain brain activity of who knows what significance for a full half minute after the guillotine.

Conclusion

Timothy Sprigge (1985) writes that in animal experimentation, the harm to animals is certain, while the benefits of research are potential, unknowns that may or may not be realized. He argues that in any sort of comparative cost analysis, different weighting should accompany different levels of certainty.

At one level, Sprigge has characterized the situation correctly: It is certain that rats are decapitated and die in some projects and that the fruits of their sacrifice may or may not amount to much. But how much of a harm is death to a rat? How much does decapitation hurt? This case study suggests that things are not so simple; the harms to animals may not be nearly so certain or defined as we would like them to be. Twenty years of controversy have left us with little narrowing of that range of uncertainty, with no consensus whether the guillotine inflicts excruciating pain for up to half a minute or whether it is a fast and painless death. And we do want and need some degree of certainty if we are to compare and choose among several candidate techniques for an experimental task.

Assessing the comparative humaneness of animal experimental techniques is inescapably fraught with value judgments. There is no scientific answer to questions such as, How strong a justification does a particular painful procedure require? or How long must a painful stimulus persist to be considered unacceptable? These sorts of questions do contain empirical components; for example, we want to know how painful a procedure might be before we assess its justification. For the empirical information, we turn to scientific study.

As this case study of the decapitation controversy demonstrates, truly objective assessment may be impossible. Differing theoretical commitments lead to flexible and often contradictory interpretations of data. When strong political and policy implications ride on the interpretation of data, we may expect that controversies will be particularly resistant to closure and consensus. This controversy may close as scientists at institutions with a more stringent reading of the AVMA Panel find that other, less controversial, euthanasia techniques yield satisfactory tissue samples for their work. Ironically, these less controversial techniques may be even less well studied than decapitation. The face of this controversy changed only slightly with the 2000 AVMA Panel report, not because of new data but because of new interpretations of existing data.

Study design and protocol review remain as value-laden as ever. The best that IACUCs may be able to hope for from scientific investigations of the painfulness of research procedures is some narrowing of the range of interpretation, some rough comparison of different techniques or variations of techniques. Protocol review and study design would then always have to be seen as working in the face of greater or lesser uncertainty. This uncertainty should be factored into whatever ethical deliberations IACUCs conduct.

In the face of competing interpretations of the data, IACUCs at different institutions evaluate the justification for the guillotine with little guidance from federal policy. A national consensus on the permissibility of this procedure may arrive one day, but it will come slowly. I predict that it will come with no significant new addition to our empirical database; rather, it will represent a consensus of value, not of data.

10

Dog walkers and monkey psychiatrists

IN 1985, CONGRESS SINGLED OUT OUR BEST FRIENDS, THE DOGS, AND OUR CLOSEST cousins, the monkeys, for special rights under the Animal Welfare Act. Senator Robert Dole inserted language into the pending Animal Welfare Act amendment to give laboratory dogs the opportunity for exercise, while his colleague, Senator John Melcher, pushed for the psychological well-being of nonhuman primates.

Anyone who thought the Animal Welfare Act was all about whether animals would be subjected to painful experiments is deeply mistaken. Yes, animals will suffer experimentation, and that decision long precedes the rules writing that the USDA embarked on in 1986. What's surprising are the particular issues that caused so much controversy, and none more so than the simple question of whether laboratory dogs should get out of their cages for some daily exercise. That controversy sputtered out after a few years. When it was still hot, it encompassed all the issues this book has been describing: the interplay between expertise and advocacy in speaking for animals; the differences between performance-based and engineering-based standards; the differences among animal protectionists, animal researchers, and veterinarians; and the ambivalent role of laboratory animal veterinarians.

Even before the USDA projected a price tag of a billion dollars nationwide to meet the new dog and monkey standards, research advocates were alarmed and annoyed. "I think it is fair to say that these regulations are an example of bureaucracy run amok," wrote one biologist to the USDA. "What other process could conceive of the . . . creation of a veterinary specialty, monkey psychiatry, to treat 'signs of psychological distress . . . to prevent the development of psychological disorders?' This fanciful speculation on the mental well-being of monkeys is absolutely bizarre" (Regulatory Analysis and Development 1987).

Just what did the USDA and Congress have in mind with these new provisions? Would scientific institutions have all their research funds siphoned off for a staff of monkey psychiatrists and dog walkers? The USDA counted some 36,000 public comments from research advocates, animal protectionists, veterinarians, patient advocacy groups, and others over the five years it spent crafting Animal Welfare Act regulations in the 1980s; whatever other issues they addressed, most of these commenters had something to say about dog exercise or primates' psychological well-being. Research advocates resisted the expansive provisions the USDA had initially proposed, while animal protectionists urged the USDA (unsuccessfully, as it came to pass) to stand firm. As the USDA abandoned the detailed standards it had started with and shifted more toward self-regulation, flexibility, and performance standards, the competition increased to be the one who could speak most authoritatively for dogs and their exercise needs and for monkeys and their emotional needs.

In resisting the USDA's proposals for dog exercise and primate psychological well-being, research advocates faced a challenge: how to rebut the common sense presumption that larger cages, social grouping, contact with human caregivers, room to run, and a varied diet were not in fact advances in welfare that animals would want. Only scientific data could provide such a powerful antidote to common knowledge, empathy, and anthropomorphism.

Most of the 1985 Animal Welfare Act amendment related to scientists' use of animals in experiments. But the 1985 Improved Standards for Laboratory Animals (as the Animal Welfare Act amendment was being called) also brought changes in the rules for animal care, changes the animal protectionists had pressed for for years: Cages sizes were modified, but more significantly, the dog and monkey provisions were added.

Remember the distinction between the law as Congress passes it (the Animal Welfare Act and its amendments) and the regulations it authorizes the USDA to write. The new dog and monkey rules were an act of law that the USDA could only dodge so far. The language of the act is general: "The Secretary [of Agriculture] shall promulgate standards to . . . include minimum requirements . . . for exercise of dogs, as determined by an attending veterinarian in accordance with general standards promulgated by the Secretary, and for a physical environment adequate to promote the psychological well-being of primates" (U.S. Congress 1985a).

Several observers cried foul at inclusion of this sentence. Representative George Brown of California and his staff had slowly crafted the legislative proposals for both the House of Representatives and the Senate, consulting extensively with organized animal protection and research advocacy interests and finding an amendment that all could accept. At the eleventh hour, senators Dole and Melcher added their amendments to the Senate bill; introduced on a Friday, they were voted on on Monday, bypassing much of the consensus building of previous months, side-stepping any debate in hearings. The House had passed no comparable provisions, but exercise and psychological well-being survived intact the House–Senate conference and became law (U.S. Congress 1985a).

The dual provisions for dog exercise programs and monkeys' psychological well-being were easily the most controversial issues in the mid-1980s of the Animal Welfare Act regulations, whether measured by the projected price tag, volume of mail to the USDA, time lag in determining final regulations, or number of lawsuits brought against the USDA for its alleged failure to meet congressional decree.

Despite the two senators' apparent last-minute maneuver, neither exercise nor psychological well-being were new issues in animal welfare policy. Exercise for dogs was explicitly discussed (and dismissed) in the early editions of the *Guide for*

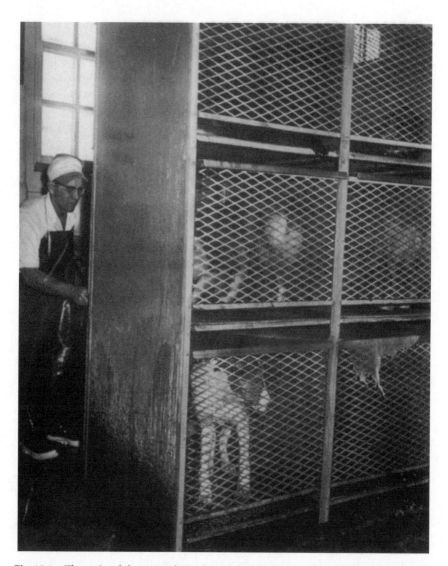

Fig. 10.1 Three-tiered dog cages, being hosed clean without removing the animals.
PHOTO: UNITED STATES DEPARTMENT OF AGRICULTURE, ANIMAL WELFARE INFORMATION
CENTER.

the Care and Use of Laboratory Animals, right from the first 1963 edition. In those
days, cages such as those depicted in figure 10.1 may not have been the norm, but
they certainly were in use in some facilities (Brewer 1961). Mandated exercise was
part of the Washington, D.C., local regulations of the 1950s that allowed for use of
dogs from pounds, provided certain minimum standards were met (Morgan 1954),
and it was part of Dole's proposed legislation in 1983, the direct forerunner of the
1985 Animal Welfare Act amendment (Scientists Center for Animal Welfare 1983).

The USDA had received so much correspondence on the subject in 1971 that
it promised to publish proposed regulations within 60 days. Three years later,

it published its 1974 exercise proposal, standards which were never finalized and which were eventually overshadowed by Congress's 1976 Animal Welfare Act amendment. When Congress failed to include dog exercise in its 1976 law, the USDA was able to let the matter drop for a while (Animal and Plant Health Inspection Service 1974; Animal and Plant Health Service 1971). When dog exercise returned in 1981 congressional hearings, the USDA explicitly opposed it: "We do not favor adding 'space for normal exercise' as a required standard of care and treatment because of the difficulty in making a determination on what exercise would be considered 'normal'" (Lee 1981, p. 146).

As for psychological well-being, people had been groping for years for the right words to describe what they were looking for for caged primates. In 1971, the USDA tried the word "anxiety," proposing standards to minimize "pain and anxiety" in animal handling, experiment, and euthanasia (Agricultural Research Service 1971). But many scientists complained to the USDA that the term might be misinterpreted. "It was stated the word anxiety is a psychiatric term that is only applicable to humans," the USDA reported, even though it believed that common usage of the word "would appear to make such term applicable in evaluating the psychological well-being as an integral part of 'humaneness.'" The USDA deferred to its critics, and replaced "anxiety" with "distress," "which is more descriptive of the physical visible state of the animal" (Animal and Plant Health Service 1971, p. 919).

The USDA drew this distinction between anxiety and distress to forestall getting too deep into animal psychology, even as it tried to go beyond the animals' physical needs. It tried to avoid going into the animals' minds by choosing a word that it believed could keep things in the realm of the physical, the visible, the objective, and the scientific. John Melcher, a veterinarian turned senator, set this attempt on its head with his 1985 amendment. Psychological well-being was back, the best term he and his USDA advisors could come up with to move away from primate cages he had described as "extremely efficient, extremely expensive, and extremely cruel" (Stevens 1990, p. 81). Once in the congressional act, the USDA could not erase it, and the battle shifted to fine-tuning the standards that the USDA would write.

The agenda of animal protectionists for dogs was clear and simple: They wanted to move away from housing dogs singly in small cages. They wanted to get dogs out of cages frequently to romp and play with each other and with their human caregivers. Construction costs (to build exercise pens) and labor costs (for the dog walkers) drove some of the resistance of research advocates to this vision, but as I described in an earlier chapter, so did the fears of laboratory animal veterinarians that they would lose control of dog husbandry, health, and safety: packs of dogs in exercise pens would fight and spread infections, while dog walkers might similarly bring their charges to all sorts of dangers, especially, again, infections, parasites, and contagion.

The protectionists' agenda for nonhuman primates was offered in far less detail, possibly because of the greater range of species involved (from the highly arboreal squirrel-sized marmoset monkeys to five-foot-tall chimpanzees to savanna-dwelling baboons), or because of primates' lesser familiarity in American life. Again, the protectionists sought to abolish single small cages as much as possible, moving laboratories more toward modern zoo standards or moving both the laboratory and the zoo closer to life in the wild. Again, cost consciousness, animal aggression, and infection control underlay most of the resistance to group housing in naturalistic enclosures, though some also feared the research logistics of having to catch semi-wild primates from large group pens when scientists needed blood samples, physiological measurements, or other data.

The dog and monkey issues have similarly long histories and roughly similar agendas and concerns for the stakeholders. The place of expertise, convincingly claiming to know what animals want, is what sets the two apart. The need of dogs for exercise and love of companionship are common knowledge; the burden of proof was on those who would limit these goods, and science was the tool to show that common sense assumptions of dogs' needs, wants, and desires were mistaken. In contrast, monkeys, apes, prosimians, and marmosets are strange animals from faraway places. Whereas animal protectionists might use common sense to wrest control of dog care out of the hands of the laboratory animal professionals, they might be on shakier ground with primates. Instead, they sought to define a cadre of primate experts who would be more sympathetic to the animals than laboratory facility managers had heretofore seemed. Instead of moving animal care management out of the hands of the laboratory animal veterinarians and scientists into the hands of the public and the USDA, they strived to move it in the other direction, into the hands of specialists—their specialists.

Dogs and exercise

Everyone knows that dogs need exercise and that they love to run and play. Just take a walk to a local park or beach and watch the dogs in action. See how eagerly they greet each other, chase their tennis balls, romp with their human companions, how rich and full of fun their lives can be. What could convince you that anything short of this sort of dog's life is a sad miscarriage of humanity? Could science convince you? Could veterinary experts?

The nascent profession of laboratory animal medicine developed throughout the 1950s at a time when impounded dogs (and their associated fleas, ticks, worms, and viruses) were the mainstay of the postwar boom in biomedical research. These motley strays were transformed into suitable experimental subjects only though lengthy conditioning periods in which the weak were culled and the strong were bathed, dipped, vaccinated, and dewormed in preparation for life in the laboratory. Solitary housing in small metal cages allowed animal facilities in even the most crowded urban medical centers to house such dogs with minimal losses to fighting and infections. Nor was this merely a matter of money: Then as now, metal cages that could stand up to strong dogs were expensive to buy, and caged dogs were labor-intensive to maintain (White et al. 1974; Whitney 1950).

Animal protectionists have long chafed at the penitentiary style of dog housing—tiers of metal cages two or three high—sometimes for the solitary confinement, sometimes for the lack of exercise, but usually for both. The Animal Welfare Institute (an animal protection organization and not any sort of research institute), for example, has published its own guidelines for animal housing since the early 1950s. In updating their *Comfortable Quarters for Laboratory Animals* in 1958, they included designs from dog-housing facilities of which they approved, writing how acceptable designs give compatible groups of dogs "room for a moderate amount of exercise instead of keeping them closely confined in metal cages. Such confinement, unfortunately for the dogs, is routine practice in far too many laboratories" (Animal Welfare Institute 1958, p.1).

As the USDA worked to accommodate the 1985 call for dog exercise programs, it simultaneously worked on several interrelated issues. Once of those was just how broad or narrow a definition of "exercise" to use. The broader definition of exercise went beyond the physical and included proposed rules for dogs' social lives. Now sociality and exercise are not synonyms. For the most part, professional guidelines for laboratory dog housing had ignored social versus solitary caging as a matter of much importance. But expertise and common sense concur in labeling dogs as social animals, even in the face of the occasional dog fight.

Despite the known sociality of dogs, social housing received relatively little attention in animal welfare policy before the 1980s. Veterinarian Leon Whitney praised that "good and faithful servant," the "adaptable dog," who is happy in a cage or roaming over acres, who can live alone or in a group (Whitney 1950, p. 182). The Animal Welfare Institute suggested that "Whenever possible, it is best to give dogs companionship by housing them in pairs" (Animal Welfare Institute 1953, p. 24), but apparently did not push this point strongly enough to draw a reaction from the research defense organizations. Thus the *Guide for the Care and Use of Laboratory Animals* in its first several editions (1963–1978) asserted that research priorities should determine group or single housing and made no recommendation, other than to watch for compatibility and overcrowding, for instances where research needs were indifferent to social or solitary caging (Animal Care Panel 1963; Committee on Laboratory Animal Housing 1976; ILAR 1965, 1972). Absent good data, Dr. Nathan Brewer had polled his veterinary colleagues on their preferred housing for laboratory dogs and concluded that dogs were optimally housed in small compatible groups (Brewer 1961).

Exercise has always been more controversial than single or group caging. As the 1950s Washington, D.C., regulations reflected, animal protectionists could see value in singly housing dogs in some circumstances, in a way that they probably never saw value in restricting dogs' freedom to exercise.[1] So the USDA veterinarians may well have been surprised at the reaction when they piggybacked proposed regulations for meeting dogs' social urges onto Congress's mandate of canine exercise.

The USDA did its best to avoid the whole issue of dog exercise for as long as possible. It had gotten right on the job in 1986 (two months after passage of the Animal Welfare Act amendment), asking for public comments on exercise and psychological well-being, but then waited until 1989 for its first published attempt at setting standards (Animal and Plant Health Inspection Service 1986, 1999). By the time it got to this stage of regulation writing, the whole business had been recast by research advocates and the Office of Management and Budget into the language of performance standards. Nonetheless, the USDA put forth a highly detailed set of standards. In them, "exercise and socialization" replaced the congressional "exercise" as the centerpiece of dog care law:

> In accordance with the 1985 amendments to the Act, we have developed standards for the exercise and socialization of dogs. . . . We would require that all dogs . . . be maintained in compatible groups. . . . Because of the social nature of dogs, we are also proposing to require, with similar exceptions, that all dogs be able to see and hear other dogs. [Where this is not possible] we would require that it receive positive physical contact with humans. . . . petting, stroking, or other touching which is beneficial to the well-being of the animal. . . . at least 60 minutes each day. (Animal and Plant Health Inspection Service, 1989b, p. 10904)

They further went on to propose that dogs in cages under a certain size be released into an exercise area for at least half an hour a day, either in groups, or at least with the ability to have social contact such as the ability "to nuzzle another dog through a chain link fence" (p. 10905). So impressed was the USDA by dogs' sociability and its own license to police it that it threw in the possibility of housing compatible dogs and cats together, as so many pet owners do, in contradiction to the *Guide for the Care and Use of Laboratory Animals*' long-standing discouragement of mixing species (p. 10906).

Mandatory group housing, nuzzling through fences, mixing of species, enforced dog petting—this was more than many laboratory animal professionals could stomach. One veterinarian wrote:

> This is the most amazing proposed change and would only make sense for pet owners or some behaviorist. The probability of a research facility having a compatible dog and cat is less likely than hitting the lotto. . . . Group housing is much more likely to lead to injury and psychological distress to some. . . . To take [dogs on leash] around the campus would create a field day for animal activists and would subject the animal to temperature extremes, exposure to endo and ecto parasites and predispose it to infectious diseases and fights. (Regulatory Analysis and Development 1989)

The first step in resisting this expansion of Animal Welfare Act standards required no claim to animal expertise, but rather legal understanding. Research advocates pointed out that the USDA was overstepping its congressional mandate by converting exercise into exercise and socialization. A few laboratory animal professionals had liked that substitution. The American Association for Laboratory Animal Science wrote in 1986 that socialization with dogs or people might better serve dogs' welfare than release into a large exercise paddock would. But few research advocates welcomed expansion of the USDA's heavy-handed, rigidly formulated approach to regulations; if Congress mandated exercise, so be it, but adding socialization into the mix was unacceptable. The National Association for

Biomedical Research reminded the USDA of the Animal Welfare Act's legislative history and how Senator Melcher's original language to provide for the "psychological well-being of research animals, particularly primates" was scaled back to "psychological well-being of primates." Dogs' psychological well-being, including their social interests, were emphatically not part of the congressional mandate, and must be "dropped entirely" from the USDA's proposed regulations (Regulatory Analysis and Development 1989). Some animal protectionists also balked, fearing that some wily research institutions might substitute socialization for exercise, doubling dogs up in small cages and calling it welfare.

Ultimately, the USDA retreated on dog socialization, though not entirely. Admitting that socialization was not what Congress mandated, it nonetheless believed that "the research data available, and in large measure, simple observation," concur that social interaction leads dogs to exercise more and, in fact, that socialization of dogs, including sensory contact, is the single most effective means of providing the opportunity for exercise (Animal and Plant Health Inspection Service 1990a, pp. 33467–33468). It dropped the presumption of social housing, removed any suggestions of ways in which to exercise dogs, kept the requirement that dogs housed without any sensory contact with other dogs must receive "positive physical contact with humans at least daily," and changed the section heading in the regulations from "Exercise and socialization for dogs" to "Exercise for dogs" (Animal and Plant Health Inspection Service 1991, pp. 6490–6491).

Most of the jockeying on regulations for canine socialization involved no competing claims about what matters to dogs. Some warned of fighting, but few claimed that dogs don't care about companionship. The laboratory animal veterinarian who wrote that purpose-bred laboratory dogs "should not be looked upon as pets who need socialization anymore than a purpose bred rat or mouse," was in a lonely minority (Regulatory Analysis and Development 1989). The socialization issue was mostly limited to the question of USDA jurisdiction or, as another laboratory animal veterinarian wrote, "We were told that we were supposed to exercise dogs. We are not supposed to make them happy" (Regulatory Analysis and Development 1990).

Exercise and expertise

In addition to its initial proposal linking exercise and socialization, the USDA proposed rigid and specific standards for exercise pens and for frequency of exercise periods. Ultimately those standards were scrapped with the shift to performance-based standards. On the way to this resolution, however, research advocates and the USDA came the closest it ever did to matching up specific scientific reports with proposed standards. Though ultimately the scientific arguments may have been totally peripheral to the policy settlement, they are well worth a closer look for the lessons they teach about this whole approach to animal welfare.

The USDA came on strong in 1989 with its proposed exercise standards. It began by reaffirming its complicated 1967 dog-cage minimum sizes, as I have described in chapter 5, that a dog's cage should be six inches longer than his body (minus the tail) on each side. The USDA supplemented this with a complicated formula to determine which dogs were being housed in big enough enclosures not to require out of cage exercise (Animal and Plant Health Inspection Service 1989b).[2] Dogs housed in smaller cages or pens must be released for exercise for at least 30 minutes daily (half of what most animal protectionists were calling for at the time), into an exercise pen of at least 80 square feet (with another complicated formula to figure out whether some groups would need even more, for note that 80 square feet is only 8 by 10).

While one dog breeder wrote to tell the USDA that larger pens with half an hour of "loving and petting" each day were "unnecessary and is disgusting," the scientific community was not so crude or callous (Regulatory Analysis and Development 1989).[3] It did not need to be, for it had science on its side. Science was the weapon of choice for those who would ward off overly expansive (and expensive) exercise provisions.

Plenty of animal protectionists writing to the USDA did not believe that science was the key to animal welfare. This writer's sentiments were typical: "Dogs need at least ONE HOUR of exercise and companionship daily . . . Scientific studies are not needed to understand that primates, and ALL animals, have basic physical and psychological needs—for space, for companionship, for stimulating activity; this is obvious to all" (Regulatory Analysis and Development 1989).

But is this obvious to all? Do all dogs need a full hour of exercise? What happens to dogs if this need is not met, if they only get, say, twenty or thirty minutes of exercise? Or might they actually need two hours of exercise? Could breed, or age, or prior experience, or what's happening in the exercise yard influence this need? With a multimillion-dollar price tag riding on the final form of the regulations, perhaps there was a role for scientific data on dog exercise after all.

The USDA had long been in pursuit of scientific information that would make its policy decision for it. In 1974, having already noted the dearth of data three years earlier, it published standards for dog exercise on its own initiative comparable to what it published fifteen years later under congressional mandate (Animal and Plant Health Inspection Service 1974). Public comments to the USDA on that proposal are no longer available for review, but ILAR of the National Academy of Sciences published its response to the USDA in its newsletter. ILAR had taken on publication of the *Guide for the Care and Use of Laboratory Animals* in the 1960s and convened a panel of laboratory animal professionals (two of whom who had served on the 1972 *Guide* committee) to address the USDA's proposal (ILAR 1974).

The ILAR group did not like the USDA's 1974 exercise proposals, published without objective evidence of their validity, or their potential price tag. The ILAR group members continued the *Guide*'s long-standing insistence that exercise be narrowly defined in physiological terms, noting with suspicion that the USDA seemed to be construing it as "releasing the animal from confinement for the sake of release rather than for exercise per se (muscle tone, stretching, etc.)" (ILAR 1974, p. 6). As such, they could offer assurance that "there is no valid scientific evidence for the necessity of exercise for the health or safety of the animal" (p. 6). They noted that "the lack of opportunity to defecate [since some former pets might be reluctant to defecate in a small laboratory cage] over a period of several days has not caused demonstrable adverse physiological effects" (p. 6), that studies show that caged animals lived longer than animals "allowed to run free of confinement" (p. 6), that blood pressure and stress hormone levels would rise during periods of exercise and contact with their canine peers, and that caged dogs and cats even have higher reproductive rates.[4]

As with the early editions of the *Guide,* the committee provided a short list of references but did not explicitly tie any particular claim in its report to any specific study in its bibliography. The critical reader would be challenged to take a closer look, for example, at the increased longevity of caged life; how big or small a cage leads to long life? How free of confinement are the animals to which they are compared—free enough to be hit by cars or to suffer the other traumas and infections of the feral life, or are they dogs in spacious but sheltered kennel runs? Or are they dogs at all? As I read this bibliography, the only support for this claim is a 1966 article in which the subject animals were albino rats (Retzlaff 1966). The ILAR committee did not make this explicit, absolving itself of defending this extrapolation to dogs.

The ILAR group was clearly interested in presenting expertise as its basis for dismissing the USDA's proposal, but claims to expertise must be established and defended before the audience at hand. The ILAR group clearly had the credentials to presume expertise: convened by the prestigious National Academy of Sciences, the members listed their doctoral degrees and university affiliations (one was a veterinarian with the American Animal Hospital Association; the remainder were in academia). As scientific experts, however, they wanted more than to rest on their credentials: they wanted to base their informed and expert opinion on the scientific record. This is how scientists write for each other, in scientific journals. They do not simply report the results of their individual experiments, but enlist other credible experts, by citing their work in peer-reviewed journals, as they build their case that their methods, observations, and interpretations are credible, significant, and in line with theory. Writing for a critical audience of other scientists, they may find the need to buttress virtually every statement they make with its source in the published record. The more controversial the science, the more likely they will be to enlist expert support in this way.

The response of laboratory animal professionals writing the early editions of the *Guide for the Care and Use of Laboratory Animals* to exercise standards and other such documents was to use the scientific record in a different way to establish their expertise. Rather than defend specific claims with their source in the scientific database, these experts line up their witnesses in extensive bibliographies, none of which is cited directly. No skeptic could sort through such an extensive reading list (seven pages of books, articles, and periodicals in the selected bibliography in the 1972 *Guide,* for instance) to raise objections to particular points, but then, how could he voice dissent without having done that homework? By combining this oblique relationship to the published science with claims of "expert opinion, and experience with methods and practices that have proved to be consistent with high quality animal care," these experts bought themselves the right to define "humane animal care in professional terms" without credible interference from other quarters (ILAR 1972, pp. v, 1). Thus the authors of the 1960s editions of the *Guide* were able to deflect calls for canine exercise as misguided and uninformed:

> The concept of "exercise" frequently is confused with that of cage size by animal welfare groups. A "small" cage is equated with lack of "exercise" and physical discomfort; while a "large" cage, a pen, or a run is equated with "exercise" and physical well-being. Scientists know that the size of the cage does not necessarily influence the amount of "exercise" an animal receives, or its well-being. Nevertheless, this semantic confusion is widely fostered by some lay groups. (Animal Care Panel 1963, p. 18)

The dog exercise controversy persisted into the 1980s (and beyond), when Senator Dole took it up and forced it on the USDA and the research industry. Its persistence is testimony both to the deep commitment animal protectionists obviously felt, as well as to the rhetorical power of images of caged dogs to move public and congressional opinion; in other words, it was an issue animal protectionists both deeply cared about and felt that they could win. In the 1980s, as earlier, research advocates wanted regulations to be based on scientific information, but their presentation of that information shifted, possibly because animal protectionists themselves had increased their own use of scientific studies to bolster their arguments. The trend in the 1980s was to cite specific studies, rather than a general appeal to science, in arguing for particular policy settlements. In earlier chapters, we saw how single studies of guinea pig cage utilization and brain wave patterns in decapitated rats found their way into policy documents. Canine exercise requirements brought forth the most extensive enrollment of published studies of any issue in animal welfare public policy during the 1980s, though even that amounted to only half a dozen studies.

Research advocates who hoped to limit the financial, staffing, and even animal health costs that they foresaw in the USDA's exercise regulations faced an uphill battle against common sense and common knowledge of dogs. For "everyone knows" that dogs need exercise, and common sense tells us that the bigger the enclosure, the more likely they are to get that exercise. But what if the scientific record shows otherwise? Aren't there myriad examples of science serving as a corrective to common sense and common observation? Contrary to everyday observation, for instance, it took science to convince us that the earth is round, that animal species change over time, that organisms too small to see cause rabies, cholera, and other diseases. Surely science can correct the confusion of animal welfare groups about dogs, cages, and exercise.

One route to casting the exercise controversy as exclusively a matter of science was to reduce exercise to a purely physical entity with an exclusively physical purpose. Several commenters to the USDA spoke of "physiological exercise," while some laboratory animal veterinarians asserted that they could find no physical evidence of lack of exercise in their caged laboratory dogs. Some sent reprints of three articles from the mid-1970s (when the USDA's first proposed exercise regulations were under consideration) that found no differences between dogs in different-sized cages and pens, in terms of physical factors such as hemoglobin levels, electrocardiograms, mineral metabolism in bone, muscle fiber size, or ophthalmoscopic examination (Hite et al. 1977; Neamand et al. 1975; Newton 1972).

Just as with the guinea pig cage space studies described in chapter 5, the authors explicitly linked their canine science to its regulatory context. In Hite et al.'s (1977) study, one of two papers from the pharmaceuticals firm Merck Sharpe and Dohme, beagle dogs were compared in USDA-regulation size cages of 6.25 square feet (30 by 30 inches, legal for small beagles of 24 inch body length or shorter) with those in a cage three times that size, which was the proposed size of an exercise pen in the USDA's 1974 proposal. But this tight linkage of their study to the USDA's regulatory proposal could have later limited its power. In light of the USDA's 1989 proposal of an 80-square-foot exercise yard, Hite et al.'s selection of a 18.75-square-foot cage as their "large cage" is of little use. If 80 square feet is the minimum acceptable exercise area by 1989 standards, then Hite et al. must have been comparing a small cage (18.75 square feet) with a very small cage (6.25 square feet), with no way of saying how dogs would differ in a large exercise pen.

Such publications on the significance of exercise in dogs to their physiological status are as rooted in their theoretical assumptions as any other scientific work is, though the role of context may be more apparent when the political implications of the work are so obvious. Nonetheless, scientists working in this arena can be quick to claim political meaning in their work, even when it seems to contradict other studies. Hite et al. (1977) found no physical difference between dogs in 6- and 18-square-foot cages, and so proclaimed 6-square-foot cages adequate for laboratory beagle dogs. A dozen years earlier, Yoder and colleagues (1964), similarly siting their work in the context of defining standards for dog care, did find physical differences between dogs, though they were comparing caged dogs with dogs exercised on treadmills (p. 727). Arguing that "canine organs are not built for the resting state but for a higher level of activity," they believed that a caged dog with limited opportunities "might not be considered a 'healthy, normal' individual of the species" (p. 727). With this as their starting point, a normal physical examination of a caged dog would be meaningless; only the techniques they were developing (blood lactate levels, muscle fiber size, post-exercise pulse rate) would be meaningful indicators of fitness, which confined dogs, almost by definition, could not have.

Competing data on canine exercise fitness, though they continued to appear in the literature, never really escalated. Few were content to leave animal welfare in the 1980s exclusively in the realm of physical fitness, and besides, animal protectionists had never really pushed for exercise merely on grounds of cardiovascular or musculoskeletal fitness. Animal *behavior* increasingly became the language of animal welfare throughout the 1980s, but observable, quantifiable canine exercise behavior still offered some hope of replacing the perceived emotionalism of protectionists with something approaching idealized, objective science.

We veterinarians are prone to speak in terms of pathology; that inclination was particularly strong when talking of primate psychological well-being, but it was applied to dog exercise as well. Concerned laboratory animal veterinarians found no physical deterioration in dogs caged for long periods, and they saw no behavioral pathology either. Some suggested a performance standard in which USDA inspectors would be charged to look for behavioral abnormalities as evidence of adequate dog exercise. Related to this pathology model of animal welfare, several laboratory animal veterinarians suggested that exercise standards only apply once dogs had been housed for more than three months in a facility, for exercise "clearly would serve no useful purpose" for dogs held short term, before pathologies might develop.

While some veterinarians were dismissing the idea that dogs need exercise at all, others were developing a different theme: that dogs can and do get their exercise in small dog cages. One laboratory animal veterinarian believed the "claim of need for extra cage exercise to keep dogs healthy and 'happy' is ridiculous," noting that in his experience, dogs placed in exercise pens would get caught in fencing, or roll in their own urine or feces, but "the majority would just sit in one corner of the run for the entire exercise period and tremble. . . . Dogs placed in these runs do not jump about, spin around, or exhibit nearly as much activity as those kept in smaller cages" (Regulatory Analysis and Development 1989). Some others agreed, noting, for instance, caged beagles "racing in circles around the cage with ease" and even "doing complete somersaults," despite the apparent confinement (Regulatory Analysis and Development 1989).

With the right video equipment, such anecdotal information could be translated into scientific data. Thus, the laboratory animal professionals at Smith Kline and French laboratories documented this same observation that dogs in small cages can be highly active. Reprints of their articles and conference proceedings quickly found their way to the USDA in 1989. Like Hite and colleagues a decade earlier, Hughes and Campbell (1990) placed their work squarely in the regulatory context by comparing their study cages to the USDA-proposed mandates for exercise pens and for housing. The work is notable for its apparent success in standing common sense on its head: the most startling finding they reported was that dogs seemed to exercise most when paired in cages that were 25% of the USDA's minimum cage size (Hughes and Campbell 1990).

Hughes and Campbell were not the first to add behavioral data to the assessment of exercise programs; Neamand et al. (1975) and Hite et al. (1977) had also used time-lapse photography to record how often dogs chose to lie down, sleep, sit, or stand, in addition to the physiological measures they were taking. Whereas Neamand et al. (1975) had found no behavioral differences between the two dogs (one in a small cage, one in a larger cage), and Hite et al. (1977) felt the observed differences (that caged dogs sat more, while dogs in runs lie more) were "not large enough to be of any practical concern" (p. 60), Hughes et al. (1989) did find that dogs in different social and spatial environments chose different levels of activity. This work came at a crucial regulatory moment and ultimately spared the research industry considerable expense; it warrants a close reading.

Hughes et al. (1989) chose four study groups: beagles housed alone, in cages either of the USDA minimum or twice that (i.e., either approximately 10.8 or 22 square feet), or paired, in either the USDA minimum, or slightly smaller (22 vs. 15 square feet for the pair). They did not compare dogs in the USDA's proposed 80-square-foot exercise pen. Their findings were that singly caged dogs spend less time moving when in the smaller cages, but they move a significantly greater distance, obviously not any one direction in a 39-inch-long cage. For paired dogs, the findings were more remarkable: in the smaller cage (~39 by 59 inches), "the distance traveled and the amount of time spent moving increased significantly" (p. 303). For all dogs, activity increased when human activity, either in or near the dog room, was high. Their conclusions: "dogs move in response to human presence" and "artificial mechanisms such as doubling the cage size do not increase exercise. In fact the reverse is true" (p. 304). The implication for policy: larger cages should be "considered only as one of the several options and not necessarily the best or the only option to promote exercise," and "emphasis needs to be placed on human-animal interactions" (Hughes et al. 1989, p. 305).

The counterintuitive finding is not that dogs respond to human activity; that conclusion fits well with common experience as well as other empirical studies and could stand unchallenged (except legally: Congress mandated exercise, not human contact, for the USDA to regulate). But the finding that dogs exercise more in a smaller cage contradicts common sense and invites skepticism, and animal protectionists and others might well ask why they should believe these authors. The key rhetorical challenge for the authors is to convincingly argue that what they measured truly represents "exercise," a rhetorical move that they strengthened by making their work as objective as possible in its data collection, in hopes that their interpretation might shine in the light of the objective glow.

Hughes et al. (1989) claimed that the major problem with all previous studies of dog-cage space utilization and exercise was their reliance on behavioral observations that were empirical and subject to bias. Though Neamand et al. (1975) and Hite et al. (1977) had used time-lapse photography, Hughes et al. apparently went even further to minimize investigator bias by using closed-circuit television with computerized image analysis. Exercise was measured as distance traveled, which the computer records as the number of pixels changed in the image when the dog moves 10 centimeters or more. The computer can add these up (distance traveled in the cage, as well as amount of time spent moving) without human interference.

But the computer cannot make the determination that skeptics would find most significant: How and why the dogs in the most confined space are "traveling" as much as they are. And so the authors reinsert the human element at the crucial moment, hoping to thwart the common-sense interpretation of the data that increased movement in a confined space must reflect increased anxiety in the dogs. They write:

> Although assertion could be made that the higher level of activity in the smaller cages could be due to stress since there was less space available, this does not seem likely. In previous studies with the same size cages using the same dogs, there were no elevations in serum cortisol or reduction of T-cell or B-cell functions. These are all excellent indicators of stress and would have detected adverse biochemical changes. (Hughes et al. 1989, p. 305)

For their final assault on common-sense interpretation, they raise the specter of just what might be happening with dogs in larger cages, who spend more time moving about, but at a sufficiently slower pace that they travel less than dogs in smaller cages: "Also, it may be that a dog in the larger cage may be restless and uncomfortable and pace slowly about the area" (Hughes et al. 1989, p. 305). For this latter possibility, they fail to offer the physiological (cortisol) or immunological (B-cell and T-cell function) data that might support such a nonobvious interpretation. What data, for instance, suggest that dogs who are "pacing" (or walking?) *slowly* are "uncomfortable?"

The attempt to use computerized video systems to remove human bias from dog exercise studies may be commendable and may have met some rhetorical success in creating the authority of objectivity. But as with all science, theoretical considerations are part and parcel of all data collection and interpretation. Computerized video cannot remove the human element—wasn't it a human hand that told the computers what to recognize as movement, and told them *not* to distinguish types of motion? Did the computers decide that dogs spinning (and that's my word choice, for remember that the authors only reported the computers' video analysis) in small cages were "traveling" or that dogs moving more slowly in larger enclosures were "pacing"? I think the authors mistook removing human stimulation of the six dogs under observation for their stated goal to minimize investigator bias.

As a veterinary clinician, I, too, have put video cameras on dogs to see how much they travel in small cages when human activity has quieted down in their environment, but with an opposite set of assumptions. On a behaviorist's advice, we used videography to help determine whether certain dogs were displaying stereotypical circling behavior, from which we would infer, regardless of what cortisol levels or T-cell measures we could have found, psychological and welfare problems that we would hope to alleviate. Seen from that perspective, the more and faster a dog traveled in a small cage with no place to go, the more welfare problem we would diagnose. And if cortisol data had failed to confirm that, then that is just one piece of evidence that cortisol levels are not a good indicator of welfare. Same data, opposite interpretation, and no computer is going to remove the human element that determines the interpretation.

Several letter writers alerted the USDA to these dog exercise studies. And though Hughes et al. (1989) had concluded both that cage size is irrelevant and human interaction deeply relevant to how much dogs exercise, the USDA had already been roundly scolded for attempting to slip socialization into its exercise regulations. Another author had made similar statements about exercise and social interaction. Michael W. Fox was a canine ethologist and one-time laboratory animal veterinarian then working for the Humane Society of the United States, one of the largest animal protection organizations lobbying on the Animal Welfare Act regulations in the late 1980s. His writings on exercise were among the small handful of more-or-less scientific materials submitted to the USDA. Ironically, though Fox self-identified as "fundamentally opposed to the use of animals in biomedical research for primarily human purposes," research advocates rather than animal protectionists used his work to bolster their cause against expanded exercise requirements (Fox 1990). Fox had written, in 1971 and again in 1986 and 1990, on the "unnaturalness" of exercise. In his 1986 book *Laboratory Animal Husbandry*, he wrote:

> Many people claim that exercise is important for animals, but animals in nature that are well-fed, warm, not afraid of predation, and not sexually frustrated do not exercise. Exercise per se is an anthropomorphic concept, an unbiological activity at variance with the law of conservation of energy. Wild animals either play with each other, by themselves, or with appropriate inanimate objects, engage in grooming or other social activities, or they sleep. No drive to exercise has been recognized by ethologists, although the basic drives to be active and explore may be anthropocentrically misinterpreted as exercise. (M. W. Fox 1986, p. 68)

He went on to propose stimulation such as social interaction rather than enforced exercise on a treadmill for caged dogs and to advocate for leash-walking and objects such as toys to explore and manipulate. At a conference in 1989, he added the quest for novelty, plenty of human contact, the ability to get distance from their own urine and feces, and the opportunity to engage in mutual care-giving behavior as other important considerations in dog housing (Fox 1990). Though Fox does little to support these claims with scientific citations, one might expect animal protectionists to seize upon them as the strongest scientific argument in favor of the enriched and enlarged housing they sought for dogs. They did not, so convinced were they that everyone knows what dogs need.

Research advocates, however, used Fox's claims to argue *against* expansive and expensive exercise regulations. The American Physiological Society (1987), for example, left out Fox's descriptions of how wild animals behave, as well as his suggestions of what dogs should get in their housing, when it wrote to tell the USDA that "exercise, per se, is neither natural nor beneficial for dogs and in some cases could be detrimental." Fox's failure to offer his own definition of exercise allowed this repackaging of his words counter to his policy preferences. Fox (1986) saw value in giving dogs "sufficient space to satisfy basic locomotor activity needs" (p. 68; whatever that phrase may mean) and believed that dogs' needs to explore, have social interactions, play, and even to get distance from their own excrement all required more space than the USDA minimum size dog cage. Rather, he seemed to be concerned with motivation to exercise for its own sake, offering comparison with the "compulsive joggers running down the street," as he declared that dogs feel no such motivation. Perhaps the fault lies with Senator Dole and the animal protectionists for choosing the word "exercise" in the first place to describe what they sought for dogs.

What dogs want and what dogs need

Without a stable definition of exercise, the decades-long controversy over how much of it dogs need dragged on.

The simplest definition is physical activity that promotes health, vigor, and physical fitness. Animal protectionists sometimes used that definition but rarely limited their concerns to physiological exercise. Rather, they spoke of dogs' psychological needs as well. The Fund for Animals and the Society Against Animal Research Abuse wrote to tell the USDA that "exercise in any species serves two purposes: (1) Maintenance of physical fitness, and (2) perhaps most importantly, an outlet for psychological stress" (Regulatory Analysis and Development 1986).

But the language of "need," whether physical or psychological, invited rebuttal in a language of pathology. If dogs need exercise that they are not currently receiving in research caging, why are laboratory animal veterinarians finding no loss of muscle mass or physical fitness; why are they reporting no behavioral stereotypies? A laboratory animal veterinarian wrote the USDA:

> I have been in laboratory animal medicine for 18 years. . . . Never, during that period of time, have I seen a need or time that dogs confined in cages of USDA minimum size or larger require any exercise outside of those cages. The dogs maintained their weight, had normal appetites, and didn't appear to be psychologically abnormal because of continuous confinement. Those investigators that did "exercise" their dogs did so to make themselves feel better. (Regulatory Analysis and Development 1989)

Another wrote:

> We are dealing with basically two distinct animals, the purposebred dog and the random source dog . . . dogs in general are very adaptable, even the random source dog will easily adjust to a cage or a run with no apparent stereotyped behavior. . . . I contend that exercise is an unproven need and the cost-benefit ratio does not correlate.[5] (Regulatory Analysis and Development 1989)

Neamand's and Hite's studies at Merck in the 1970s anticipated the shift in discourse from what dogs *need* to what dogs *want*. Both supplemented their physical and physiological examinations of dogs with time-lapse photography of dog behavior. They were not looking for behavioral needs or resultant pathology of thwarted needs, but more simply they were examining how dogs chose to spend their time. Their studies were the direct precursors of Hughes et al.'s work a decade later, which found dogs in small cages choosing to travel far and fast. Laboratory animal professionals had assured themselves through individual observation and formal study that dogs had a low level of need, either physical or psychological, for exercise. They then took canine welfare a step further, asking what dogs want, and here too, found that they did not seem to want all that much.

As the USDA was formulating its exercise regulations, most animal protectionists were demanding one-half to one hour of exercise per dog per day. By 1990, research advocates who found this excessive had convinced the USDA that "additional space provided to certain dogs would be underutilized," because of the choices dogs themselves make: "even if released into a relatively large run, many dogs will find a corner to lie down" (Animal and Plant Health Inspection Service 1990a, p. 33467).

Animal protectionists had sought to speak for dogs, but Hughes and other researchers had asked dogs, as directly as they could, what they wanted. The answers they got, that dogs were generally content to lie around unless stirred, failed to meet the protectionists' experiences and expectations of canine nature. The controversy did not close because the two camps did not share a definition of behavior or a way to observe and interpret it. The attempt of Hughes and colleagues to exclude the human element from his study of dog behavior (by resorting to computer-analyzed video images free of investigator bias) is the key to understanding the incommensurate understanding of behavioral information by the two groups.

Is behavior emitted or elicited? Is behavior what animals do when environmental influences are reduced to a minimum, or is it what they do in response to their environment? Dozens of research advocates and laboratory animal veterinarians told the USDA how dogs, left to their own devices, quickly explore a large exercise pen for ten or fifteen minutes, and then lie down. Most readily asserted that dogs act differently when people are available for interaction, but they saw this, as Hughes et al. (1984) did in formal studies, as a distraction, noise in the system, an artifact that masks what dogs *really* want, what they do when they think they're alone with no one watching. But start with the assumption that dogs are highly social by nature, intelligent and inquisitive, interactive with their social and physical environment, and it makes no more sense to study dog behavior isolated from environmental and social stimuli than it would make to study respiratory physiology without the "distractions" of oxygen and carbon dioxide.

In the sort of pop anthropomorphic anecdotal report guaranteed to make many scientists cringe, Elizabeth Marshall Thomas (1993) set off on her bicycle to find out what one dog, a husky named Misha, really wanted, and by extension, what dogs want. Confident that her constant noninteractive (at least, as far as the human eye could tell) presence ceased to influence Misha's behavior, she watched his hidden life, what he did when he assumed no human was watching. Misha did not lie down in a corner after ten minutes, but then, he was not confined to a barren eight-by-ten foot exercise pen. Rather, he covered a range of 130 square miles in Cambridge, Massachusetts, interacting with other dogs in his environment, both directly, but also through the high drama of competitive urine marking (Thomas 1993).

While researching this chapter, I watched competing notions of what dogs want. At work, on campus, I saw dogs seeming to be both well adapted to their penned lives *and* always eager for human interaction. At home, I sat with a stack of scientific studies of what dogs want, papers by Hughes and Neamand and others, leaving my Boston terrier, Freddie, to his own devices. With snow piled high outside, he spent most of his day interacting with his environment—asleep! However, he changed his resting place frequently, now seeking the sun, now lying by the wood stove, sometimes on the floor and sometimes on cushy furniture. He might seek out the company of Vito, the retired laboratory cat with whom we lived (figure 10.2). Occasionally he would watch at the window for what might be around, or solicit play from me (or was I projecting anthropomorphically?) by dropping his tennis ball in my lap. Other times, he would play with his toys by himself. Even this uneventful day at home struck me as far richer than the small solitary cages that the scientific literature seemed to support. Was I so misreading this dog whom I thought I knew, or was the science missing the significance of a spacious and varied environment?

Now, laboratory beagles are not huskies or Boston terriers; perhaps Thomas's and my anecdotal observations are irrelevant on genetic grounds. Several people sought to convince the USDA that laboratory beagles were sufficiently a breed apart as to have different, that is, lower, exercise needs. I have to disagree. I recall Dolly Griffiths and other "retired" laboratory beagles that I have placed as pets, dogs who showed as much joy and mettle as any others I have known, despite their laboratory rearing. No fence could stop Dolly from her escapades through upstate New York—so much for her purpose-bred happy-to-be-caged genes! Harry Ake's (1996) survey of 59 beagles from the University of Pennsylvania supports my experience: Most owners reported their beagles made excellent pets, though housebreaking these adult dogs took some time.

What the animal protectionists are seeking for dogs is not welfare as the absence of pathology. It is not merely the satisfaction of basic needs. They are really not impressed by how small a cage the adaptable dog will learn to live in, to settle for. They want what no legislature or regulations will give them: the richest possible life for the animals. Inclusion of exercise in the 1985 Animal Welfare Act amendment after decades of campaigning was their success, but with the focus on physiological exercise and canine behavior in a vacuum, it fell far short of what the animal protectionists sought. "Exercise" was shorthand for the wide range of activities and experiences that animal protectionists want for a dog's life—fun and social contact, affection and novelty, the busy work of marking territory, and, yes, running around; but in the law, exercise is exercise and no more.

From this perspective, it is not enough to ask dogs what they want, especially if the only alternative to a small, barren cage is a slightly larger, barren run. If dogs

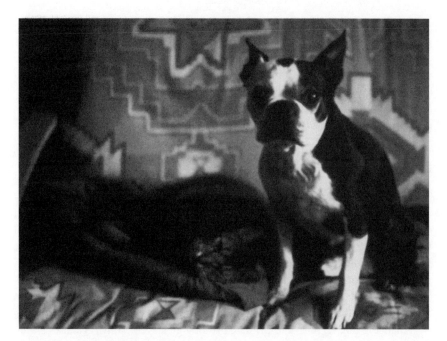

Fig. 10.2   A shelter dog and a laboratory cat, adopted as companion animals, learn a new range of options for their lives.

behave significantly differently when people are present or absent, why should we privilege videotaped data? Why is that more real than what they do in our presence? What counts is what dogs are capable of, what they can learn to enjoy, and all of the studies and observations converge on the realization that domestic dogs, our best friends, thrive in the company of people. Only rarely do the protectionists themselves depart from the language of need, but whether they realize it or not, what they are talking about is what dogs *deserve*. "Some dogs may be shy or timid," wrote one veterinarian and animal rights proponent, urging the USDA to develop strong exercise requirements, "Exercise should be encouraged in them and others by the use of toys, presence of conspecifics or positive human interaction" (Regulatory Analysis and Development 1986). The Animal Legal Defense Fund defended dogs' rights to decide how much of the opportunity for exercise to take: "If a dog has arthritis, he or she should nevertheless be afforded the opportunity for exercise, if that only means the opportunity to fully stretch limbs and walk around quietly without interference from other dogs" (Regulatory Analysis and Development 1990). How can scientific studies of how little dogs will settle for possibly undercut what we know from our lives with them of how much potential they have?

   This notion of animal welfare that goes beyond both what animals seem to need and what they seem naively to want may be part of what the philosopher Bernard Rollin (1995) is getting at when he speaks of respecting animals' *telos*, the "dogness of the dog," the "genetically based" nature of animals. "Social animals need to be with others of their kind;" he writes. "Animals built to run need to run"

(Rollin 1995, p. 159). But this formulation may overlook the plasticity of intelligent animals' behavior in its language of genetics, nature, and need. If human and canine *telos* is realized through a life of interaction and education, what do people or dogs lose when denied these goods, when they learn to accept a life of isolation and limited opportunity? And if scientific study, with its computer-driven video cameras that eliminate humanity from its observation, cannot identify this loss, perhaps it is the wrong, or an insufficient, tool for the job.

Exercise standards in the 1990s

The rest of the story is a bit of an anticlimax, at least in the policy arena. The animal protectionists never got much beyond demanding that dogs need x hours of exercise and social contact per day, sensing perhaps that the language of animal need would carry more weight with regulators. Research advocates brandished the handful of studies that showed no physical need or behavioral choice for so much activity. The story lost its drama because the new emphasis on performance standards at the end of the 1980s allowed the USDA to sidestep its uncomfortable role of adjudicating the claims of protectionists and the researchers.

Finalizing dog exercise and primate psychological well-being regulations were the USDA's last tasks after the 1985 Animal Welfare Act amendment. It published its final rule-making on February 15, 1991. The USDA reviewed the half dozen scientific reports that research advocates had sent it and decided that:

> The scientific evidence available to us now leads us to conclude that space alone is not the key to whether a dog is provided the opportunity for sufficient exercise. . . . it appears that additional space provided to certain dogs would be underutilized . . . certain dogs can receive sufficient exercise even in cages of the minimum size mandated by the regulations, if they are given the opportunity to interact with other dogs or with humans. (Animal and Plant Health Inspection Service 1990a, p. 33467)

However, the USDA disagreed that exercise would serve no useful purpose for dogs held only weeks or months, and so made no exercise exemption for them.

The USDA also listened to the federal Office of Management and Budget and others who complained that its initial proposal, with mandated group housing, human contact, and specified exercise pen dimensions and schedules, was too rigid and too expensive. Ultimately, its version of general standards by which laboratory animal veterinarians would exercise their dogs was scaled back to specifying those dogs who must be exercised (specifically, those in anything smaller than twice the minimum dog housing cage) and leaving virtually all details to the laboratory animal veterinarian and the IACUC to determine.[6] Research advocates and laboratory animal professionals debated languidly whether the institution, IACUC, or laboratory animal veterinarian was the proper determinant of the exercise program, but mostly they were relieved with the USDA's move. Animal protectionists, of course, were livid and were forced to shift their demands from particular exercise standards to trying to salvage the notion of government-mandated standards at all. The Humane Education Network urged members to write to the USDA, "the good guys," not to scrap their original half-hour exercise requirements, or to cave in to the "unholy alliance" of animal dealers, the biomedical research industry, the NIH, and the Office of Management and Budget:

> The "Unholy Alliance" has succeeded in changing this to read that each facility (many thousands of them) can write its OWN rules. No record-keeping is even required to show that exercise has been provided. There is no way they [the 63 USDA inspectors then working nationwide] can protect the animals as Congress intended, unless there are specific enforceable regulations and records to check. (Regulatory Analysis and Development 1990)

Animal protectionists charged, ultimately, in court, that these performance standards were no standards at all. A mid-1990s internal survey of the USDA's animal welfare inspectors supported this concern. While most of those participating in the survey felt that animal welfare was improving since the 1985 Animal Welfare Act amendment (more for primates than for dogs), 25% felt that the "criteria for dog exercise plans do not make clear what facilities need to do to meet them" (USDA 1996, p. 3). About 40% felt that they as inspectors found little usefulness or support in the current standards when evaluating difficult regulatory situations. This should come as no surprise when the inspectors themselves report a wide range of definitions of exercise and of methods for determining compliance (USDA 1996).

Judge Charles Richey also knew what animals want and agreed with the animal protectionists' lawsuit. Deciding in 1993 that the USDA's choice of performance standards had been arbitrary and capricious, he ordered them to write more specific standards written without delay. He wrote, "'A dog is man's best friend' is an adage the defendants have either forgotten or decided to ignore" (Labaton 1993; Richey 1993). A court of appeals, however, decided that the Animal Legal Defense Fund and its co-plaintiffs had no legal standing on which to sue (and neither would the dogs), and overturned Richey's ruling (Shalev 1994b). The flexible performance standard stands today.

The psychological well-being of monkeys and apes

In many ways, the Animal Welfare Act provision that standards should be promulgated for a physical environment that promotes the psychological well-being of primates followed the same course as the dog exercise provision. So closely linked were the two concerns that the USDA barely distinguished them in its initial 1989 rule-making proposal, just as the Animal Legal Defense Fund would link them in its 1993 lawsuit before Judge Richey four years later.

Just as the USDA had expanded dog exercise to include a mandate for social housing and human interaction, so, too, did it fold exercise into its conception of primates' psychological well-being. Its 1989 proposal included a list of enrichments (perches, swings, toys, foraging devices) and mandated housing in social groups with compatible conspecifics. For those primates who must be housed singly, the USDA required "positive physical contact or other interaction" with people and release into an exercise area (three times the area and twice the height of the minimum housing cage for the individual) "for a minimum of four hours of exercise and social interaction per week" with humans, others of their species, or with individuals of a different but compatible species. Their diet must consist of "varied food items" and even the method of feeding "must be varied daily in order to promote their psychological well-being" (Animal and Plant Health Inspection Service 1989b, pp. 10948–10949). The keen reader can readily imagine the research advocates' response to this expansive, and potentially expensive, regulatory proposal.

The primate proposal followed the same trajectory the dog exercise proposal did. The USDA recanted its extensive and detailed standards and called instead for performance standards for primate psychological well-being. In its 1990 reproposal, it required research facilities, dealers, and exhibitors to "develop, document, and follow a plan for environmental enhancement adequate to promote the psychological well-being of nonhuman primates" (Animal and Plant Health Inspection Service 1990a, p. 33525). Such plan "must be in accordance with currently accepted professional standards, as cited in appropriate professional journals or reference guides, and as directed by the attending veterinarian" (p. 33525). In other words, the plan consisted of flexible performance standards (make your own plan) with a jurisdictional component (the attending veterinarian makes the plan) embedded in it (Animal and Plant Health Inspection Service 1990a, p. 33525).

In the spirit of more flexible performance standards, the USDA replaced mandatory social housing with the requirement that the plan "include specific provisions to address the social needs of nonhuman primates known to exist in social groups in nature" (p. 33525). The four hours of mandated exercise were dropped. So was the mandated daily variety in food and food presentation, demoted to one of the approaches to environmental enrichment among which primate facilities might choose.

On the other hand, some specific provisions remained intact, though always, in research facilities, with the dual provisos that the IACUC could allow research needs to supersede welfare considerations when necessary, and the veterinarian could alter standards on behalf of an animal's health. The USDA continued to prohibit more than twelve consecutive hours in a primate restraint chair without an hour of unrestrained exercise. And it continued its broadly worded requirement that "the physical environment in the primary enclosures must be enriched by providing means of expressing noninjurious species-typical activities" (Animal and Plant Health Inspection Service 1990a, p. 33525).

So dogs and monkeys had a lot in common in the late 1980s: both were singled out for special treatment in the 1985 Animal Welfare Act amendment, and both were subjects of expanded and detailed regulatory proposals in 1989 that later gave way to flexible performance standards. The same people who argued for getting dogs out of the cages as much as possible had the same agenda for primates, while those defending institutional flexibility and less rigid standards for dogs made the same case for primates. The same people who argued that the USDA's canine mandate was limited to exercise for dogs (not socialization, play, or happiness) argued that the primate mandate was limited to a physical environment to promote psychological well-being (not social interaction, physical contact, or exercise), but devoted little effort to sustaining this legalistic move.

The striking difference between the dog and monkey debates is in the deployment of expertise in the two different cases. While people debated what the expert information on dogs is, they debated who the experts on primates were.

Scientists and veterinarians had faced an uphill battle in trying to refute what "everyone knows" about dogs, with their evident joy in running and playing. Their strategy was to cite specific studies and experiences that showed dogs' disinterest and lack of need for out-of-cage exercise. But animal protectionists were on shakier ground with what "everyone knows" about monkeys and apes and relied more on a strategy of calling for real primate experts to counter the assertions of the professionals—laboratory animal veterinarians, comparative psychologists—who work with them in laboratories. The response was not so much to cite specific studies and data as to argue, sometimes together and sometimes against each other, that scientists and laboratory animal veterinarians indeed had all the necessary expertise.

The primate case is confounded by its complexity. "Psychological well-being" was every bit a term in need of definition as "exercise" ever was, but was a bit further removed from common parlance and common experience. The USDA steadfastly refused to list a statutory definition of either term among the dozens of definitions it provides (such as *animal, cat, pet animal, positive physical contact, business hours, major operative experiment* and others), stating: "We believe the standard dictionary meanings of the two words [exercise and socialization] would be sufficient in complying with the regulations" (Animal and Plant Health Inspection Service 1990a, p. 33470) and "what actually constitutes psychological well-being in each species and each primate, however, is difficult to define. As an agency, we are mandated by Congress to establish standards to promote the psychological well-being of nonhuman primates, even though there is disagreements [*sic*] as to the meaning of the term and how best to achieve it" (Animal and Plant Health Inspection Service 1990a, p. 33496).

However, it is not simply that psychological well-being is a complex concept, but that primates are a complex and varied group. Though occasionally I hear mention of the "six species" identified by Congress for Animal Welfare Act coverage, in fact, the order Primates comprises several dozen very different animals.[7] I have mentioned chimpanzees, marmosets, and baboons as some of the widely varying primates. Several commenters and the USDA felt that brachiating species (animals like gibbons and spider monkeys whose locomotion includes swinging by the arms) were significantly different in their space utilization from other primate groups as to warrant special consideration. Even within a single genus, the genus *Macaca* familiar to researchers and zoo goers, including the rhesus monkeys, crab-eating macaques, Japanese snow monkeys, and others, there can be a wide range of sizes, temperaments, and behaviors. Could the USDA write specific psychological well-being standards that fit all of these varied animals, or must they elaborate a lengthy document defining standards separately for each species? Imagine the relief at being able to define a performance standard—in essence, that IACUCs and laboratory animal veterinarians develop their own psychological well-being plan—even if it might come back to haunt the USDA inspectors as largely unenforceable.

Reflecting the complexity of the animals and of the concept of psychological well-being, the database on primates is voluminous and complex. Just as the USDA's early 1970s and late 1980s proposals to set standards for dog exercise were accompanied by small flurries of published studies on (or, for the most part, against) dog exercise, so, too, does most of the literature on primate psychological well-being date only from the mid-1980s. Individual reports as well as review articles, symposia, and doctoral dissertations on the topic proliferated. As with much of the dog exercise and other animal welfare science reports, most of these quite explicitly set aside the scientists' ideal of impartiality or objectivity and site their work squarely in its political context. For example, a 1989 scientific literature review in *Life Sciences* described the cost of new regulations, the authors' concern that USDA regulations would be useless and damaging, and their major conclusion—too late, they feared—that there was "little or no scientific justification for changing current regulations" and that "anthropomorphic guesses" were threatening to upstage "observable, objective, and quantifiable" behavioral measurements of psychological well-being (Woolverton et al. 1989, pp. 913, 913, 903).

Who knows what about monkeys?

Dogs may be our best friends, but monkeys and apes are our closest living relatives. As such, they are popular research animals, though the expense and difficulty of keeping them has always kept their numbers in the laboratory relatively low. For Westerners, however, they are distant relatives, in terms of geography if nothing else. Monkeys live side by side with people over most of the globe, but for Americans, they are exotic. We see them in zoos or on television programs, but few of us have enough contact with them to break through the media stereotypes. Whether we view them as loveable and comical caricatures of ourselves or as fiercely intelligent foreigners, they are as much outside of Americans' daily experience as dogs are inside.

Whether through pity or respect, popular support for monkey welfare ran high. Nearly 5000 of the USDA's 36,000 public comments on its proposed regulations were signatures on a survey of people in Philadelphia's Rittenhouse Square (conducted by Bernard Migler, president of Primate Pole Housing Inc., a commercial supplier of monkey caging) asserting the need for taller primate cages (Regulatory Analysis and Development 1990). Another 3500 were signed postcards that the Animal Legal Defense Fund had collected, protesting the USDA's "failure to protect chimpanzees from painful laboratory research of dubious scientific value," and urging the Secretary of Agriculture to quickly finalize Animal Welfare Act regulations to "help protect these gentle and intelligent creatures" (Regulatory Analysis and Development 1989). But these petitions could not write the specific regulations for animal care; that is where the competition to speak as experts on the primates behalf comes in.

Once performance standards became the buzzword halfway through the USDA's rule-writing exercises of the late 1980s, the monkey debates focused almost exclusively on locating, defining, and defending expertise. The USDA had proposed that laboratory animal veterinarians write their own in-house psychological well-being plans, and, for the most part, the veterinarians liked that idea. Many scientists did not and wanted to see other experts vested with authority instead, while animal protectionists believed that a national committee of primate experts should write the rules, and even come in on a case-by-case basis to evaluate variances and exemptions.

So focused was this debate on experts and authority that I have had difficulty divining in the public record just what rules each of these constituencies would enact, like an election campaign in which the issues are hidden behind the personalities.

As a group, the laboratory animal veterinarians' plans were the most clearly identifiable, though I find little consensus among them in their letters to the USDA beyond their call for freedom of professional judgment. Many articulated their fears of infection and aggression among group-housed primates just as they had for dogs. Wild-caught monkeys are comparable to random-source dogs and similarly outnumbered their purpose-bred relatives in the formative years of laboratory animal medicine. Taken from the plains and jungles of Africa, Asia, or Latin America, they carry an impressive array of parasites and infections. For most species, mixing unfamiliar adults can quickly elicit life-threatening aggression. Specialized caging and handling is required to prevent human injury as well. The argument for single caging in small, sanitizable steel containers was at least as strong for monkeys as it was for dogs.

Many laboratory animal veterinarians saw a need to defend their priorities of hygiene and safety against intrusions from the USDA and animal protectionists, with their free-for-all plans for group exercise pens and human playtime. The threats to order were not all external, however, for their own investigators, the scientists whose research animals they managed, were problematic too. One laboratory animal veterinarian wrote: Some primate behaviorists and psychologists resist all efforts to have a clean, rodent and roach free environment. . . . It is stated that 10 non-human primate experts were selected [to advise the USDA]. It is apparent that those selected were not veterinarians who have the responsibility for attending to traumas, diarrheas, infectious diseases . . . sanitation, vermin, and pest control. . . . Those without knowledge or experience in crucial areas were excluded or their advice ignored (Regulatory Analysis and Development 1990).[8]

The Association of Primate Veterinarians (APV) likewise tried to rein in the USDA's proposals, though without disparaging scientists in the process. Citing the combined experience of this organization of 200 veterinarians and reference to a small handful of scientific studies, the APV urged the USDA to scale back its proposals for larger cages for baboons and chimps, for exercise, mandatory dietary variety, and especially, physical contact with humans, fraught as it is with the potential for spread of zoonotic infections from which primate keepers have died, and from the billion dollar price tag on the new rules. The APV extolled social interaction (for social species) but not mandatory social housing (like many in the field, it believed that monkeys have extensive social interaction even when singly caged in a room), increased complexity in cages (judicious use of toys, perches, and visual barriers) and other enrichments. It noted the wide diversity of primates in its case against the USDA's proposed standards, even as it cited studies of rhesus monkeys for its claims that adult primates choose toys over exercise or that larger cages can be harmful. Its bottom line was that the USDA should tap into the expertise it was offering: at the national level, by using the APV's expertise in writing regulations, and at the local level, by embracing performance-oriented standards for the professional judgment of veterinarians and IACUCs (Regulatory Analysis and Development 1989).

Efforts to empower veterinarians met resistance from scientists and from animal protectionists, as this 1989 letter from a neurobiology and physiology professor illustrates, in his criticism of

> the creation of a veterinary specialty, monkey psychiatry, to treat "signs of psychological distress . . . to prevent the development of psychological disorders"? This fanciful speculation on the mental well-being of monkeys is absolutely bizarre. . . . On top of this imaginative attribution of human mental capacities to animals, the regulations then go on to set up the veterinarian as a god in this fictive world, all-knowledgeable, above the scientist or medical practitioner. (Regulatory Analysis and Development 1989)

Animal protectionists and scientists often had opposing priorities for primate care. They shared the conviction, however, that veterinarians simply did not know enough about primate behavior to carry such authority. The American Psychological Association (APA) was clear on this in its letters to the USDA:

> If decisions are to be based upon "observation" of the animals during a brief visit by the veterinarian, the important influence of the observer in modifying the primate's behavior is overlooked, thereby limiting the value of data obtained by such informal observation. . . . Veterinary contact with nondiseased primates is normally very limited, making it difficult for them to assess subtle behavioral changes over time. (Regulatory Analysis and Development 1989)

The solution?

> Since the expertise in animal behavior lies with animal psychologists, we recommend a requirement that institutions consult with a behavioral

primatologist when evaluating the psychological well-being of nonhuman primates . . . a member of the American Society of Primatologists, the International Primatological Society, and/or the American Psychological Association. (Regulatory Analysis and Development 1989)

The APA points out *why* veterinarians get it wrong—lack of training in animal behavior, insufficient time for formal observation of animals—but never *how*. What specific policies would veterinarians institute that the APA would find so objectionable? Since the APA defended the use of primate restraint chairs and solitary caging, it is surely not the veterinarians' old reliance on solitary caging as the antidote to contagion and violence that rankled it.

The response of animal protectionists to veterinarian-empowering performance standards was virtually indistinguishable from the response of the APA. The Animal Legal Defense Fund, not the APA, wrote to the USDA:

The exemptions [to USDA minimum standards] for primates allow a veterinarian, trained in physiology, to make a determination in regard to the species-typical behavior or the psychological well-being of a primate. This is most inappropriate and it makes as much sense as hiring a plumber to install the electrical wiring. . . . Decisions . . . should be left to experts in *primate behavior,* such as ethologists or behavioral comparative psychologists who have expertise with regard to the particular species at hand. (Regulatory Analysis and Development 1990 [emphasis in original])

The Animal Legal Defense Fund would not empower the laboratory animal veterinarian, whose "allegiance is to the facility not the animal," but rather USDA "veterinarians, who are impartial, objective and charged with promoting animal welfare should determine what factors in a physical environment are needed to promote the psychological well-being of primates." Others echoed this concern, pointing out that veterinary colleges provide little or no training in either primate care or in animal behavior (Regulatory Analysis and Development 1990).

Animal protectionists called for mandatory consultation with experts, but probably not the comparative laboratory psychologists that the APA might enlist. Just as research advocates had used animal rights proponent Michael Fox's (1986) words (with his quote that contented dogs do not engage in exercise) to argue against exercise requirements for dogs, so, too, did animal protectionists seize on a statement they attributed to neuroscientist (and then Yerkes Primate Center's director) Frederick King: "We don't know what makes primates happy" (Regulatory Analysis and Development 1990). While King surely meant that *none* of us know what makes primates happy (and therefore, none of us has a basis for regulation), protectionists quickly concluded that King and the other experts did not know and so must have the decision of how to treat primates taken out of their hands.

When animal protectionists called for enlistment of primate experts, they were often quite clear on who would meet their criteria. "Only *field* primatologists, and those who have observed adequately primates in their wild environments can comment knowledgeably on what constitutes enriched and enhanced housing for nonhuman primates," wrote the Association of Veterinarians for Animal Rights in 1990 (Regulatory Analysis and Development 1990 [emphasis in the original]). The famed chimpanzee specialist Dr. Jane Goodall was most frequently mentioned as the paradigm of such an expert.

But what does a person who has spent her life in the field studying presumably normal animals know about normal or abnormal responses to captive care? Possibly very little. A laboratory animal veterinarian wrote in 1989: "Housing and other requirements based upon what pet owners say they should be, Jane Goodall says they should be based upon observation of wild chimps in Africa, or what zoos say they should be are frequently incompatible with what the scientific community and veterinarians trained and/or experienced in the specialty of laboratory animal medicine would say they should be" (Regulatory Analysis and Development 1989).

What does an ethologist like Goodall know about infection control, medical research procedures, or even adaptation to a 25-square-foot cage? Does her intimate familiarity with normal free-living chimpanzees give her any insight into how to help animals cope with caging and isolation?

Goodall's nomination for the role reflects the common assumption among animal protectionists that *natural* equals *good*. As countless critics have pointed out, natural may not be entirely benign, especially for bottom-ranking individuals, who may get the least food and the most bullying in times of stress (Rosenblum and Andrews 1995). "Natural" can include vagaries of weather and of food availability; it can include predation and rates of infection, disease, and mortality that no primate center or zoo would find acceptable.

Even in the attempt to provide animals just the good parts of nature, condensing primate care into the laboratory requires some selection (for space, for financial and research considerations) of which features of nature to bring in with the animals. In some species, low-ranking animals choose to be near the group, but on the periphery, with plenty of chance to escape from aggressors. In a restricted environment, "near" may not be an option: The animals can live in pairs or groups or in solitary cages.

In interviews with laboratory primate veterinarians, I learned some of the small tricks, the craft knowledge, of captive monkey management, things that an ethologist might never learn studying animals in the wild. It is not enough, for instance, to put barrels in a pen into which low-ranking monkeys can scurry when attacked (not that monkeys in the wild have barrels available); there must be an anchored bar inside the barrel for the monkey to grab, lest the aggressor simply pull him out of the barrel and continue the attack (Henrickson 1995). Primate behaviorist/veterinarian Viktor Reinhardt (1990, 1994) has written extensively on strategies for pairing macaque monkeys in small cages; pairing a young juvenile with a previously solitary adult may seem unnatural and even dangerous, yet he reports a low incidence of violence and a high incidence of "species-typical" behaviors. This is precisely the sort of trial-and-error learning about monkeys that proponents of flexible standards extol, and it has very little to do with knowing what's natural about monkeys.

Dogs and monkeys: Divergent tracks

Exercise for dogs and psychological well-being for nonhuman primates went on opposite trajectories once the USDA finalized its regulations in 1991. Research into dog exercise ended (research for dog welfare, not as a model of human exercise physiology), and there are no primary studies of dog exercise in the laboratory animal literature after 1991. Not only had consensus been reached that social interaction was important to dogs in ways that increased cage size did not seem to be, but the USDA's low requirements for exercise programs were easy enough for research facilities to reach, making further research to refute them unnecessary. Dogs must be in pretty small cages for the USDA's requirement for supplemental exercise to apply, and merely taking them out to run around—on the floor, in a pen—while their cage is being cleaned can easily meet a facility's obligation to develop an exercise plan. In fact, that may be all Senator Dole envisioned with his amendment in the first place, a chance to get out of their small cages once a day or so and stretch their legs for a bit (Melcher 1991).

Nor did exercise beome a concern for other species. A few people told the USDA in the 1980s that cats needed exercise too. The USDA neither believed that about cats, nor felt it had the congressional mandate to enact it. Even the handful of studies now coming out of Europe suggesting that lack of exercise in American-sized rabbit cages may result in osteoporosis or other physical pathologies have failed to find much of an American audience (Drescher and Loeffler 1991; Gunn and Morton 1993; Kalagassy et al. 1999). The case is pretty much closed on exercise, but not on environmental enrichment or primate psychological well-being.

Primate psychological well-being has grown and become mainstreamed as a professional field of study since the mid-1980s. Conferences have been held and research studies and reviews published (Segal 1989; Woolverton et al. 1989). The National Academy of Science's Institute for Laboratory Animal Research, whose handbooks on laboratory management of primates in 1968 and 1973 contained not a whisper about welfare, well-being, or environmental enrichment, has recently published a 160-page book on the subject (Committee on Well-Being of Nonhuman Primates 1998; Subcommittee on Primate Standards 1968; Subcommittee on Revision of Nonhuman Primate Standards 1973). Similarly, laboratory animal medicine texts in the 1970s glossed over the issue, or relegated it to concern mainly if it might affect animal behavior during psychological studies; now psychological well-being gets its own chapter in the American College of Laboratory Animal Medicine's text on primate medicine and care (Keeling 1974; Rosenblum and Andrews 1995; Whitney et al. 1973). A busy Primate Enrichment Forum, hosted by the Wisconsin Regional Primate Center, fosters on-line communication among zoo and laboratory workers, and laboratory animal and primatology journals continue to publish primary studies of primate enrichment and psychological well-being (Boinski et al. 1999; Crockett et al. 2000; Martin et al. 2002; Schapiro 2002). The USDA even published its own detailed summary of environmental enrichment for primates, though its initial plans for 29 species-specific appendixes has stalled, with detailed information provided only for spider monkeys and brown capuchin monkeys (Animal and Plant Health Inspection Service 1999b).

The 1985 law for a physical environment that promotes the psychological well-being of primates has clearly spurred the drive to develop and to professionalize this expert knowledge. And the drive has been multidisciplinary, with the APA, laboratory animal veterinarians, and animal protectionists at the Animal Welfare Institute all contributing. Zoo professionals have spawned a newsletter, *The Shape of Enrichment*, one early hallmark of a budding new profession. Beyond the monkeys, this concern for enriched environments has trickled down to other laboratory species as well, including rodents, frogs, birds, and most others.[9]

Human primates interested in the psychological well-being of their wild cousins now face an information overload, but how much of this really affects the lives of laboratory monkeys? Answering that question will take vigilance and vigor, critical distance and healthy skepticism—and may all of that pay off with the best possible answer for the animals. Concerns are not restricted to primate psychological well-being but to animal welfare generally. Philosophical challenges remain: how to define welfare and well-being, for instance. The philosophical challenges are intimately related to professional boundaries and competition, such as when applied ethologists (as good a name for the emerging profession of behavior-focused animal welfare specialists as any) challenge the inclination of veterinarians and stress physiologists to define welfare as simply the absence of pathology (Fraser 1995; Mench 1994). Is "well-being" a neutral condition, the absence of psychopathology, or is it something larger, such as the animals' ability to maximize their potential?

At present, skeptical outsiders have little chance to see whether the vibrant exchange of ideas and information reflects similar vibrancy in the animal quarters. The first question: are people treating their monkeys and other animals differently now that providing for their psychological well-being is the law? Anecdotally, I know that they are. Many campuses now have an environmental enrichment staff who make the rounds providing toys for the cats and monkeys, take the dogs out for walks, and distribute nesting material for the mice. Quantitative assessments are harder to come by: Are all animals recipients of these efforts? Do all campuses have enrichment staffs or enrichment programs? Before-and-after assessments are even more elusive. Though the USDA shut down its on-line Freedom of Information access to inspection reports almost as soon as it had started it, reports are still available with enough effort. But the USDA was not commenting on inspections on psychological well-being before the law went into effect, so older inspection reports would not even touch on this.

The regulations have indeed changed human behavior. Monkeys are now housed in pairs, for instance, in situations where they would never have been in

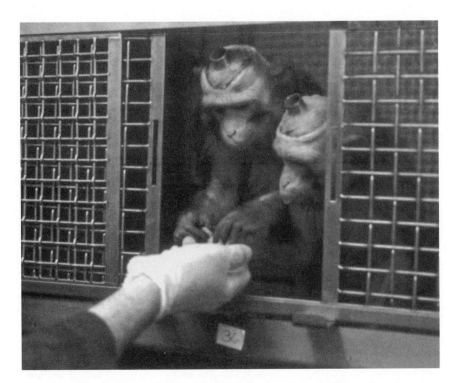

Fig. 10.3   With patience and training, monkeys can be pair-housed even when they are on study and can learn to cooperate with research procedures. COURTESY OF VIKTOR REINHARDT.

the past. Behaviorist Viktor Reinhardt has developed techniques for pair-housing monkeys even after they have had electrode implants placed (figure 10.3). Monkeys like this can cost several thousands of dollars to purchase and maintain, and the electrode surgeries represent many hours of delicate work. How many scientists would risk their animals' safety and their research usefulness in this pursuit of animal sociality, were the USDA inspector not demanding to see results?

But the important question, of course, is not whether people are thinking and doing new things, but whether the animals are actually happier now in research laboratories than they were fifteen years ago. Can an inspector look at these animals and their records for ten minutes once or twice a year and make that determination? Is it really that simple? Are both animals in the pair happier than they would be living solo, or is one animal there at the expense of the other? If there is an occasional spat, and blood is drawn, does that mean they're better off alone?

There is much we do not know about animals and their welfare. Systematic scientific studies of animals can supplement and correct common-sense approaches to animals, that anthropomorphic "How might I feel if I were this animal in this cage, in this experiment?" But scientific studies and the people who wield them are not innocent, objective, neutral bystanders, and they must not be given more authority than they warrant. Sometimes common sense must serve as the corrective to science. Systematic observation of how much attention monkeys pay to various treats, toys, and enrichments have a place in learning how best to care for the animals we have subjected to our science, but when videotapes of six dogs spinning and traveling in their small cages can shape public policy, something is amiss.

The information gaps leave plenty of space in which scientists and veterinarians and animal caregivers and animal protectionists and government officials all vie to speak for what animals want. The challenge is charting the humane course—humane to the animals in laboratories and to the people who need what the laboratories produce—in the face of our uncertainty.

11

SOMEDAY, ANIMAL EXPERIMENTATION WILL COME TO AN END. I WOULD LIKE TO live to see that day.

A hundred years from now, people may look back with dread at the way we now treat animals and will see a book such as this one as an exercise in denial, a hollow apologetic, meaningless platitudes. I have presided over the deaths of thousands of laboratory animals and have seen more pain and suffering than I care to recall, yet I make no call to stop animal experimentation now, only to make it better.

But animal research cannot continue for much longer. It may end, as American slavery did, because of shifting political and ethical vicissitudes. It may end, as hand-setting type did, as the technology becomes obsolete. Most likely the two will reinforce each other. Morality and politics will continue to spur the search for replacement technologies. Technological advances will strengthen the moral arguments against animal use. These dual processes are already in progress.

In the short term, animal numbers will continue to increase, but not uniformly. Mice, rats, and other small animals (e.g., zebrafish) have "job security" for several reasons (figure 11.1). First, they are easily genetically modified, either by removing one or more of their native genes ("knock-out" animals) or by inserting one or more genes from humans, other rodents, or even fireflies and jellyfish.[1] Second, as with computers, technological advances have allowed the miniaturization of many animal research projects: microsurgical instruments and assays that require minute microliter blood samples now allow mice and rats to replace dogs, cats, sheep, and rabbits for many uses. Third, rodents and fish lack the political capital and public concern that larger mammals have; their exclusion from Animal Welfare Act coverage is itself sufficient to push many research institutions to deal exclusively in rodents and "lower" animals.

As small rodents ascend and large animals such as dogs become scarcer in laboratories, primates alone will buck the trend. Despite their cost, scarcity, and the health and safety risks in working with monkeys, their place in the lab is assured by their close phylogenetic relationship to people. But their numbers, too, will decline. Monkeys will only get more expensive to purchase and house, and the regulations governing their use will be more stringently enforced. Public unease about the ethics of experimenting on monkeys and apes is likely to grow as well. And

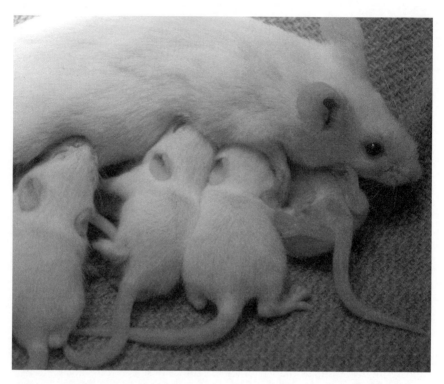

Fig. 11.1 The future of laboratory animal care is mouse medicine. A mother mouse tends her litter.

here, too, technology will reinforce the political, ethical, and economic incentives to move from primate studies. Transgenic mice carrying a host of human genes or receiving human bone marrow or stem cells will be more similar to humans in some important ways even than our closest kin, the chimpanzees.

For the rest of my career in laboratory animal medicine, laboratory animal veterinarians will be mostly mouse and monkey doctors. For this book, I have studied the scientists who study animals and the veterinarians and animal protectionists who want to tell them what to do. In the process, I have refined my own agenda and concerns for how we should respect what animals want. Throughout these pages, I've illustrated these lessons—how I learned them, what they signify. This is my summary of what I have learned, and my guide to how we can improve animals' lives in the laboratory.

Animal welfare must be seen as more than the absence of suffering

There is so much potential for animal suffering in the laboratory. Those of us who work with animals sometimes find comfort just in successfully blocking the pain. Veterinarians examine animals for signs of pain and for physical health. Animal behavior specialists go beyond this, through observation of spontaneous animal behavior and through laboratory experiments in which animals demonstrate their preferences. These are sophisticated experiments, and their results are subject to a range of interpretation; no single study can result in policy prescriptions. What does it mean when we find guinea pigs lined up together along a wall for several hours a day? Does it mean we can take away the less-used space in the cage? That we must provide them more walls and corners for huddling? Do we need to know more about what they do in different areas of the cage, how hard they would work to get the chance to huddle together? Studies of dogs must account for their behavioral plasticity. If they can learn to live in small cages without distress, have we done our best by them? If they can learn to expect a life of companionship and novelty and fun and exploration, do we harm them by denying them that glimpse of a better life? I think we do. As I've argued throughout this book, animal welfare is bigger and more complicated than simply keeping animals fed, free of infections, free of pain, free of pathology—something best described by words like "fun," "happy," "fulfilled," and "thriving." Mice are overwhelmingly the laboratory animal of the future and are just as amenable to the study of their wants and their potential as are dogs and guinea pigs.

Individual animals must count

Inbred white mice are all but indistinguishable, huddled together in their cage. Genetically near-identical and raised in the same environment, they have little individuality to the human observer. But they can indeed have different life experiences. For whatever reason, one will outrank another in the cage, and life as a winner can differ radically from life as a loser. Moreover, they will respond differently to what humans do to them (handling, experimental procedures, euthanasia methods), if only because humans can only be standardized so far. As our animal wards become increasingly identical (mice *will* be cloned from each other in great numbers in the near future) the challenge is even greater to assess how each animal in a cohort is responding to the experiment and how each can be treated to minimize pain and distress. Veterinarians are trained to treat animals both as populations (herds, flocks, gaggles, etc.) and as individual patients. They can take the lead in keeping the focus on individuals when it's needed.

Legal protections matter and should be extended

The Animal Welfare Act excludes the majority of American laboratory animals from its protections. It is true that in some states, a state veterinarian inspects the rats, mice, and others excluded from federal protections. And on those campuses that seek voluntary accreditation, site visitors from the Association for the Assessment and Accreditation of Laboratory Animal Care look in on the rodents every three years. On the rest of the campuses, however, self-reporting is the strongest oversight of rat and mouse care, and not all campuses are even required to self-report. This is not sufficient oversight. Animal Welfare Act inspections can be vexing when inspectors fixate on regulatory minutiae that have no impact on animal welfare. But the inspectors are learning, and the inspection process has room for flexibility and for addressing realistic concerns. Lessons learned from inspections of monkeys and even hamsters do not necessarily trickle down; as long as campus IACUCs and administrators have the luxury of distinguishing regulated species from the others, they have the luxury of deciding some welfare rules simply do not apply to mice and rats.

Mice and rats and, yes, birds and frogs and fish deserve this level of federal oversight.

Death should be seen as a serious harm to animals

I may be alone among laboratory animal professionals in the belief that animal death is a harm to be avoided, but I don't think so. Death is preferable to serious, untreatable pain, and when our experiments cannot exclude all possibility of pain, euthanasia is an important welfare safeguard. It is the ultimate opiate for refractory pain. But while it is preferable to intractable pain, death is not welfare neutral, at least, not for those animals (all mammals and birds?) possessed of a certain degree of consciousness. Most primate scientists know this, and if their work must include killing animals, they take the time to see who else can use the animal tissues that will be available. Killing a monkey is a significant event, one not taken lightly.[2] I have also known scientists to develop studies and classroom exercises around the potential to leave healthy, intact, well-trained dogs and cats ready to be placed as pets. When individual animal lives are invested with this much gravity (or even sanctity), scientists rise to the occasion. I would have deaths of mice, rabbits, and frogs invested with similar care.

Not all ethical questions have technical fixes

Those of us trained in the sciences look first at how we can fix things, and often we are successful. We can avoid deep questions about causing pain to animals when we know we're doing our best to develop less painful techniques and to develop the best painkillers. It is the technical expertise of scientists, not the goading of animal protectionists, that has made it possible to produce monoclonal antibodies in tissue culture flasks instead of in distended mouse abdomens. Veterinarian and information specialist Ken Boschert, for instance, has earned my deepest respect for developing a worldwide Internet forum of laboratory animal specialists. On it, more than 2000 veterinarians, scientists, technicians, and others vibrantly exchange information and experiences in fine-tuning and refining animal experiments. If I want expert advice and anecdotal experiences on the best painkillers for a particular type of monkey surgery, I post my question and within a day receive a wealth of information.

Expertise and technology have their limits, though, and cannot answer the value questions embedded in most animal welfare assessments. Not all pain or distress is currently treatable with drugs, for instance. What level of pain calls for terminating an experiment? Do we have any right to conduct experiments that could cause untreatable pain? What trade-offs in hygiene and safety are justified by our desire to house monkeys in social groups? And what do we do when the technology or knowledge might someday meet the animals' needs, but has not gotten there yet? How do we proceed in our animal use when the experts have not found agreement on the welfare impacts of different research methods? How do I kill mice or rats when the science of evaluating the painfulness (or painlessness) of decapitation, carbon dioxide inhalation, and cervical dislocation remains controversial among the experts? In the face of uncertainty, where do we place the benefit of the doubt?

Veterinarians can and should be animal advocates

As I have stated earlier, work as a laboratory animal veterinarian has convinced me of the enormous potential of that profession to be the strongest possible in-house advocates for research animals; I will not drop my conviction that this is what laboratory animal veterinarians should strive to be. They *should* have the best combination of institutional authority, daily contact with animals and animal caregivers, high level professional knowledge, clinical focus on the experiences of individual patients, and personal commitment for that role, and they *should* do everything in their power to minimize any conflicts with that role.

Political, social, professional, and philosophical factors have shaped this advocacy potential and must be reckoned with. Veterinarians have been allowed their place in the halls of science for good and bad reasons. Our job as veterinarians is to watch out for animal health and welfare; that's a good reason to be there. Conscripted to the politics of keeping animal protection agendas at bay, we risk compromising our professional commitments; that is not so good. Veterinarians swear an oath to relieve animal suffering, but the oath is conflicted. We swear also to promote public health and to benefit society: does that mean political advocacy to promote biomedical research, even at the cost of animal welfare?[3]

Veterinarians cannot be the sole advocates for animals. Scientists must design their studies to minimize the welfare costs to animals; technicians who most closely work with the animals must be empowered to speak up for them; IACUC members must carefully review every proposed use of animals and every ongoing use of animals; protectionists and watchdog groups must keep up their pressures to hold animal research to the highest standards and to public scrutiny.

Moreover, we must be careful about defining advocacy in a meaningful way in a setting in which animals are routinely injected, infected, irradiated, and killed, in which their bodies are invaded by surgery, and in which even their very genes are manipulated. No scientist I know wants to think of himself or herself as someone

244 WHAT ANIMALS WANT

who callously inflicts pain with no regard to the animals. But the choice to argue animal pain away with fancy theory and language or to roll up our sleeves to really improve procedures, no matter the cost or inconvenience, will have real impacts on those animals. Because we are working to refine rather than abolish animal research, we must never rest too comfortably with the balance we've struck at any particular moment. Good animal care and good science do *not* always go hand in hand; working together as animal advocates, we must pledge that when conflicts arise, good science cannot always override good animal care.

We need to respect the many ways of knowing about animals

Who will speak for animals and what they want? Everyone. Everyone has some idea what animals think, want, feel, suffer, know, enjoy, hate, fear, or long for. We variously speak for animals, for our own version of animals, because we are animals, we watch animals, we study animals, we heal animals, we live with animals, we hunt animals, we love animals, we fear animals.

Scientific studies of animals are valuable as a corrective to the limits of common-sense observation and assumptions. If scientific studies had no human lens, perhaps we could leave it at that: out with superstition and anecdote, in with unbiased science. If computerized videography of dogs truly yielded unimpeachable data on what dogs want, how helpful that might be. But scientific data are not stone tablets handed down from on high; they are gathered by human hands, shaped by human hands and interpreted through thick lenses of theory and ideology. Human scientists cannot invent a "human-free" way to know animals; it is disingenuous to pretend we can. The corrective? Common sense, anecdotal observation, empathy, and imagination all serve to balance what we learn from scientific studies.

Some versions of knowing what animals want are surely more correct than others. Trouble is, we don't always know which ones. And so I argue to respect a plurality of voices, to recognize some strengths and weaknesses of every word we put in animals' mouths. Speaking for animals is a blend of knowledge and advocacy, expertise and authority, worthy of our most serious concern.

AAALAC   Association for the Assessment and Accreditation of Laboratory Animal Care. The only organization recognized by the NIH to accredit animal research facilities.

AALAS   American Association for Laboratory Animal Science, an organization of laboratory animal professionals and scientists (originally the Animal Care Panel, formed in 1950)

ACLAM   American College of Laboratory Animal Medicine, the organization that certifies veterinarians as specialists in laboratory animal medicine

ALDF   The Animal Legal Defense Fund, a legal advocacy and animal protectionist organization

analgesic   A drug that decreases pain

anesthetic   A drug that decreases sensation, with or without general unconsciousness

Animal Care Panel   Formed in 1950; renamed AALAS in the 1960s

animal protectionist   My inclusive term for members of animal rights, animal welfare, and/or antivivisection organizations

anthropomorphism   Attributing human characteristics (correctly or incorrectly) to nonhuman animals

antivivisectionist   A person who advocates abolition of animal research

APA   The American Psychological Association

APHIS   The Animal and Plant Health Inspection Service, a division of the USDA with responsibility for Animal Welfare Act enforcement (formerly called the Animal and Plant Health Service)

AVMA   The American Veterinary Medical Association

AWI   The Animal Welfare Institute, an animal protection organization founded in 1950; its lobbying wing is the Society for Animal Protective Legislation

cervical dislocation   A method of killing very small animals (without using euthanasia drugs) by stretching the neck beyond its natural extension and thus severing the spinal cord

Draize test   Standardized ocular or skin contact toxicity test, in which test substances are applied to restrained rabbits' eyes or skin and the reaction and damage scored

engineering standards   Regulations that define means rather than outcomes. Example: dogs under 15 kg receive 8 ft^2 of cage floor; contrast "performance standards."

environmental enrichment Provision of toys, companions, or other items that provide caged animals more opportunities to engage in a range of activities than if they were housed in a barren cage or enclosure

euthanasia Killing an animal with minimum pain or distress, regardless of the reason for killing the animal

***Guide*; NIH *Guide*.** *Guide for the Care and Use of Laboratory Animals* (originally the *Guide for Laboratory Animal Facilities and Care*). Published in 1963 (by the Animal Care Panel), 1965, 1968, 1972, 1978, 1985 (by NIH), and 1996 (by ILAR).

HREA Health Research Extension Act of 1985, Public Law 99-158, which authorizes continued funding of the NIH with mandates for humane laboratory animal care and use

IACUC Institutional Animal Care and Use Committee; IACUCs oversee animal care and use on most campuses

ILAR Institute for Laboratory Animal Research (originally Institute of Laboratory Animal Resources), a unit of the National Academy of Sciences National Research Council, a nongovernmental science advisory organization

Improved Standards for Laboratory Animals Public Law 99–198, the 1985 amendment of the Animal Welfare Act

laboratory animal professional Laboratory animal veterinarians, animal care staff, technicians, and others involved in laboratory animal care

laboratory animal veterinarian A veterinarian who oversees care of research animals for a research institution

Laboratory Animal Welfare Act (LAWA) The initial 1966 version of the Animal Welfare Act (Public Law 89–544)

LD$_{50}$ Lethal dose 50% test; toxicity test to determine the dose of a substance that kills half of the animals that receive it

multiple major survival surgery Surgery that enters a body cavity (abdomen, chest) or has the potential to create serious deficits, performed repeatedly on a single animal, after which the animal is expected to awake from anesthesia

NABR The National Association for Biomedical Research, a major animal research advocacy organization throughout the 1980s and 1990s

NIH The National Institutes of Health (a division of the United States Public Health Service)

nonaffiliated member An IACUC member who has no other affiliation with the institution (e.g., is not an employee); also the "community member" or the "unaffiliated member"

Office of Laboratory Animal Welfare The NIH office that oversees care of animal subjects and human subjects at institutions receiving Public Health Service research funding

performance standards Regulations that emphasize outcomes rather than means. Example: dog cages must be big enough to allow dog to stand or lie comfortably and to walk normally; contrast "engineering standards"

PETA People for the Ethical Treatment of Animals, a large animal protection/animal rights organization

PHS The U.S. Public Health Service

PHS *Policy* Animal care and use guidelines for institutions receiving PHS/NIH funds

primate A member of the order *Primates* that includes lemurs, monkeys, apes, and people; also nonhuman, subhuman, or infrahuman primates

protocol Animal Care and Use Proposal; a researcher's proposal, for IACUC review, to use animals in research, teaching, or ethics

psychological well-being The mental health of an animal. Since 1985, the Animal Welfare Act has mandated housing primates in an environment that is "adequate to promote the psychological well-being"

purpose bred A laboratory animal bred and raised specifically for laboratory use

random-source A laboratory animal from virtually any other source: donation, auction, animal pound, assorted dealers, pet store, etc.

research advocate Organizations such as NABR as well as individuals who lobby for minimal restrictions and maximal support for biomedical research

sacrifice To kill an animal for a scientific procedure

Secretary The Secretary of Agriculture, who is the head of the USDA

Silver Spring Monkeys Monkeys from Bernard Taub's lab who were the subject of a PETA exposé in 1981

terminal surgery Experimental procedure in which an animal is anesthetized and undergoes surgery, but then is killed before recovery from anesthesia

USDA The United States Department of Agriculture, which enforces the Animal Welfare Act

vivisection Invasive experimentation on a living animal (with or without anesthesia)

Notes

1: Introduction

1. For a nice exposition on the damaging effects of this sort of rhetoric, from a primate researcher-turned-philosopher, see Gluck and Kubacki (1991).
2. Animal welfare policy studies most closely approximate environmental policy in this respect. Note, though, that many environmental policy discussions are really about impacts on people and need not incorporate concern for what is good for the environment for its own sake.
3. As with so many words, "realist" and "realism" have both common meanings and formal definitions within a particular academic arena. Here I use realist to identify a theory within the philosophy of science, not to distinguish realistic people from idealistic people. See Sergio Sismondo (1996) for an in-depth discussion of the different flavors of realism and constructivism in the philosophy of science.
4. In this context "nature" does not refer exclusively to the wild and untamed world of field and forest, but to anything a scientist may focus his or her gaze upon, including the animals, cells, DNA, genes, and chemicals of the modern biomedical laboratory.
5. Abbott calls his model "ecological," emphasizing the contextual history of professionalization of various fields and the competition for limited resources (jurisdiction over socially valued tasks) that determines which professions are fittest for survival.
6. Thomas Gieryn (1995) has developed the concept of "boundary work" in science studies to describe this active policing by professionals.
7. Ethologists (such as Jane Goodall and her field studies of chimpanzee behavior or Konrad Lorenz with his greylag geese) capture the public eye and are popularly called animal behaviorists. As Rollin and others draw the professional distinction, behaviorists and their work are better exemplified by Pavlov and his salivating dogs or B. F. Skinner and his lever-pressing rats. They study animals in highly unnatural laboratory settings, collecting behavioral data as a means of discovering basic processes of brain function, learning, and so on. Ethologists tend to observe animal behavior in more natural settings, often with a focus on ecological and evolutionary questions, rather than questions of mechanism or neurology.
8. The *Guide* has been primarily funded in most of its editions by the National Institutes of Health, a division of the federal government. It has been written and pub-

lished, however, by the National Academy of Sciences (specifically, the Institute of Laboratory Animal Resources within the NAS National Research Council).

9. In keeping with that tradition, I should write instead, "The impersonal voice is used" to place the actors (scientists) and their actions (choosing and writing) backstage, where the reader cannot see them.

2: Life in the animal laboratory

1. Dr. John Draize developed a system for testing chemical warfare agents for eye irritancy (Draize et al. 1944). After an incident in 1933 in which a woman was blinded by mascara, the Food and Drug Administration acquired authority to assess safety testing of cosmetics. See Rowan (1984) and Parascandola (1991) for a history of the test and of Spira's efforts to replace it.

2. Frederick Grant Banting and Charles Herbert Best shared the Nobel Prize in 1923 for their discovery of the role of insulin in diabetes mellitus. The work required removing the pancreas from dogs to create the diabetic condition, then restoring the active insulin hormone (Best 1974; Gay 1984) A twenty-first century version of this approach of inferring function from absence is the use of "knockout" transgenic mice. The gene to produce a specific hormone or enzyme is removed, and that missing compound's role in fighting infection, directing embryonic development, or promoting some other process is studied (Quimby 2002).

3. "SCID-hu" mice are severe combined immune-deficient mice whose poorly developed immune systems tolerate grafting of human fetal cells. As these cells grow in the mouse, a near-human immune system develops, which can then harbor the HIV virus (Carballido et al. 2000; McCune 1997).

4. Antibodies are the immune proteins that bind to infectious invaders to eliminate them from the body. In laboratories, antibodies are induced to recognize specific proteins that the scientist is interested in studying. For example, to tell if a person has a particular parasite in his or her blood, you might use a rabbit antibody that would bind to some of the parasite's proteins in a blood sample. You would get these antibodies by vaccinating the rabbit with a killed extract of the parasite and then collect blood samples from the rabbit over several months.

5. In addition to technological limits to how quickly animals are being replaced, there is regulatory inertia as well. The Food and Drug Administration has relied on animal safety testing before allowing drugs to proceed to human clinical trials. The FDA (as well as the Environmental Protection Agency, which evaluates safety testing of compounds released into the environment) must be convinced that alternative methods have been sufficiently validated to reliably replace animal testing.

6. For a history of the legislative events (including failed bills), see Christine Stevens's (1990) account. Stevens and her Society for Animal Protective Legislation were key figures in passing the early legislation; her narrative makes no pretense of impartiality, but is rich in detail and even intrigue.

7. The professional standards are found in the *Guide for the Care and Use of Laboratory Animals,* which I usually refer to as either the NIH *Guide,* or more simply, the *Guide.* The voluntary accreditation program is administered by a private nonprofit agency, the Association for the Assessment and Accreditation of Laboratory Animal Care (AAALAC). The most current regulatory documents are available on websites maintained by the USDA Animal and Plant Health Inspection Service, the

Animal Welfare Information Center of the National Agriculture Library, the NIH Office of Laboratory Animal Welfare, and the Association for Assessment and Accreditation of Laboratory Animal Care International. For printed versions, see Animal and Plant Health Inspection Service (1991); Institute of Laboratory Animal Resources (ILAR, 1996); Office of Protection from Research Risks (1986); and U.S. Congress (1985a, 1985b).

8. Much of the public correspondence to the USDA serves to ratify the leadership of the Animal Welfare Institute, the National Association for Biomedical Research, and other organizations and strengthens the impression that they are diametrically opposed on all issues. As I learned in my interviews, most of the fine detail of the 1985 legislation involved compromise between these groups in meetings with congressional staff. The provisions for dog exercise and for psychological well-being of primates were two major issues that sidestepped this negotiation process.

9. The Institute for Laboratory Animal Research, housed within the National Research Council, is part of the National Academy of Sciences, and thus technically not a government agency. The NAS holds a government charter (like the Boy Scouts of America), is housed in Washington, D.C., and does much of its work under contract with government agencies. This technical independence from the government ostensibly enhances its claims to scientific objectivity and political neutrality.

10. The complicated inclusion/exclusion of birds and rodents results from the 1970 expansion of the act to cover warm-blooded animals in research, followed by a 2002 amendment specifically excluding birds and laboratory rats and mice. Chapter 4 covers some of the controversy surrounding this exclusion.

3: Animal welfare

1. David DeGrazia (1996) uses the term "animal ethics" and seems to think it is the term of choice for the ethical study of animals or the study of human obligations toward animals. The term seems as useful as any. It embraces the notion that how we treat animals is a question of ethics, without implying a particular philosophy such as animal rights, contract theory, utilitarianism, and so on.

2. Singer (1975) credits Richard Ryder for initially developing the concept and significance of speciesism. Ryder (1998) distinguishes weaker versions of speciesism from this stricter definition and example: "A human may seek to justify discrimination against, say, an armadillo on the grounds that the armadillo cannot talk, is not a moral agent, has no religion, or is not very intelligent; such an attitude is often described as speciesist. But more strictly, it is when the discrimination or exploitation against the armadillo is justified solely on the grounds that the armadillo is of another species that it is speciesist" (p. 320).

3. In the language of laboratory animal welfare policy, we are talking about "multiple survival surgery" versus "terminal surgery." To really map this case onto regulations, we would also need to distinguish whether the survival surgeries under consideration were major or minor surgeries. Major surgeries are those that enter major body cavities (chest, abdomen, braincase) or that have the potential to induce serious defects, such as blindness, lameness, or organ or limb removals.

4. Albert Schweitzer was very influential with the Animal Welfare Institute and with the animal liberationist-journalist Ann Cottrell Free. The Schweitzer quotes here are from her book *Animals, Nature, and Albert Schweitzer* (1982).

5. Based in Australia, the Great Ape Project is an international organization of scientists, philosophers, activists, and others whose goal is a United Nations "declaration of the rights of great apes." This would mean including the great apes (chimpanzees, bonobos, gorillas, and orangutans) as persons in a community of rightsholders equal to the other members of the family Hominidae, the human beings (Cavalieri and Singer 1993).

6. This important philosophical question has narrowly circumscribed policy implications in animal research ethics, however, given that great apes comprise roughly only 0.005% or fewer of American research animals.

7. Cohen is interesting in that his major contribution on animal ethics appeared not in a philosophical journal, but in the *New England Journal of Medicine* (1986, whence it has been reproduced for countless veterinary and laboratory animal science conferences and readers). He gets it partly wrong when he proudly claims to be a speciesist; he is, but not for the reasons he cites. He elaborates on his self-identification as a speciesist by citing attributes of people and animals—specifically, who can enter into a moral contract and who cannot as his reason to limit rights holders to humans. That claim is actually not speciesist in the Ryder/Singer sense, as he is basing his moral divide on rationality, not species membership. Only later in his article does he embrace strict speciesism when he argues to include nonrational, nonautonomous humans (such as infants or the severely retarded) in the human moral community as members of the human kind, they "count" morally because their human relatives possess autonomy, not because of their own attributes. Similar attempts by Cohen, Carruthers, Morrison, Fox, and others to justify morality by species are actually more attempts to base morality on other attributes, attributes of mental capacity that are primarily restricted to our own species (so far as we know). Their sentiments may be speciesist, but their arguments, for the most part, are not.

    In contrast to Cohen, Raymond Frey is a medical ethicist who has written against animal liberation philosophies from a utilitarian rather than contractarian or rights-based perspective. Unlike Cohen, who locks out nonautonomous animals from rights, but lets various nonautonomous humans in the back door, Frey (1987) simply bites the bullet and puts marginal humans pretty much with the animals, deserving of some protections in their capacity for suffering, but hardly on a par with functioning autonomous adult humans. Though Singer and Frey have been described as two utilitarians drawing opposite conclusions about animal research (the former quite restrictive and the latter more permissive), their positions are not so very different, either in the use of animals or in the use of marginal humans in medical research.

8. Descartes's theory of mind was often interpreted to equate animals with senseless machines, allowing their free use for human purposes. "My thesis is not so much cruel to animals as lenient to men . . . since it absolves them from the suspicion of crime when they eat or kill animals," he wrote in 1649. Wallace Shugg (1968) writes, though without indicating how he obtained the data, that "soon after Descartes's *Discours de la Methode* was translated and published in England (1649), experimentation on animals increased greatly, and as a result, scores of dogs, cats, and birds were slaughtered" (p. 228). Other historians believe that Descartes has

been unduly demonized and that he was neither so cruel to animals himself (though he did perform his own animal experiments) nor correctly interpreted as giving people free rein to do howsoever they please to them (Cottingham 1978).

9. Behaviorism and ethology represent two ends of the spectrum of studies of animal behavior. B. F. Skinner and J. B. Watson are two prominent figures in the early days of behaviorism. Interested in animal behavior as a model of how the human brain works, they focused on mechanistic stimulus–response patterns (as in the highly refined "Skinner box" in which a rat learns to press a lever and receive a reward). Ethologists (Konrad Lorenz, Niko Tinnbergen, and Jane Goodall, for example) tend to be more interested in evolutionary developments in animal mental functions and tend more toward observation of animals in more-or-less natural situations.

10. The elephant swaying back and forth in the zoo, the mouse chewing all night long on cage bars—these are examples of animals displaying stereotypical behaviors. "A stereotypy is a repeated, relatively invariant sequence of movements that has no obvious function" (Broom 1998, p. 325). The causes of stereotypies are not always identified, though in both humans and animals mental illnesses and poor (frustrating, confined) environments need to be considered. For a fuller discussion, see Toates (2000).

11. Rowan and DeGrazia deserve credit for bringing the scientific literature on animal anxiety to the attention of animal ethicists. Anxiety, like pain, seems a blend of physical and emotional, which animals may possess to differing degrees. Most vertebrates (but not sharks) possess benzodiazepine receptors in the brain, capable of binding to the class of anxiety-reducing medicines that include diazepam and midazolam (commonly known by their tradenames, Valium and Versed). If the receptors are there in reptiles or frogs, it seems likely they are there to help modulate the degree of anxiety the animal experiences (unless they have some other functions, on top of which anxiolysis has developed over the course of evolution). If they are not present, chances seem good that animals such as sharks have little or no capacity for anxiety and therefore little or no need for chemicals and receptors to diminish it (DeGrazia and Rowan 1991).

12. In this chapter, I have restricted my coverage to those philosophers who put animal ethics on a strong footing (Singer and Regan), those most influential among veterinarians and animal professionals (Rollin and Tannenbaum), the contractarians who present the strongest case against animal liberation (Cohen, Michael A. Fox), and DeGrazia, whose work builds on all of these and whose synthesis and review I have found most enlightening. Any serious student of animal ethics should also start with the cluster of books that emerged in the active period of the early 1980s to the early 1990s, including Steve Sapontzis (1987), James Rachels (1990), Mary Midgley (1983), and Carol Adams (1990).

4: A rat is a pig

1. We cannot get bogged down in this chapter with analyzing all the different levels of treatment of that these categories entail. Following the order they are mentioned in the main text, these are some species-related policy considerations for animal use: Work with endangered species requires special permits under the Endangered Species Act, as administered by the U.S. Department of the Interior. The Public Health

Service Policy on Humane Care and Use of Laboratory Animals covers animals with backbones while excluding invertebrate animals. Warm-blooded animals are covered (with notable exceptions) under the Animal Welfare Act. Pet animals (at least, dogs and cats) have special coverage for how and whence they may be obtained for laboratories and are the subject of the 1990 Pet Protection Act. Work with local wildlife may require state permits (especially if they are a species favored by hunters), while work with exotic wildlife entails international permits and, often, special quarantine procedures. "Cute and cuddly" are in the eye of the beholder, and vary by culture and over time, as rats, mice, and dogs amply demonstrate. The Class B animal dealer provisions of the Animal Welfare Act do not cover dogs and cats specifically bred for laboratory use, as they are usually going directly from breeding facility to the laboratory. Mice and rats specifically bred for research are excluded from Animal Welfare Act protections, though wild-caught members of their kind are covered. The Animal Welfare Act likewise excludes agricultural species when they are used in food and fiber research (such as how to get sheep to birth more lambs) but covers them when they are in biomedical research (such as studying pregnant sheep as models of fundamental processes of human and other pregnancies). I know of no laws covering treatment of wild mice invading a laboratory's food storage area, other than that this must be prevented (for the safety of the resident animals) and that their deaths (such an intruder's typical fate) would hopefully conform to the recommendations of American Veterinary Medical Association's Panel on Euthanasia. And finally, the Public Health Service rules and regulations only apply to animals in federally supported programs, not small commercial laboratories or small teaching colleges.

2. The Health Research Extension Act (HREA) of 1985 gave legal weight to the NIH *Guide for the Care and Use of Laboratory Animals*, then in its twenty-second year. The HREA does not actually say which animals count under its provisions (mice? cockroaches?). But the related policies that that law empowers, the *Public Health Service Policy on Humane Care and Use of Laboratory Animals* and the NIH's *Guide*, are explicit that they cover all live vertebrate animals.

3. The Helms amendment to exclude rats, mice, and birds also calls on the National Research Council to submit a report to Congress on the implications, especially the financial implications, of including rats, mice, and birds within the definition of "animal" under the regulations promulgated under the Animal Welfare Act. The NRC was granted one year from the date of enactment of the law (May 2002) to prepare this report, but received no funding from NIH or USDA to act on it. It is likely this report will never be written.

4. The USDA files contain one 1977 letter on the subject, submitted not by an animal protection organization, but by the National Society for Medical Research (NSMR). NSMR said the USDA was tampering with Congress's definition of "animal" "in a manner that alters the intent of the basic law." Their expressed reason for concern, however, was neither animal welfare nor regulatory burden, but the potential challenge of USDA regulations conflicting with Food and Drug Administration rules already in place.

5. As testimony to the political weight of these magazine stories, the USDA put a picture of Pepper on participant nametags at its 1996 symposium honoring the first thirty years of the Animal Welfare Act.

6. Domitian and Sarah are two of the "Silver Spring Monkeys." This was PETA's inaugural exposé of an animal laboratory, in 1981. Coupled with videotapes stolen during a 1984 Animal Liberation Front break-in at a University of Pennsylvania laboratory, the Silver Spring exposé spurred passage of the Improved Standards for Laboratory Animals (Animal Welfare Act amendment) and the Health Research Extension Act (which made NIH's animal welfare guidelines legally binding) in 1985. For fuller treatments of these two historical events, see Blum (1994).

7. In 1930, legislative initiatives were introduced to ban the use of dogs in research within the District of Columbia. In 1945, the National Society for Medical Research was formed primarily to focus on assuring a continued source of dogs for research. Minnesota passed a law in 1948 forcing tax-supported shelters to provide animals for research, and several states followed suit, with some later repealing those laws. In 1990, an Animal Welfare Act amendment, the Pet Protection Act of 1990, was passed to further tighten the flow of dogs from questionable sources to laboratories (Jones 2003; Lederer 1987; Stevens 1990).

8. The late Christine Stevens founded the Animal Welfare Institute and its political affiliate, the Society for Animal Protective Legislation, in the early 1950s and was influential in shaping both the 1966 Laboratory Animal Welfare Act and its 1985 amendment. Ingrid Newkirk was cofounder and president of People for the Ethical Treatment of Animals. Known for her outspoken rhetoric, one of her statements gave the name to this chapter: "When it comes to having a central nervous system and the ability to experience pain, hunger, and thirst, a rat is a pig is a dog is a boy" (quoted in Feldman 1996). F. Barbara Orlans founded the Scientists Center for Animal Welfare in the 1970s, while working as a research scientist at the NIH. She moved on to Georgetown's Kennedy Center for Ethics, expanding that group's focus to include issues of laboratory animal welfare. These three important leaders have worked with other notable women scientists within the animal welfare movement, including the ethologist Joy Mench, the veterinarian W. Jean Dodds, and others.

9. I went to this source of data expecting that parents of seriously ill children, writing to urge minimal restrictions on animal research, would be the most likely to invoke the biblical primacy of human over animal. I found none conforming to this expectation, while the rare mention of religion in the USDA's 30,000-plus letters was always in service of kindness to animals. One woman, for instance, wrote that she had "gotten a saintly Catholic nun to organize a number of her students to make novenas to stop the satanic proposal to override the reproposed rules" (Regulatory Analysis and Development 1990).

10. Many feminists, especially ecofeminists, are skeptical of limiting moral concern to animals with certain cognitive capacities, or of limiting moral concern to people and animals at all (Plumwood 1991; Warren 2000).

11. In 1978 and 1979, first India and then Bangladesh cut off the supply of wild-caught rhesus monkeys to United States research laboratories after learning that the United States was using some of them, in violation of treaty agreements, in nuclear weapons research (M. A. Fox 1986).

12. Both authors readily admit the pitfalls inherent in such an artificial test: they are not reviewing their peers' but some imaginary scientists' protocols; they may give little attention in their busy day to a hypothetical case; or conversely, they may scru-

tinize the protocol particularly thoroughly, knowing that they are being watched. Any study of how IACUCs function must also be careful not to conflate rejection of protocols with careful consideration—in my experience, the vast majority of the work of an IACUC rests in careful negotiation and planning with a scientist to minimize harm to animals, not in simple votes to approve or disapprove. In Dresser's study, outright disapproval of hypothetical protocols and unconditional approval on initial submission were equally uncommon.

5: Performance standards

1. The USDA published its proposals, along with its response to public commentaries and its final rules, in the *Federal Register* (Animal and Plant Health Inspection Service 1987; Animal and Plant Health Inspection Service 1986, 1989a, 1989b, 1990a, 1990b, 1991).
2. None of these documents arose de novo as book-length treatises on animal care. The Animal Welfare Institute, the Animal Care Panel, and various government agencies had been producing smaller sets of guidelines and handbooks throughout the 1940s and 1950s (Animal Welfare Institute 1953; Earl 1955; Farris 1950).
3. As in the American scene, the European trend is toward increasingly explicit explanations of how they base their recommendations. For example, a 1993 British report on refinements in rabbit husbandry called for increased cage sizes for rabbits based on medical information (disuse osteoporosis in rabbits housed in American-sized cages) and behavioral data (such as that young rabbits are more active than adults). Along with specific sizes (engineering standards) they articulate performance standards as well: rabbits should be housed in compatible groups whenever possible; rabbits should be able to "stretch fully along the length, width and diagonal" of a cage; a cage should be tall enough for a rabbit to sit upright "to perform typical lookout behavior" (Morton et al. 1993, pp. 24, 25).
4. Among other critiques of this one guinea pig study is the feminist challenge to the authors' equation of a vasectomized harem as a "breeding group." They were a breeding group in terms of gender composition, with sexual activity divorced from reproduction. Females in such a group never go through the dramatic size changes of guinea pig pregnancies, nor do the breeding groups, if they're successfully producing babies, remain at a static population.

6: Centaurs and science

1. Alas, for the veterinary historian, Abbott (1988) does not more fully explicate his understanding of the professional status of veterinary medicine to justify his claim of a limited jurisdiction. Legally, physicians are *more* restricted in the species on which they are licensed to practice than vets are. The jurisdiction is split along species lines, with physicians licensed to treat the single higher-status, higher-paying, third-party-insured human species, while vets are left with all the others. Other than the species split, in most states veterinarians and physicians enjoy the same privileges to diagnose, prescribe, and treat.
2. Another lesson in laboratory animal science: Animals are sold by species and sex and weight and infection status. Specific-pathogen-free (SPF) animals, for example, have tested negative for infection with various microorganisms and com-

mand a higher price than untested or known-infected animals. SPF laboratory rabbits, for example, are kept free of infection with *Pasteurella* and coccidia, which cause pneumonia and diarrhea, respectively, in backyard pet rabbits.

3. Technically, most research animals are the legal property of the institution, not of the individual working with them, even when that individual has written the grant application funding their purchase. Nonetheless, it has been rare for me to encounter individuals in my years of practice who did not think of the animals as their own.

4. "Spontaneous disease" in the laboratory animal medicine context refers to diseases and infections which the animals acquire accidentally, spontaneously, "on their own," as opposed to diseases intentionally induced by scientists for the express purpose of studying them.

5. After nine years, they dropped "facilities" and added "use" to the title, for the *Guide*'s fourth edition, further breaking down the care/use dichotomy. The title of the fourth through the seventh editions (the seventh, in 1996, being the most current) is the *Guide for the Care and Use of Laboratory Animals*.

6. Research surgery was the companion of pain in undermining care/use jurisdictional divisions. Surgical manipulations of animals was seen as part of experimental animal use, not as a medical or therapeutic aspect of animal care. Students, physiologists, human physicians, and other scientists perform these surgeries, not veterinarians. Research surgery as the researcher's domain—the image of scientist, scalpel and animal, alone and unwatched in the laboratory—has long been under assault.

7. Following the Melcher amendment for an environment to "promote the psychological well-being of nonhuman primates," the USDA assembled a panel of ten primate specialists, including chimpanzee specialist Jane Goodall, the director of the Yerkes Primate Center in Georgia, and three veterinarians (U.S. Congress 1985a).

8. I distinguish behaviorists from animal behaviorists (see note 7, chapter 1). Behaviorism was a prominent school of experimental psychology and of learning theory in the first half of the twentieth century, often associated with B. F. Skinner and his "Skinner boxes" in which rats press levers to receive rewards or avoid shock. Rollin (1989) has written on how the focus of behaviorists on animals as stimulus–response mechanisms rather than thinking, feeling, motivated individuals has actually worked against progress in promoting animal welfare. In contrast, the animal behaviorists (also known as applied animal behaviorists) prominent at the end of the century are an assortment of ethologists, biologists, veterinarians, and even animal trainers who focus on how and why animals act the way they do and how to shape the behaviors they perform, often with an eye to improving their welfare. Prominent leaders in this field include (but are certainly not limited to) Hal Markowitz and Scott Line (1990), Joy Mench (1994, 1998), Ian Duncan (1993; Duncan and Mench 2000; Duncan et al. 1993), Temple Grandin (2000; Gregory and Grandin 1998), and Marc Bekoff (2002; Bekoff et al. 1992), along with veterinary behaviorists Katherine Houpt (1998) and Tom Wolfle (1987, 2002).

7: The problem of pain

1. The monkeys had been surgically deafferentated (i.e., the sensory nerves that would normally bring information from the arm to the brain had been cut [under

anesthesia] to simulate injuries that some people sustain) for study of nerve regeneration and limb reuse.

2. Though they took some time to develop, current professional definitions of pain include both the neurological events (often called nociception) as well the conscious subjective unpleasant emotional experience associated with them. The International Association for the Study of Pain describes the dual physical/emotional quality of pain:

> The inability to communicate in no way negates the possibility that the individual is experiencing pain. . . . Pain is always subjective. . . . Pain is that experience we associate with actual or potential tissue damage. It is unquestionably a sensation in a part or parts of the body, but it is also always unpleasant and therefore also an emotional experience. Experiences which resemble pain but are not unpleasant, e.g., pricking, should not be called pain. (Merskey and Bogduk 1994, p. 210)

3. The reporting requirements were modified in 1977 into the format still used twenty years later (and described in chapter 2). In addition to reporting animal experimentation in which painkillers are withheld, facilities now also report numbers of animals in experiments in which no significant pain is induced and numbers of those in which potentially painful experiments are accompanied by anesthetics or painkillers. Thus we now have a tripartite reporting system of no pain/pain with drugs/pain without drugs. Procedures that are considered minor and/or momentary—routine blood collection, inoculations, tattooing, for example—are generally excluded from this reporting requirement.

4. The USDA's requirements for classifying animals into "pain categories" in research facilities' annual reports are described in chapter 2.

5. In addition to supplying the most detailed catalog of painful procedures, the ALDF's submission was unique in addressing the other side of the coin, the justification for performing painful procedures without anesthetic in the first place. It did not address just how a scientist would make the case that anesthetics would interfere with his or her project, other than to put the burden of proof on the scientist, rather than on those who would push for painkillers. Instead it cited the insistence of several members of Congress that the new Improved Standards for Laboratory Animals would not interfere with research, but gave those words a bit of a twist: Congressman Montgomery was careful that the Animal Welfare Act would not tie the hands of researchers working to "unlock the secrets of *dread diseases*"; Senator Moynihan cited Parkinson's disease, heart disease, and cancer as examples of the research that must not be curtailed; and the conference report on the bill made clear the intent "that *essential research* not be impeded" (Regulatory Analysis and Development 1986). As ALDF read these congressional comments, they were not just the dramatic examples of why Congress should keep its hands off the conduct of animal experiments. Rather, they were the indication that only "essential research" on "dread diseases" could justify inflicting pain on animals. Following this reasoning, the ALDF submitted a second list, of procedures that should almost never be allowed, including several psychological studies (maternal deprivation, electric shock as a form of punishment, induction of psychosis) and LD_{50} toxicity tests. Research programs in this category failed to meet the criteria of essential studies of dread diseases.

6. The Scientists Center for Animal Welfare's proposed system was:

Category A: procedures that did not involve vertebrate animals at all.

Category B: experiments on vertebrate animal species that are expected to produce little or no discomfort.

Category C: experiments that involve some minor distress or discomfort (short-duration pain) to vertebrate animal species.

Category D: experiments that involve significant but unavoidable distress or discomfort to vertebrate animal species.

Category E: experiments that involve inflicting severe pain near, at, or above the pain threshold of unanesthetized, conscious animals.

See Orlans (1993, pp. 87–88) for the examples of procedures that exemplify each category.

7. The notion of "chemical restraint" is more common in veterinary medicine than in human medicine. Drugs (usually injected, and often at some distance, via blow-darts, guns, or pole syringes) replace lassos and nets in capturing and holding wild or difficult-to-control animals. In such situations, such as apprehending an animal for relocation to another site, but without performing surgeries or other invasive procedures in the process, safety, ease of delivery, degree of immobility induced, and duration of action may be of higher priority than the degree of pain relief, amnesia, or unconsciousness induced. In these situations very light doses of anesthetics or even muscle-paralyzing drugs with no known effect on consciousness or pain perception may be used. Rollin's veterinary correspondent seems to be claiming that a dog is anesthetized for abdominal surgery, for instance, not because abdominal surgery hurts, but because otherwise she will squirm and wriggle the whole time, presenting the scalpel with a constantly moving target during delicate operations.

8: The animal advocates

1. The Nuremberg Code's third principle is that the experiment should be so designed and based on the results of animal experimentation . . . that the results will justify the performance of the experiment." The Declaration of Helsinki declares that "the welfare of animals used for research must be respected," and goes on to elaborate its first basic principle: "Biomedical research involving human subjects must conform to generally accepted scientific principles and should be based on adequately performed laboratory and animal experimentation and on a thorough knowledge of the scientific literature."

2. In this study, rural African-American men were left untreated to chart the course of syphilis in humans, despite the advent of penicillin during the course of the study. Public exposure of this study in 1972 led to the formation of a national commission to develop standards for human experimentation (Jones 1981).

3. As of this writing, human subjects requirements, like the NIH's jurisdiction over research animals, only applies to federally funded projects and research. There is no human subjects equivalent of the Animal Welfare Act to cover research in privately funded settings, such as at drug companies. If it weren't for the fact that animal welfare regulations allow the infliction of severe pain, distress and death, the animals might actually be enjoying greater protection of their interests than do human subjects.

4. I thank Professor Robert Veatch for the insight that consideration of animals as "vulnerable subjects" would be an interesting, if disturbing, way to explore research animal ethics.

5. Note that since his ethic is primarily individualistic in focus, Sapontzis would not be inclined to harm or kill individual dogs in research, even though that may benefit their species, any more than he would allow serious harm to individual humans for projects that would only benefit other humans. Rather he has in mind experimental therapeutic research that could help the individual animal with a medical condition (as well as providing data of use to the individuals species, and possibly other species as well).

9: Death by decapitation

1. This chapter is an expansion of ideas I first published in 1997 in *Society and Animals* (Carbone 1997c).

2. I have found David DeGrazia's (1996) and Steven Sapontzis's (1987) treatments of these discussions particularly thoughtful, readable, and helpful. Philosophers debate such questions as whether death's preclusion of potential good things to come is a harm, and whether animals (while still alive) would need enough of a sense of the future for early death to be a harm.

3. "Animals that would otherwise experience severe or chronic pain or distress that cannot be relieved will be painlessly sacrificed at the end of the procedure or, if appropriate, during the procedure" (Office of Protection from Research Risks 1986, p. 27).

4. I find Tannenbaum's justification of meat eating to be the weak spot in his excellent text on veterinary ethics. He finds justification for meat eating in its long history in human culture, overlooking many of the spiritual leaders over the centuries who have promoted vegetarianism as one of several forms of nonviolence (Tannenbaum 1995).

5. The American Veterinary Medical Association has made a similar move in its contrast of animal rights and animal welfare, linking animal welfare and animal use as roughly synonymous in the face of anti-exploitation animal rights philosophies: "The AVMA cannot endorse the philosophical views and personal values of animal rights advocates when they are incompatible with the responsible use of animals for human purposes" (quoted in Tannenbaum 1998, p. 153).

6. Some of this separation of individual ethics and scientific assessment of well-being went away with the 2001 revision of the AVMA's position (American Veterinary Medical Association 2002).

7. The rats they studied had been paralyzed with gallamine (a drug that paralyzes muscles, but not believed to tranquilize or to blunt pain perception) to assure proper placement in the guillotine and to "reduce artifacts of motion and muscle twitching" (Mikeska and Klemm, 1975, p. 175). Paralytic drugs render rats incapable of displaying much behavior to be observed or interpreted, and so behavioral data (and the threat of subjective observer biases) are not part of the study. Neither were stress hormone analyses included. Stress hormones are measured after the pituitary gland (in the brain) sends hormones through the bloodstream to the adrenal glands (in the abdomen), which then release corticosterone and

other stress-induced hormones. But the act of decapitation severs the bloodborne communication between pituitary and adrenal, and so even the most stressed and activated of pituitary glands could not reach the adrenal glands to induce corticosterone production.

8. Atropine, or belladonna, affects the parasympathetic nervous system, but it is not considered a painkiller or anesthetic.

9. Though the USDA was continuing its exclusion of laboratory-bred rats and mice and mice from Animal Welfare Act coverage, the AVMA's panel recommendations could prohibit guinea pig or hamster decapitation and so could still impact research practices.

10. Though not the primary focus of this chapter, Andrew Rowan (1992) has raised the question of how good a gold standard conscious decapitation is. Tissue collection through decapitation is not completely artifact free: there is a time lag from decapitation to tissue collection, a time lag with demonstrable data artifacts (Faupel et al. 1972; Nishihara and Keenan 1985; Veech et al. 1972), as well as the effects of handling and positioning as potential sources of stress and distress.

11. The standard error is a statistical calculation that gives some indication of how tightly the data cluster around the average versus how widely they range.

10: Dog walkers and monkey psychiatrists

1. These were the Washington, D.C., regulations in the 1950s assuring that the availability of pound dogs for research were linked to government standards for animal care, including the provisions that "dogs must be caged individually" and that "large animals" should be given daily exercise (Morgan 1954, p. 18). Detailing these regulations to his fellow laboratory animal professionals, Charles Morgan added, "These safeguards to the animals' health are satisfactory to the people who were previously opposed to animal experimentation" (p. 118).

2. These were the proposed rules for determining which dogs did *not* need to taken out of their enclosures for exercise: singly caged dogs in cages four times the dog-plus-six-inches minimum, or, if group-housed, dogs "in pens or runs that provide the greater of 80 square feet or 150 percent of the space each dog would require if maintained separately under the minimum floor space requirements" (Animal and Plant Inspection Service 1989b, p. 10935).

3. A few small-scale dog breeders explained that raising dogs was a way to supplement a limited income, and resisted anything that would increase the expense (even calling a veterinarian for a sick dog) of that enterprise.

4. Some of their concerns seem specious in retrospect, or disingenuous, especially their dismissal of the USDA's proposal that exercise regulations would only apply to dogs held twenty-one days or longer. After extolling dogs' ready adaptability (such as to life in a cage) they cautioned darkly of the effects of allowing previously cage-adapted dogs "sudden" release for exercise after twenty-one days: "Having once adapted to 21 continuous days of confinement, it is highly probable that sudden release may actually be detrimental to his physiological as well as psychological well-being. . . . The dog is then abruptly introduced to a new pattern with a resultant stress to having to readjust to a new situation" (ILAR 1974, p. 6). They offered no explanation of why dogs could adapt to cage confinement so readily, but

not to release for exercise, nor why institutions acquiring dogs for long-term projects would go through twenty-days of cage adaptation if dogs would not be housed
that way long term. Perhaps they thought the USDA was *prohibiting* exercise of
dogs until their twenty-first day in the laboratory? This caution seems particularly
odd given that the 1972 *Guide* that they had written just two years earlier had also
suggested the use of "pens, runs, or other out-of-cage space" in all dog housing
areas and limited claims to the necessity and usefulness of smaller cages to "short-
term holding of dogs (one to three months)" (ILAR 1972, p. 5). That edition of the
Guide contained no warnings of the stress of letting dogs out of their cages after
three months of such confinement (ILAR 1972).

5. Laboratory dogs may be bred in-house for use, purchased from commercial breeders, or obtained as "random source" animals. Per the USDA's definition: "*Random
source* means dogs and cats obtained from animal pounds or shelters, auction sales,
or from any person who did not breed and raise them on his or her premises" (Animal and Plant Health Inspection Service 1989a, p. 36122). Use of random source
dogs and cats has been controversial for several decades, but it was not a major
controversy connected with the 1985 Animal Welfare Act amendment. In1990,
however, Congress passed the fourth amendment to the act, Protection of Pets, further specifying (but by no means eliminating) the identification and care of animals
at pounds and shelters if they are to be sold or released to dealers or to research institutions (Debra Beasley, unpublished manuscript [1996]; U.S. Congress 1990).

6. This involves the complicated USDA cage size determination based on the dog's
body length (minus her tail) plus six inches. A single dog housed in anything less
than twice that must receive supplemental exercise; grouped dogs must be housed
in a cage that provides each dog that minimum cage size but do not require additional exercise. In the USDA's final rule:

§ 3.8 Exercise for dogs.

Dealers, exhibitors, and research facilities must develop, document, and follow
an appropriate plan to provide dogs with the opportunity for exercise. In addition, the plan must be approved by the attending veterinarian. The plan must
include written standard procedures to be followed in providing the opportunity for exercise. The plan must be made available to APHIS upon request, and,
in the case of research facilities, to officials of any pertinent funding Federal
agency. The plan, at a minimum, must comply with each of the following:

(a) *Dogs housed individually.* Dogs over 12 weeks of age, except bitches with litters, housed, held, or maintained by any dealer, exhibitor, or research facility, including Federal research facilities, must be provided the opportunity
for exercise regularly if they are kept individually in cages, pens, or runs
that provide less than two times the required floor space for that dog, as indicated by § 3.6(c)(1) of this subpart.

(b) *Dogs housed in groups.* Dogs over 12 weeks of age housed, held, or maintained in groups by any dealer, exhibitor, or research facility, including Federal research facilities, do not require additional opportunity for exercise
regularly if they are maintained in cages, pens, or runs that provide in total
at least 100 percent of the required space for each dog if maintained separately. Such animals may be maintained in compatible groups, unless:

(1) Housing in compatible groups is not in accordance with a research proposal and the proposal has been approved by the research facility Committee;

(2) In the opinion of the attending veterinarian, such housing would adversely affect the health or well-being of the dog(s); or

(3) Any dog exhibits aggressive or vicious behavior.

(c) *Methods and period of providing exercise opportunity.* (1) The frequency, method, and duration of the opportunity for exercise shall be determined by the attending veterinarian and, at research facilities, in consultation with and approval by the Committee.

(2) Dealers, exhibitors, and research facilities, in developing their plan, should consider providing positive physical contact with humans that encourages exercise through play or other similar activities. If a dog is housed, held, or maintained at a facility without sensory contact with another dog, it must be provided with positive physical contact with humans at least daily.

(3) The opportunity for exercise may be provided in a number of ways, such as:

(i) Group housing in cages, pens or runs that provide at least 100 percent of the required space for each dog if maintained separately under the minimum floor space requirements of § 3.6(c)(1) of this subpart;

(ii) Maintaining individually housed dogs in cages, pens, or runs that provide at least twice the minimum floor space required by § 3.6(c)(1) of this subpart;

(iii) Providing access to a run or open area at the frequency and duration prescribed by the attending veterinarian; or

(iv) Other similar activities.

(4) Forced exercise methods or devices such as swimming, treadmills, or carousel-type devices are unacceptable for meeting the exercise requirements of this section. (Animal and Plant Health Inspection Service 1991)

7. The six species since 1970 are dog, cat, monkey (nonhuman primate mammal), guinea pig, hamster, and rabbit. These six have separate sections and specific regulations (such as for cage and transport crate size), whereas other covered species, such as gerbils, swine, or wild nonprimate mammals, receive only general treatment and standards.

8. The 11-member advisory committee that met to review the USDA's initial draft included three primate center veterinarians, and its one meeting was attended by veterinarians from USDA, the Institute of Laboratory Animal Resources and NIH. Seven additional members were laboratory primatologists/primate behaviorists. Dr. Jane Goodall, a field ethologist with little formal work in the captive setting, rounded out the committee, though she did not attend its sole meeting. The committee reported to the USDA in April 1987. They suggested greater flexibility than the USDA was proposing, with responsibility on the IACUC to develop and document a program for psychological well-being at existing facilities. They also recommended "that a Standing Advisory Committee be appointed to develop

regulations for facilities yet to be constructed" (Regulatory Analysis and Development 1987).

9. The Animal Welfare Act amendment of 1985 established the Animal Welfare Information Center (AWIC) at the National Agriculture Library. AWIC's staff of information specialists publish occasional literature reviews, including their 294-page book on enrichment for dogs, rodents, farm animals, and other nonprimate laboratory animals. The Smithsonian Institution's contribution to this field focuses more on zoo animals (Baer 1998).

11: A look to the future

1. Scientists can insert genes for bioluminescent proteins (luciferase from fireflies, or green fluorescent protein from jellyfish) into mice. These genes will distribute with another mouse gene (native, or also inserted) so that when and where the mouse genes of interest are turned on to function, the luminescent reporter genes will light up. So, for instance, if you wanted to know when a particular protein was expressed during normal spinal cord development, you could collect a series of mouse embryos and see at what embryonic age the fluorescence is first detected.

2. One could argue that scientists conserve monkeys because they are so expensive and so hard to come by. I am sure that cost and availability do drive some of the economy in sharing primate bodies among scientists, but my experience of primate users is that they do indeed, as a group, see these animals' lives as inherently valuable and not to be taken lightly.

3. The American Veterinary Medical Association publishes, and occasionally updates, its Veterinarian's Oath, working to walk the line of protecting animals in an animal-exploiting world. The current version was updated in 1999:

> Being admitted to the profession of veterinary medicine, I solemnly swear to use my scientific knowledge and skills for the benefit of society through the protection of animal health, the relief of animal suffering, the conservation of animal resources, the promotion of public health, and the advancement of medical knowledge.
>
> I will practice my profession conscientiously, with dignity, and in keeping with the principles of veterinary medical ethics.
>
> I accept as a lifelong obligation the continual improvement of my professional knowledge and competence. (American Veterinary Medical Association 2003)

References

Abbott, Andrew. 1988. *The System of Professions.* Chicago: The University of Chicago Press.

Achor, Amy Blount. 1996. *Animal Rights: A Beginner's Guide.* Yellow Springs, OH: WriteWare, Inc.

Adams, Carol J. 1990. *The Sexual Politics of Meat.* New York: Continuum.

Agricultural Research Service, USDA. 1966. Notice of proposed rule making, laboratory animal welfare. *Federal Register* 31: 16110–16119.

Agricultural Research Service, USDA. 1971. Proposed rule making, laboratory animal welfare. *Federal Register* 36:20472–20180.

Ake, Harry J. 1996. Laboratory beagles as pets: Follow-up analysis of 59 beagles placed through an adoption program. *Contemporary Topics in Laboratory Animal Science* 35(3):51–53.

Allred, John B., and Gary G. Berntson. 1986. Is euthanasia of rats by decapitation humane? *Journal of Nutrition* 116:1859–1861.

Allred, John B., and Gary G. Berntson. 1987. Reply to the letter of Dr. Brown (letter to the editor). *Journal of Nutrition* 117:1313.

American Dietetic Association. 1997. Position of the American Dietetic Association: Vegetarian diets. *Journal of the American Dietetic Association* 97(11):1317–1321.

American Medical Association. 1992. *Use of Animals in Biomedical Research: The Challenge and the Response. An American Medical Association White Paper.* Chicago: American Medical Association.

American Veterinary Medical Association. 1961. First AVMA Panel on Euthanasia convenes. *Journal of the American Veterinary Medical Association* 138(7):395.

American Veterinary Medical Association. 1975. New directives for Animal Welfare Act. *Journal of the American Veterinary Medical Association* 167(4):260.

American Veterinary Medical Association. 1980. Pain relief for laboratory animals. *Journal of the American Veterinary Medical Association* 177(1):28–29.

American Veterinary Medical Association. 1998. AVMA Policy Statements and Guidelines. In *AVMA Membership Directory and Resource Manual.* Schaumburg, IL: American Veterinary Medical Association. pp. 51–92.

American Veterinary Medical Association. 2002. Positions on Animal Welfare. In *2002 AVMA Directory and Resource Manual.* Schaumburg, IL: American Veterinary Medical Association. pp. 73–77.

American Veterinary Medical Association. 2003. Veterinarian's Oath (updated November 1999). In *AVMA Membership Directory and Resource Manual.* Schaumburg, IL: American Veterinary Medical Association. p. 399.

Andrews, Edwin J., B. Taylor Bennett, J. Derrell Clark, Katherine A. Houpt, Peter J. Pascoe, Gordon W. Robinson, and John R. Boyce. 1993. 1993 Report of the AVMA Panel on Euthanasia. *Journal of the American Veterinary Medical Association* 202 (2):229–249.

Animal and Plant Health Inspection Service, USDA. 1974. Proposed veterinary care, space and exercise, and audio-visual requirements. *Federal Register* 39:34335–34336.

Animal and Plant Health Inspection Service, USDA. 1986. Proposed rules. *Federal Register* 51(45):7950.

Animal and Plant Health Inspection Service, USDA. 1987. Proposed rules. *Federal Register* 52(61):10292–10322.

Animal and Plant Health Inspection Service, USDA. 1989a. Animal welfare; final rules. *Federal Register* 54(168):36112–36163.

Animal and Plant Health Inspection Service, USDA. 1989b. Animal welfare; proposed rules. *Federal Register* 54(49):10822–10954.

Animal and Plant Health Inspection Service, USDA. 1990a. 9 CFR Part 3. Animal welfare; standards; proposed rule. *Federal Register* 55(158):33448–33531.

Animal and Plant Health Inspection Service, USDA. 1990b. Animal welfare; guinea pigs, hamsters, and rabbits. *Federal Register* 55(136):28879–28883.

Animal and Plant Health Inspection Service, USDA. 1991. 9 CFR Part 3. Animal welfare; standards; final rule. *Federal Register* 56(32):6426–6505.

Animal and Plant Health Inspection Service, USDA. 1996. *USDA Employee Opinions on the Effectiveness of Performance-Based Standards for Animal Care Facilities.* Rockville, MD: U.S. Department of Agriculture.

Animal and Plant Health Inspection Service, USDA. 1999a. Animal welfare; petition for rulemaking. *Federal Register* 64(18):4356–4367.

Animal and Plant Health Inspection Service, USDA. 1999b. *Final Report on Environmental Enhancement to Promote the Psychological Well-being of Nonhuman Primates.* Rockville, MD: U.S. Department of Agriculture.

Animal and Plant Health Inspection Service, USDA. 2001. *Animal Welfare Report Fiscal Year 2001.* Rockville, MD: U.S. Department of Agriculture.

Animal and Plant Health Service, USDA. 1971. Title 9–Animals and animal products. *Federal Register,* 36:917–948.

Animal Care Panel. 1963. *Guide for Laboratory Animal Facilities and Care.* Washington, DC: Public Health Service.

Animal Welfare Institute. 1953. *Basic Care of Experimental Animals.* New York: Animal Welfare Institute.

Animal Welfare Institute. 1955. *Comfortable Quarters for Laboratory Animals.* New York: Animal Welfare Institute.

Animal Welfare Institute. 1958. Dogs' need for space stressed in new animal quarters designs. *Animal Welfare Institute Information Report* 7(4):1.

Animal Welfare Institute. 1979. *Comfortable Quarters for Laboratory Animals,* 7th ed. Washington, DC: Animal Welfare Institute.

Annis, John R., Nicholas H. Booth, L. Meyer Jones, T. C. Jones, Ralph L. Kitchell, and

Richard L. Ott. 1963. Report of the AVMA Panel on Euthanasia. *Journal of the American Veterinary Medical Association* 142(2):162–170.

Anzaldo, A. J., P. C. Harrison, G. L. Riskowski, L. A. Sebek, R.-G. Maghirang, W. R. Stricklin, and H. W. Gonyou. 1994. Increasing welfare of laboratory rats with the help of spatially enhanced cages. *Animal Welfare Information Center Newsletter* 5(3):1.

Arluke, Arnold. 1993. Trapped in a guilt cage. *Animal Welfare Information Center Newsletter* 4(2):1–8.

Arluke, Arnold. 1994. The ethical socialization of animal researchers. *Lab Animal* 23(6): 30–35.

Arluke, Arnold, and Julian Groves. 1998. Pushing the boundaries: Scientists in the public arena. In *Responsible Conduct with Animals in Research,* edited by L. A. Hart. New York: Oxford University Press. pp. 145–164.

Arluke, Arnold, and Clinton R. Sanders. 1996. *Regarding Animals.* Philadelphia: Temple University Press.

Associated Press. 1993. Rats are dissected on shuttle in first such tests in space. *The Boston Globe,* October 31, 1993, p. 11.

Baer, Janet F. 1998. A veterinary perspective of potential risk factors in environmental enrichment. In *Second Nature: Environmental Enrichment for Captive Animals,* edited by D. J. Shepherdson, J. D. Mellen, and M. Hutchins. Washington, DC: Smithsonian Institution Press. pp. 277–301.

Baier, Annette. 1985. What do women want in a moral theory? *Nous* 19:53.

Baker, J. R., and M. B. Dolan. 1977. Experiments on the humane killing of lobsters and crabs. *Scientific Papers of the Humane Education Centre* 2:1–24.

Bar-On, E., D. Weigl, R. Parvari, K. Katz, R. Weitz, and T. Steinberg. 2002. Congenital insensitivity to pain. Orthopaedic manifestations. *The Journal of Bone and Joint Surgery, British* 84(2):252–257.

Bateson, Patrick. 1986. When to experiment on animals. *New Scientist,* February 20, pp. 30–32.

Beauchamp, Tom L. 1992. The moral standing of animals in medical research. *The Journal of Law, Medicine and Health Care* 20(1–2):7–16.

Beaver, Bonnie V., Willie Reed, Steven Leary, Brendan McKiernan, Fairfield Bain, Roy Schultz, B. Taylor Bennett, Peter Pascoe, Elizabeth Shull, Linda C. Cork, Ruth Francis-Floyd, Keith D. Amass, Richard Johnson, Robert H. Schmidt, Wendy Underwood, Gus W. Thornton, and Barbara Kohn. 2001. 2000 Report of the AVMA Panel on Euthanasia. *Journal of the American Veterinary Medical Association* 218(5): 669–696.

Bekoff, Marc. 2002. *Minding Animals: Awareness, Emotions, and Heart.* New York: Oxford University Press.

Bekoff, Marc, Lori Gruen, Susan E. Townsend, and Bernard E. Rollin. 1992. Animals in science: Some areas revisited. *Animal Behavior* 44:473–484.

Bennett, B. Taylor, Christian R. Abee, and Roy Henrickson, eds. 1995. *Nonhuman Primates in Biomedical Research: Biology and Management.* San Diego, CA: Academic Press.

Bennett, B. Taylor, Marilyn J. Brown, and John C. Schofield, eds. 1994. *Essentials for Animal Research: A Primer for Research Personnel,* 2nd ed. Beltsville, MD: National Agriculture Library.

Bentham, Jeremy. 1789. Excerpt from chapter XVII, section 1. In *The Principles of Morals and Legislation*, reprint 1948 by Hafner Publishing Co., New York.

Best, Charles H. 1974. A short essay on the importance of dogs in medical research. *Physiologist* 17:437–439.

Birke, Lynda, and Mike Michael. 1995. Raising the profile of welfare: Scientists and their use of animals. *Anthrozoos* 8(2):90–99.

Birke, Lynda, and Jane Smith. 1995. Animals in experimental reports: The rhetoric of science. *Society and Animals* 3(1):23–42.

Bivin, W. Sheldon, and Edward H. Timmons. 1974. Basic biomethodology. In *The Biology of the Laboratory Rabbit*, edited by S. H. Weisbroth, R. E. Flatt and A. L. Kraus. New York: Academic Press. pp. 74–90.

Blakely, T. J. 1950. What the Animal Care Panel can contribute to the eradication of the antivivisection cult. *Proceedings of the Animal Care Panel* 1:46–47.

Blum, Deborah. 1994. *The Monkey Wars*. New York: Oxford University Press.

Boinski, S., S. P. Swing, T. S. Gross, and J. K. Davis. 1999. Environmental enrichment of brown capuchins (*Cebus apella*): Behavioral and plasma and fecal cortisol measures of effectiveness. *American Journal of Primatology* 48(1):49–68.

Bowden, Douglas, and Cathy Johnson-Delaney. 1996. U. S. primate research is alive and well in the 1990s. *Contemporary Topics in Laboratory Animal Science* 35(6):55–57.

Brewer, Nathan R. 1961. Housing for research dogs. *Federation Proceedings* 20:917–918.

Brewer, Nathan R. 1980. Personalities in the early history of laboratory animal science and medicine. *Laboratory Animal Science* 30(4):741–758.

Breyer, Stephen. 1982. *Regulation and Its Reform*. Cambridge: Harvard University Press.

Broom, Donald M. 1998. Stereotypies in animals. In *Encyclopedia of Animal Rights and Welfare*, edited by M. Bekoff and C. Meaney. Westport, CT: Greenwood Publishing Group. pp. 325–326.

Brown, Oliver M. 1987. Impact of the 1986 Report of the AVMA Panel on Euthanasia. *Journal of Nutrition* 117:1311–1312.

Budiansky, Stephen. 1992. *The Covenant of the Wild: Why Animals Chose Domestication*. New York: William Morrow and Company.

Cannon, Walter B. 1926. *The Dog's Gift to the Relief of Human Suffering*. New York: American Association for Medical Progress.

Carballido, J. M., R. Namikawa, N. Carballido-Perrig, S. Antonenko, M. G. Roncarolo, and J. E. de Vries. 2000. Generation of primary antigen-specific human T- and B-cell responses in immunocompetent SCID-hu mice. *Nature Medicine* 6(1):103–106.

Carbone, Larry. 1997a. Adoption of research animals. *Animal Welfare Information Center Newsletter* 4(3–4):1.

Carbone, Larry. 1997b. The public life of dogs: Dogs in the Animal Welfare Act. *Society for Veterinary Medical Ethics Newsletter* 3(supplement):14–16.

Carbone, L[arry]. 1997c. Death by decapitation: A case study of the scientific definition of animal welfare. *Society and Animals* 5(3):239–256.

Carbone, Larry. 1998. Euthanasia. In *Encyclopedia of Animal Rights and Welfare*, edited by M. Bekoff and C. Meaney. Westport, CT: Greenwood Publishing Group. pp. 164–166.

Carruthers, Peter. 1992. *The Animals Issue: Moral Theory in Practice*. Cambridge: Cambridge University Press.

Cavalieri, Paola, and Peter Singer, eds. 1993. *The Great Ape Project: Equality beyond Humanity.* New York: St. Martin's Press.

Clarkson, Thomas B. 1961. Laboratory animal medicine and the medical schools. *Journal of Medical Education* 36:1329–1330.

Cohen, Bennett J. 1959. The evolution of laboratory animal medicine in the United States. *Journal of the American Veterinary Medical Association* 135:161–164.

Cohen, Bennett J., and Franklin M. Loew. 1984. Laboratory animal medicine: Historical perspectives. In *Laboratory Animal Medicine,* edited by J. G. Fox, B. J. Cohen and F. M. Loew. Orlando, FL: Academic Press. pp. 1–17.

Cohen, Carl. 1986. The case for the use of animals in biomedical research. *The New England Journal of Medicine* 315(14):865–870.

Collins, Harry M. 1985. *Changing Order: Replication and Induction in Scientific Practice.* London: Sage.

Committee on Infectious Diseases of Mice and Rats, National Research Council. 1991. *Companion Guide to Infectious Diseases of Mice and Rats.* Washington, DC: National Academy Press.

Committee on Laboratory Animal Housing, Institute of Laboratory Animal Resources. 1976. *Laboratory Animal Housing.* Hunt Valley, MD: ILAR.

Committee on Pain and Distress in Laboratory Animals, Institute of Laboratory Animal Resources, Commission on Life Sciences, National Research Council. 1992. *Recognition and Alleviation of Pain and Distress in Laboratory Animals.* Washington, DC: National Academy Press.

Committee on Rodents, Institute of Laboratory Animal Resources, Commission on Life Sciences, National Research Council. 1996. *Laboratory Animal Management: Rodents.* Washington, DC: National Academy Press.

Committee on the Use of Animals in Research. 1991. *Science, Medicine, and Animals.* Washington, DC: National Academy Press.

Committee on the Use of Laboratory Animals in Biomedical and Behavioral Research, National Research Council. 1988. *Use of Laboratory Animals in Biomedical and Behavioral Research.* Washington, DC: National Academy Press.

Committee on Well-Being of Nonhuman Primates, Institute for Laboratory Animal Research, National Research Council,. 1998. *The Psychological Well-Being of Nonhuman Primates.* Washington, DC: National Academy Press.

Conahan, S. T., S. Narayan, and W. H. Vogel. 1985. Effect of decapitation and stress on some plasma electrolyte levels in rats. *Pharmacology, Behavior and Biochemistry* 23: 147–149.

Cottingham, John. 1978. A brute to the brutes? Descartes' treatment of animals. *Philosophy* 53:551–559.

Cowley, Geoffrey, Mary Hager, Lisa Drew, Tessa Namuth, Lynda Wright, Andrew Murr, Nonny Abbott, and Kate Robins. 1988. Of pain and progress. *Newsweek,* December 26, pp. 50–59.

Crockett, C. M., M. Shimoji, and D. M. Bowden. 2000. Behavior, appetite, and urinary cortisol responses by adult female pigtailed macaques to cage size, cage level, room change, and ketamine sedation. *American Journal of Primatology* 52(2):63–80.

Cunliffe-Beamer, Terrie L. 1983. Biomethodology and surgical techniques. In *The*

Mouse in Biomedical Research, Vol. 3, edited by H. L. Foster, J. D. Small and J. G. Fox. New York: Academic Press. pp. 401–437.

Cunningham, D. J. C., J. M. Patrick, and B. B. Lloyd. 1964. The respiratory response of man to hypoxia. In *Oxygen in the Animal Organism,* edited by F. Dickens and E. Neil. New York: Pergamon Press. pp. 277–293.

Curtin, Deanne. 1991. Toward an ecological ethic of care. *Hypatia* 6(1):60–73.

Dana, Charles. 1909. The zoophilic-psychosis. *Medical Record* 75:381–383.

Danneman, P. J., S. Stein, and S. O. Walshaw. 1994. Humane and practical implications of rodent anesthesia and euthanasia using different mixtures of carbon dioxide and oxygen. *Contemporary Topics in Laboratory Animal Science* 33(4):A-8.

Dawkins, Marian Stamp. 1980. *Animal Suffering: The Science of Animal Welfare.* London: Chapman and Hall.

DeGrazia, David. 1996. *Taking Animals Seriously.* Cambridge: Cambridge University Press.

DeGrazia, David, and Andrew Rowan. 1991. Pain, suffering, and anxiety in animals and humans. *Theoretical Medicine* 12:193–211.

del Mar, David Peterson. 1998. "Our Animal Friends": Depictions of animals in *Reader's Digest* during the 1950s. *Environmental History* 3(1):25–44.

Dennis, Clarence. 1966. America's Littlewood crisis: The sentimental threat to animal research. *Surgery* 60(4):827–839.

Derr, Robert F. 1991. Pain perception in decapitated rat brain. *Life Sciences* 49(19): 1399–1402.

Descartes, Rene. 1649. Letter to Henry More (1649). In *Animal Rights and Human Obligations,* edited by T. Regan and P. Singer. 1989. Englewood Cliffs, NJ: Prentice Hall. pp. 17–18.

Donnelly, Strachan. 1990. Introduction: The troubled middle *in media res. Hastings Center Report* Special Supplement (May/June): 2–4.

Dragstedt, Lester R. 1960. Ethical considerations in the use and care of laboratory animals. *Journal of Medical Education* 35(1):2–3.

Draize, J. H., G. Woodard, and H. O. Clavery. 1944. Methods for the study of irritation and toxicity of substances applied topically to the skin and mucous membranes. *The Journal of Pharmacology and Experimental Therapeutics* 82:377–390.

Drescher, R., and K. Loeffler. 1991. Einfluss unterschiedlicher Haltungsverfahren und Bewegungsmoglichkeiten auf die Kompakta der Rohrenknochen von Versuchsund Fleischkaninchen [The effects of different housing systems on the structure of long bones in Chinchilla and New Zealand White rabbits]. *Tierdarztliche Umschau* 46:736–741.

Dresser, Rebecca. 1989. Developing standards in animal research review. *Journal of the American Veterinary Medical Association* 194(9):1184–1191.

Dubner, Ronald. 1987. Research on pain mechanisms in animals. *Journal of the American Veterinary Medical Association* 191(10):1273–1276.

Duncan, Ian J., and Joy A. Mench. 2000. Does hunger hurt? *Poultry Science* 79(6):934.

Duncan, Ian J. H. 1993. The science of animal well-being. *Animal Welfare Information Center Newsletter* 4 (1):4–7.

Duncan, Ian J. H., Jeffrey Rushen, and Alistair B. Lawrence. 1993. Conclusions and implications for animal welfare. In *Stereotypic Animal Behavior: Fundamentals and Applications to Welfare,* edited by A. B. Lawrence and J. Rushen. Wallingford, UK: CAB International. pp. 193–206.

Earl, Alfred E. 1955. Care and use of dogs for research. *The Bulletin for Medical Research of the National Society for Medical Research* (March-April): 2–6.

Epstein, Steven. 1996. *Impure Science: AIDS, Activism, and the Politics of Knowledge.* Berkeley: University of California Press.

Farris, Edmond J. 1950. *The Care and Breeding of Laboratory Animals.* New York: John Wiley & Sons.

Faupel, R. P., H. J. Seitz, and W. Tarnowski. 1972. The problem of tissue sampling from experimental animals with respect to freezing technique, anoxia, stress and narcosis. *Archives of Biochemistry and Biophysics* 148:509–522.

Feldman, Bruce Max. 1996. The immorality of nonhuman animal research. *Journal of the American Veterinary Medical Association* 208(11):1798–1801.

Festing, M. F., and D. G. Altman. 2002. Guidelines for the design and statistical analysis of experiments using laboratory animals. *ILAR Journal* 43(4):244–258.

Fettman, Martin. 1995. Animals in space life sciences research: A personal perspective. *Newsletter of the International Foundation for Ethical Research* 8(3):1–7.

Finsen, Lawrence. 1988. Institutional animal care and use committees: A new set of clothes for the emperor? *The Journal of Medicine and Philosophy* 13:145–158.

Flecknell, Paul. 1995. Euthanasia. In *Laboratory Animals: An Introduction,* edited by B. A. Tuffery. West Sussex: John Wiley and Sons. pp. 375–381.

Flecknell, Paul A. 1996. *Laboratory Animal Anesthesia; 2nd ed., A Practical Introduction for Research Workers and Technicians.* London: Academic Press.

Flecknell, Paul, and Avril Waterman-Pearson. 2000. *Pain Management in Animals.* London: W. B. Saunders.

Flynn, Robert J. 1980. The founding and early history of the American Association for Laboratory Animal Science. *Laboratory Animal Science* 30(4):765–779.

Fontaine, Nicholas. 1738. *Memoires pour servir a l'histoire de Port-Royal.* Cologne.

Foster, Henry L. 1980. The history of commercial production of laboratory rodents. *Laboratory Animal Science* 30(4, Part II):793–798.

Foundation for Biomedical Research. 1987. *The Biomedical Investigator's Handbook.* Washington, DC: Foundation for Biomedical Research.

Foundation for Biomedical Research. 1990. *Portraits of a Partnership for Life: The Remarkable Story of Research, Animals and Man.* Washington, DC: Foundation for Biomedical Research.

Foundation for Biomedical Research. 1993. *Research Helping Animals.* Washington, DC: Foundation for Biomedical Research.

Fouts, Roger S. 1998. On the psychological well-being of chimpanzees. *Journal of Applied Animal Welfare Science* 1(1):65–73.

Fox, Michael Allen. 1986. *The Case for Animal Experimentation.* Berkeley: University of California Press.

Fox, Michael W. 1986. *Laboratory Animal Husbandry: Ethology, Welfare and Experimental Variables.* Albany: State University of New York Press.

Fox, Michael W. 1990. Canine behavior. In *Canine Research Environment,* edited by

J. A. Mench and L. Krulisch. Bethesda, MD: Scientists Center for Animal Welfare. pp. 21–32.

Fox, Michael W., and Marc Bekoff. 1975. The behaviour of dogs. In *The Behaviour of Domestic Animals*, edited by E. S. E. Hafez. Baltimore, MD: Williams & Wilkins. pp. 370–409.

Francione, Gary L. 1995. *Animals, Property, and the Law.* Philadelphia: Temple University Press.

Fraser, D., D. M. Weary, E. A. Pajor, and B. N. Milligan. 1997. A scientific conception of animal welfare that reflects ethical concerns. *Animal Welfare* 6:187–205.

Fraser, David. 1995. Science, values and animal welfare: Exploring the "inextricable connection." *Animal Welfare* 4:103–117.

Free, Ann Cottrell. 1982. *Animals, Nature, and Albert Schweitzer.* New York: The Albert Schweitzer Fellowship.

Frey, Raymond G. 1987. The significance of agency and marginal cases. *Philosophica* 39:39–46.

Gallup Poll. 1999. Poll on the honesty and ethics of people in different professions, November 4–7. Washington, DC: Gallup News Service.

Gay, William I. 1984. The dog as a research subject. *The Physiologist* 27(3):133–141.

Geelhoed, Glenn W. 1987. That animals might live … In *The Biomedical Investigator's Handbook*. Washington, DC: Foundation for Biomedical Research. pp. 76–79.

Gieryn, Thomas F. 1995. Boundaries of science. In *Handbook of Science and Technology Studies*, edited by S. Jasanoff, G. Markle, T. Pinch and J. Petersen. Newbury Park, CA: Sage. pp. 393–443.

Gilligan, Carol. 1982. *In a Different Voice.* Cambridge: Harvard University Press.

Gluck, J. P., and S. R. Kubacki. 1991. Animals in biomedical research: The undermining effect of the rhetoric of the besieged. *Ethics and Behavior* 1:157–173.

Grandin, Temple. 2000. *Livestock Handling and Transport*, 2nd ed. New York: CABI Publishing.

Gregory, Neville G., and Temple Grandin. 1998. *Animal Welfare and Meat Science.* New York: CABI Publishing.

Griffin, Charles A. 1952. A study of prepared feeds in relation to *Salmonella* infection in laboratory animals. *Journal of the American Veterinary Medical Association* 1221: 197–200.

Groves, Julian McAllister. 1997. *Hearts and Minds: The Controversy over Laboratory Animals.* Philadelphia: Temple University Press.

Gunn, Debbie, and David B. Morton. 1993. The behaviour of singly-caged and group-housed laboratory rabbits. Paper read at *Welfare and Science: Proceedings of the Fifth Symposium of the Federation of European Laboratory Animal Science Associations,* June 8–11, 1993, at Brighton, UK.

Hagen, Karl W. 1974. Colony husbandry. In *The Biology of the Laboratory Rabbit*, edited by S. H. Weisbroth, R. E. Flatt and A. L. Kraus. New York: Academic Press. pp. 23–47.

Harkness, Richard, and Gladys Harkness. 1956. Medicine's animal pioneers. *Reader's Digest* (October):165–168.

Harwood, William. 1993a. Shuttle becomes a biology lab for weightlessness research on rats. *The Washington Post*, October 31, p. A7.

Harwood, William. 1993b. Shuttle crew draws blood to explore disorders. *The Washington Post*, October 24, p. 26.

Heidbrink, Gail. 1987. Survey of attitudes of laboratory animal technicians. *Laboratory Animal Science* 37:104–105.

Herrick, John B. 1990. An open letter to animal rights activists: Let's get our priorities in perspective. *Journal of the American Veterinary Medical Association* 197(6):712–713.

Herzog, Harold A. 1989. The moral status of mice. *American Psychologist* 43(6):473–474.

Herzog, Harold A. 1993. "The movement is my life": The psychology of animal rights activism. *Journal of Social Issues* 49(1):103–119.

Herzog, Harold A. 1998. Understanding animal activism. In *Responsible Conduct with Animals in Research*, edited by L. A. Hart. New York: Oxford University Press. pp. 165–183.

Hite, M., H. M. Hanson, N. R. Bodihar, P. A. Conti, and P. A. Mattis. 1977. Effect of cage size on patterns of activity and health of beagle dogs. *Laboratory Animal Science* 27(1):64.

Holden, Constance. 1988. Billion dollar price tag for new animal rules. *Science* 242: 662–663.

Holmes, Donald D. 1984. *Clinical Laboratory Animal Medicine*. Ames: Iowa State University Press.

Holson, R. Robert. 1992. Euthanasia by decapitation: Evidence that this technique produces prompt, painless unconsciousness in laboratory rodents. *Neurotoxicology and Teratology* 14:253–257.

Houpt, Katherine A. 1998. *Domestic Animal Behavior for Veterinarians and Animal Scientists*, 3rd ed. Ames: Iowa State University Press.

Houri, J. M., and F. X. O'Sullivan. 1995. Animal models in rheumatoid arthritis. *Current Opinions in Rheumatology* 7(3):201–205.

Hoversten, Paul. 1993. Heads they lose—in space. *USA Today*, October 14, p. 3A.

Hughes, Everett Cherrington. 1958. *Men and Their Work*. Toronto: The Free Press.

Hughes, Howard C., and Sarah Campbell. 1990. Effects of primary enclosure size and human contact. In *The Canine Research Environment*, edited by J. A. Mench and L. Krulisch. Bethesda, MD: Scientists Center for Animal Welfare. pp. 66–75.

Hughes, Howard C., Sarah Campbell, and Cheryl Kenney. 1989. The effects of cage size and pair housing on exercise of beagle dogs. *Laboratory Animal Science* 39(4): 302–305.

Hughes, Howard C., and Charles C. Warnick. 1986. Euthanasia: A comparison of the 1978 and 1986 AVMA Panel Reports. *Lab Animal* 15:29–31.

Humane Society of the United States. 2002. *Concerns about Carbon Dioxide Use in Euthanasia and Anesthesia*. Available: http://www.hsus.org/ace/12633. Accessed April 14, 2003.

Hume, C. W. 1957. The legal protection of laboratory animals. In *The UFAW Handbook on the Care and Management of Laboratory Animals*, edited by A. N. Worden and W. Lane-Petter. London: Universities Federation for Animal Welfare. pp. 1–14.

Iadarola, Michael J., and Robert M. Caudle. 1997. Good pain, bad pain. *Science* 278: 239–240.

ILAR (Institute of Laboratory Animal Resources). National Research Council. 1965. *Guide for Laboratory Animal Facilities and Care,* 2nd ed. Washington, DC: National Institutes of Health.

ILAR (Institute of Laboratory Animal Resources). 1968. *Guide for Laboratory Animal Facilities and Care,* 3rd ed. Washington, DC: National Institutes of Health.

ILAR (Institute of Laboratory Animal Resources) National Research Council. 1972. *Guide for the Care and Use of Laboratory Animals,* 4th ed. Bethesda, MD: National Institutes of Health.

ILAR (Institute of Laboratory Animal Resources) National Academy of Sciences. 1974. ILAR comments to proposed rules. *ILAR News* 18(1):6–8.

ILAR (Institute of Laboratory Animal Resources) National Research Council. 1978. *Guide for the Care and Use of Laboratory Animal Resources,* 5th ed. Bethesda, MD: National Institutes of Health.

ILAR (Institute of Laboratory Animal Resources). 1985. *Guide for the Care and Use of Laboratory Animals.* NIH Publication no. 85–23. Bethesda, MD: National Institutes of Health.

ILAR (Institute of Laboratory Animal Resources). 1996. *Guide for the Care and Use of Laboratory Animals.* Washington, DC: National Academy Press.

International Association for the Study of Pain. 1983. Ethical guidelines for investigations of experimental pain in conscious animals. *Pain* 16:109–110.

Irving, George W. 1967. Laboratory animal welfare, rules and regulations. *Federal Register* 32:3270–3282.

Jamison, Wesley V., and William M. Lunch. 1992. Rights of animals, perceptions of science, and political activism: Profile of American animal rights activists. *Science, Technology, & Human Values* 17(4):438–458.

Jasanoff, Sheila. 1990. *The Fifth Branch: Science Advisors as Policy Makers.* Cambridge: Harvard University Press.

Jasper, James M., and Dorothy Nelkin. 1992. *The Animal Rights Crusade: The Growth of a Moral Protest.* New York: The Free Press.

Jenkins, William L. 1987. Pharmacologic aspects of analgesic drugs in animals: An overview. *Journal of the American Veterinary Medical Association* 191(10):1231–1240.

Jones, James H. 1981. *Bad Blood.* New York: Free Press.

Jones, Susan D. 2003. *Valuing Animals: Veterinarians and Their Patients in Modern America.* Baltimore, MD: Johns Hopkins University Press.

Kalagassy, Erin, Lawrence G. Carbone, and Katherine A. Houpt. 1999. Effect of castration on rabbits housed in littermate pairs. *Journal of Applied Animal Welfare Science* 2(2):111–121.

Keeling, Michale E. 1974. Housing requirements—primates. In *CRC Handbook of Laboratory Animal Science,* edited by E. C. Melby and H. C. Altman. Boca Raton, FL: CRC Press. pp. 97–106.

Kelley, Stephen T., and Arthur S. Hall. 1995. Housing. In *Nonhuman Primates in Biomedical Research: Biology and Management,* edited by B. T. Bennett, C. R. Abee and R. Henrickson. San Diego, CA: Academic Press. pp. 193–209.

Kitchell, Ralph L., Howard E. Erickson, E. Carstens, and Lloyd E. Davis, eds. 1983.

Animal Pain: Perception and Alleviation. Bethesda, MD: American Physiological Society.

Klemm, W. R. 1987. Letter to the editor. *Laboratory Animal Science* 37(2):148–151.

Klemm, William R. 1992. Are there EEG correlates of mental states in animals? *Neuropsychobiology* 26:151–165.

Kohn, Dennis F., Sally K. Wixson, William J. White, and G. John Benson, eds. 1997. *Anesthesia and Analgesia in Laboratory Animals.* San Diego, CA: Academic Press.

Kruse, Corwin R. 1998. Who said that? Status presentation in media accounts of the animal experimentation debate. *Society and Animals* 6(3):235–243.

Labaton, Stephen. 1993. Animal advocates win court ruling. *The New York Times,* February 26, p. A12.

LaFollette, Hugh, and Niall Shanks. 1996. *Brute Science: Dilemmas of Animal Experimentation.* London: Routledge.

Latour, Bruno, and Steve Woolgar. 1979. *Laboratory Life: The Construction of Scientific Facts.* Princeton, NJ: Princeton University Press.

Leader, Robert W., and Dennis Stark. 1987. The importance of animals in biomedical research. *Perspectives in Biology and Medicine* 30(4):470–485.

Lederer, Susan E. 1987. The controversy over animal experimentation in America, 1880–1914. In *Vivisection in Historical Perspective,* edited by N. A. Rupke. London: Croon Helm. pp. 236–257.

Lederer, Susan E. 1992. Political animals: The shaping of biomedical research literature in twentieth-century America. *Isis* 83:61–79.

Lederer, Susan E. 1995. *Subjected to Science: Human Experimentation in America before the Second World War.* Baltimore, MD: Johns Hopkins University Press.

Lee, James O. 1981. Testimony before the Subcommittee on Science, Research and Technology, United States House of Representatives. In *The Use of Animals in Medical Research and Testing.* Washington, DC: U.S. Government Printing Office. pp. 145–147.

Levin, Lisa Hara, and Martin L. Stephens. 1994. Appointing animal protectionists to institutional animal care and use committees. *Animal Welfare Information Center Newsletter* 5(4):1–10.

Levitt, M. 1985. Dysesthesias and self-mutilation in humans and subhumans: a review of clinical and experimental studies. *Brain Research* 357(3):247–290.

Linzey, Andrew. 1998. Sentientism. In *Encyclopedia of Animal Rights and Welfare,* edited by M. Bekoff and C. Meaney. Westport, CT: Greenwood Publishing Group. p. 311.

Lorden, Joan F. 1987. Letter to the editor. *Laboratory Animal Science* 37(2):148.

Lynch, M. E. 1988. Sacrifice and the transformation of the animal body into a scientific object: laboratory culture and ritual practices in the neurosciences. *Social Studies of Science* 18:265–289.

MacNabb, Donald G. C. 1967. Hume, David. In *The Encyclopedia of Philosophy,* vol. 4, edited by Paul Edwards. New York: Macmillan.

Mahoney, James. 1998. *Saving Molly: A Research Veterinarian's Choices.* Chapel Hill, NC: Algonquin Books.

Markowitz, Hal, and Scott Line. 1990. The need for responsive environments. In *The*

Experimental Animal in Biomedical Research, edited by B. E. Rollin and M. L. Kesel. Boca Raton, FL: CRC Press. pp. 153–170.

Marshall, Steve, and Todd Halvorson. 1993. Space to be final frontier for 5 shuttle rats. *USA Today,* May 12, p. 3A.

Martin, Brian, and Evelleen Richards. 1995. Scientific knowledge, controversy, and public decision making. In *Handbook of Science and Technology Studies,* edited by S. Jasanoff, G. Markle, T. Pinch and J. Petersen. Newbury Park, CA: Sage. pp. 506–526.

Martin, D. P., T. Gilberto, C. Burns, and H. C. Pautler. 2002. Nonhuman primate cage modifications for environmental enrichment. *Contemporary Topics in Laboratory Animal Science* 41(5):47–49.

Matfield, Mark. 1995. The public debate about animal experimentation. *Alternatives to Laboratory Animals (ATLA)* 23:312–316.

Mathias, Francis J. 1987. Decapitating animals shows insensitivity to life. *Chronicle of Higher Education,* May 6, p. 5.

McCune, J. M. 1997. Animal models of HIV-1 disease. *Science* 278(5346):2141–2142.

McDonald, L. E., N. H. Booth, W. V. Lumb, R. W. Redding, D. C. Sawyer, L. Stevenson, and W. M. Wass. 1978. Report of the AVMA Panel on Euthanasia. *Journal of the American Veterinary Medical Association* 173:59–72.

McGlone, John J. 1993. What is animal welfare? *Journal of Agricultural and Environmental Ethics* 6(special supplement 2):26–36.

Melcher, John. 1991. Enrichment strategies for dog housing and exercise: Questions and answers. Paper read at Implementation Strategies for Research Animal Well-Being: Institutional Compliance with Regulations, June 1992, Baltimore, MD.

Mench, J. 1998. Why it is important to understand animal behavior. *ILAR Journal* 39(1):20–26.

Mench, Joy A. 1994. Environmental enrichment and exploration. *Lab Animal* 23(2): 38–41.

Merskey, H., and N. Bogduk, eds. 1994. *Classification of Chronic Pain,* 2nd ed. Seattle, WA: IASP Press.

Merton, Robert K. 1942. Science and technology in a democratic order. *Journal of Legal and Political Sociology* 1:115–126.

Michael, Mike, and Lynda Birke. 1994. Enrolling the core set: The case of the animal experimentation controversy. *Social Studies of Science* 24:81–95.

Midgley, Mary. 1983. *Animals and Why They Matter.* Athens: University of Georgia Press.

Mikeska, J. A., and W. R. Klemm. 1975. EEG evaluation of humaneness of asphyxia and decapitation euthanasia of the laboratory rat. *Laboratory Animal Science* 25(2): 175–179.

Millennium Guild. 1980. Advertisement in the *New York Times.* April 15, p. 318.

Miller, Robert M. 1983. Animal welfare—yes! Human laws—sure! Animal rights—no! *California Veterinarian* 37(1):21.

Moberg, Gary P. 1985. Biological response to stress: Key to assessment of well-being? In *Animal Stress,* edited by G. P. Moberg. Bethesda, MD: American Physiological Society. pp. 27–49.

Moore, George E. 1903 (reprinted 1959). *Principia Ethica.* Cambridge, UK: Cambridge University Press.

Morgan, Charles F. 1954. The Procurement of Animals in the District of Columbia. Paper read at Fifth Annual Meeting of the Animal Care Panel, December 1–2, 1954, Chicago.

Morrison, Adrian R. 1998. Thoughts of a working scientist: Basic ethics of animal research clear within scientific mission. *Science and Animal Care* 9(2):1.

Morton, David B., et al. 1993. Refinements in rabbit husbandry. Second report of the BVAAWF/FRAME/RSPCA/UFAW Joint Working Group on Refinement. *Laboratory Animals* 27:301–329.

Muchmore, E. A. 2001. Chimpanzee models for human disease and immunobiology. *Immunological Reviews* 183:86–93.

Nace, Patrick. 1994. WARDS and the Animal Welfare Act (Part 1 of 2). *Our Animal WARDS* (Winter 1994):3–8, 17–18.

Nasto, Barbara. 1994. Space rats. *Lab Animal* 23(1):12.

National Commission for the Protection of Human Subjects of Biomedical and Behavioral Research. 1978. *The Belmont Report.* DHEW Publication OS 78–0012. Washington, DC: Department of Health, Education, and Welfare.

National Institute of Environmental Health Sciences. 1989. *With Respect to Life: Protecting Human Health and the Environment through Laboratory Animal Research.* Washington, DC: Department of Health and Human Services.

National Research Council, Institute of Laboratory Animal Resources, Subcommittee on Dog and Cat Standards, 1973. *Dogs: Standards and Guidelines for the Breeding, Care and Management of Laboratory Animals.* Washington, DC: National Academy of Sciences.

National Society for Medical Research. 1947. A review of state legislation on animal experimentation. *Bulletin of the National Society for Medical Research* 2(2):1–4.

National Society for Medical Research. 1949. How to obtain animals from local authorities. *Bulletin of the National Society for Medical Research* 3(3):1–2, 10–17.

National Society for Medical Research. 1954. March of medicine: Tells story of animal research frankly. *The Bulletin for Medical Research* 8(5):6–7.

Neamand, Janet, W. T. Sweeney, A. A. Creamer, and P. A. Conti. 1975. Cage activity in the laboratory beagle: A preliminary study to evaluate a method of comparing cage size to physical activity. *Laboratory Animal Science* 25(2):180–183.

Nelkin, Dorothy, 1992. *Controversy*, 3rd ed. Newbury Park, CA: Sage Publications.

Nesse, Randolph M. 1991. What good is feeling bad? *The Sciences* (Nov./Dec.): 31–37.

Newton, W. M. 1972. An evaluation of the effects of various degrees of long-term confinement on adult beagle dogs. *Laboratory Animal Science* 22(6):860–864.

Nishihara, Masateru, and Roy W. Keenan. 1985. Inositol phospholipid levels of rat forebrain obtained by freeze-blowing method. *Biochimica et Biophysica Acta* 835:415–418.

Nolen, R. Scott. 2000. Lawsuit settlement draws ire of research community: Congress delays agreement to regulate research on rats, mice, birds. *Journal of the American Veterinary Medical Association* 217(11):1607, 1612.

North Carolina Association for Biomedical Research. 1991. *The Lucky Puppy.* Raleigh: North Carolina Association for Biomedical Research.

The Nuremberg Code. 1949. In *From Trials of War Criminals Before the Nuremberg Military Tribunals Under Control Council Law No. 10.* Nuremberg.

Office of Protection from Research Risks. 1986. *Public Health Service Policy on Humane Care and Use of Laboratory Animals.* Bethesda, MD: National Institutes of Health.

Office of Technology Assessment. 1986. *Alternatives to Animal Use in Research, Testing and Education.* Washington, DC: U.S. Government Printing Office.

Olfert, Ernest D., Brenda M. Cross, and A. Ann McWilliam, eds. 1993. *Guide to the Care and Use of Experimental Animals,* vol. 1, 2nd ed. Ottawa, Ontario: Canadian Council on Animal Care.

O'Mara, Kevin T., William E. Hinds, and Robert W. Phillips. 1994. Euthanasia during life science research in space. *Contemporary Topics in Laboratory Animal Science* 33(1):68–72.

Orlans, F. Barbara. 1993. *In the Name of Science: Issues in Responsible Animal Experimentation.* New York: Oxford University Press.

Orlans, F. Barbara, Tom L. Beauchamp, Rebecca Dresser, David B. Morton, and John P. Gluck. 1998. *The Human Use of Animals: Case Studies in Ethical Choice.* New York: Oxford University Press.

Orwell, George. 1945. *Animal Farm.* London: Secker and Warburg.

Ott, Randall S. 1995. The natural wrongs about animal rights. *Journal of the American Veterinary Medical Association* 207(8):1023–1032.

Panel on the Recognition and Alleviation of Animal Pain and Distress. 1987. Panel Report on the Colloquium on Recognition and Alleviation of Animal Pain and Distress. *Journal of the American Veterinary Medical Association* 191(10):1186–1191.

Parascandola, John. 1991. The development of the Draize test for eye toxicity. *Pharmacy in History* 33(3):111–117.

Patton, Nephi M. 1994. Colony Husbandry. In *The Biology of the Laboratory Rabbit,* edited by P. J. Manning, D. H. Ringler and C. E. Newcomer. San Diego, CA: Academic Press. pp. 28–46.

Pavia, Audrey. 1998. Saying grace. *ASPCA Animal Watch* (Fall):27–31.

Penslar, Robin Levin, and National Institutes of Health Office for Protection from Research Risks. 1993. *Protecting Human Research Subjects: Institutional Review Board Guidebook,* 2nd ed. Bethesda, MD: U.S. Deptartment of Health and Human Services.

People for the Ethical Treatment of Animals. 1984. *Unnecessary Fuss* (videotape). Rockville, MD: PETA.

Phillips, Mary T. 1993. Savages, drunks, and lab animals: The researcher's perception of pain. *Society and Animals* 1(1):61–81.

Phinizy, Coles. 1965. The lost pets that stray to the labs. *Sports Illustrated,* November 27, pp. 36–49.

Plous, S., and H. Herzog. 2001. Animal research. Reliability of protocol reviews for animal research. *Science* 293(5530):608–609.

Plumwood, Val. 1991. Nature, self, and gender: Feminism, environmental philosophy, and the critique of rationalism. *Hypatia* (1):3–27.

Pollan, Michael. 2002. An animal's place. *The New York Times Magazine,* November 10.

Prentice, Ernest, Andrew Jameson, Dean Antonson, and Irving Zucker. 1988. Prior ethical review of animal versus human subjects research. *Investigative Radiology* 23:695–697.

Presidential Task Force on Regulatory Relief. 1983. *Reagan Administration Regulatory Achievements.* Washington, DC: U.S. Government Printing Office.

Quimby, Fred. 2002. Animal models in biomedical research. In *Laboratory Animal Medicine*, edited by J. G. Fox, L. C. Anderson, F. M. Loew and F. Quimby. New York: Academic Press.

Quimby, Fred W. 1994. Twenty-five years of progress in laboratory animal science. *Laboratory Animals* 28:158–171.

Rachels, James. 1990. *Created from Animals: The Moral Implications of Darwinism*. Oxford: Oxford University Press.

Reed, Susan, and Sue Carswell. 1993. Animal passion. *People*, January 18, pp. 34–39.

Regan, Tom. 1983. *The Case for Animal Rights*. Berkeley: University of California Press.

Regulatory Analysis and Development, Animal and Plant Health Inspection Service, USDA. 1986. Docket 86-009.

Regulatory Analysis and Development, Animal and Plant Health Inspection Service, USDA. 1987. Dockets 84-010, 84-027.

Regulatory Analysis and Development, Animal and Plant Health Inspection Service, USDA. 1989. Dockets 87-004, 88-013, 88-014.

Regulatory Analysis and Development, Animal and Plant Health Inspection Service, USDA. 1990. Docket 90-040.

Reinhardt, Viktor. 1990. Time budget of caged rhesus monkeys exposed to a companion, a PVC perch and a piece of wood for an extended time. *American Journal of Primatology* 20:51–56.

Reinhardt, Viktor. 1994. Pair-housing rather than single-housing for laboratory rhesus macaques. *Journal of Medical Primatology* 23:426–431.

Reinhardt, Viktor, and Annie Reinhardt, eds. 2002. *Comfortable Quarters for Laboratory Animals*, 9th ed. Washington, DC: Animal Welfare Institute.

Retzlaff, E. 1966. Effects of daily exercise on life span of albino rats. *Geriatrics* 21:171.

Robb, J. Wesley. 1991. Ethical aspects of the use of animals in research. *Journal of Investigative Surgery* 4:239–246.

Rollin, Bernard E. 1981. *Animal Rights and Human Morality*. Buffalo, NY: Prometheus Books.

Rollin, Bernard E. 1989. *The Unheeded Cry: Animal Consciousness, Animal Pain, and Science*. New York: Oxford University Press.

Rollin, Bernard E. 1992. *Animal Rights and Human Morality*, 2nd ed., rev. Buffalo, NY: Prometheus Books.

Rollin, Bernard E. 1995. *Farm Animal Welfare: Social, Bioethical, and Research Issues*. Ames: Iowa State University Press.

Rollin, Bernard E., and M. Lynne Kesel, eds. 1990. *The Experimental Animal in Biomedical Research*, vol. 1. Boca Raton, FL: CRC Press.

Rollin, Bernard E., and M. Lynne Kesel, eds. 1995. *The Experimental Animal in Biomedical Research*, vol. 2. Boca Raton, FL: CRC Press.

Rosenberger, Jack. 1990. Animal rites. *The Village Voice*, March 6, pp. 30–39.

Rosenblum, Leonard A., and Michael W. Andrews. 1995. Environmental enrichment and psychological well-being of nonhuman primates. In *Nonhuman Primates in Biomedical Research: Biology and Management*, edited by B. T. Bennett, C. R. Abee and R. Henrickson. San Diego, CA: Academic Press. pp. 101–112.

Roughan, J. V., and P. A. Flecknell. 2002. Buprenorphine: A reappraisal of its antinociceptive effects and therapeutic use in alleviating post-operative pain in animals. *Lab Animal* 36(3):322–343.

Rowan, Andrew N. 1984. *Of Mice, Models, and Men: A Critical Evaluation of Animal Research.* Albany: State University of New York Press.

Rowan, Andrew. 1992. More on decapitation and scientific research. *Science and Animal Care: The WARDS Newsletter* (Summer 1992):3.

Rowan, Andrew N. 1998. Silver Spring monkeys. In *Encyclopedia of Animal Rights and Welfare,* edited by M. Bekoff and C. Meaney. Westport, CT: Greenwood Publishing Group. pp. 317–318.

Rowan, Andrew N., Franklin M. Loew, and Joan C. Weer. 1995. *The Animal Research Controversy: Protest, Process and Public Policy.* N. Grafton, MA: Center for Animals and Public Policy, Tufts University School of Veterinary Medicine.

Royal Society and the Universities Federation for Animal Welfare. 1987. *Guidelines on the Care and Use of Laboratory Animals and their Use for Scientific Purposes.* London: Wembley Press.

Rudwick, Martin J. S. 1985. *The Great Devonian Controversy: The Shaping of Scientific Knowledge among Gentlemanly Specialists.* Chicago: University of Chicago Press.

Rupke, Nicolaas, ed. 1987. *Vivisection in Historical Perspective.* London: Croon Helm.

Russell, W. M. S., and R. L. Burch. 1959. *The Principles of Humane Experimental Technique.* London: Methuen.

Russow, Lilly-Marlene. 1995. Protocol review: Too much paperwork? Paper read at Current Issues and New Frontiers in Animal Research, December 8–9, 1994, San Antonio, TX. Greenbelt, MD: Scientists Center for Animal Welfare.

Russow, Lilly-Marlene. 1998. Institutional Animal Care and Use Committees. In *Encyclopedia of Animal Rights and Welfare,* edited by M. Bekoff and C. Meaney. Westport, CT: Greenwood Publishing Group. pp. 204–206.

Ryder, Richard D. 1998. Speciesism. In *Encyclopedia of Animal Rights and Welfare,* edited by M. Bekoff and C. Meaney. Westport, CT: Greenwood Publishing Group. p. 320.

Sapontzis, Steve. 1987. *Morals, Reason, and Animals.* Philadelphia: Temple University Press.

Sapontzis, Steve F. 1990. The case against invasive research with animals. In *The Experimental Animal in Biomedical Research,* vol. 1, edited by B. E. Rollin and M. L. Kesel. Boca Raton, FL: CRC Press.

Saulmon, E. E. 1970. Implementation of laboratory animal laws. *Journal of the American Veterinary Medical Association* 157(11):1964–1968.

Schapiro, S. J. 2002. Effects of social manipulations and environmental enrichment on behavior and cell-mediated immune responses in rhesus macaques. *Pharmacology, Biochemistry and Behavior* 73(1):271–278.

Schwindaman, Dale, Mark Conner, Charles McPherson, Joseph Pierce, John C. Norman, Julius Cass, Harold R. Parker, and Lowell T. Harmison. 1973. The use of animals in medical research and experimentation. In *Research Animals in Medicine,* edited by L. T. Harmison. DHEW Publication no. 72-333. Washington, DC: U.S. Department of Health, Education and Welfare.

Scientists Center for Animal Welfare. 1983. Update: Animal welfare legislation. *Scientists Center for Animal Welfare Newsletter* 5(2):1–2.

Scientists Center for Animal Welfare. 1987. Consensus recommendations on effective institutional animal care and use committees. *Laboratory Animal Science* 37:11–13.

Segal, Evalyn F., ed. 1989. *Housing, Care and Psychological Wellbeing of Captive and Laboratory Primates.* Park Ridge, NJ: Noyes Publications.

Shalev, Moshe. 1994a. Appeals court dismisses ruling requiring regulations for laboratory-raised rats, mice and birds. *Lab Animal* 23(7):4.

Shalev, Moshe. 1994b. Court of appeals overturns "Primates and dogs" ruling. *Lab Animal* 23(10).

Shugg, Wallace. 1968. Humanitarian attitudes in the early experiments of the Royal Society. *Annals of Science* 24(3):227–238.

Silva, Michel. 1966. Concentration camps for dogs. *Life,* February 4, pp. 22–29.

Singer, Peter. 1975. *Animal Liberation,* 1st ed. New York: Avon Books.

Singer, Peter. 1990. *Animal Liberation,* 2nd ed. New York: Avon Books.

Sismondo, Sergio. 1996. *Science Without Myth: On Constructions, Reality, and Social Knowledge.* Albany: State University of New York Press.

Smith, A. W., K. H. Houpt, R. L. Kitchell, D. F. Kohn, L. E. McDonald, M. Passaglia, J. C. Thurmon, and E. R. Ames. 1986. 1986 Report of the AVMA Panel on Euthanasia. *Journal of the American Veterinary Medical Association* 188(3):252–268.

Smith, Alvin W. 1988. Euthanasia (letter to the editor). *Journal of the American Veterinary Medical Association* 193(2):161–162.

Smith, C. R., N. H. Booth, M. W. Fox, B. S. Jortner, W. V. Lumb, A. F. Moreland, and W. M. Wass. 1972. Report of the AVMA Panel on Euthanasia. *Journal of the American Veterinary Medical Association* 160(5):761–772.

Smith, David R. 1990. Comment. *Journal of the American Veterinary Medical Association* 196:1738–1739.

Smith, Jane A., and Kenneth M. Boyd. 1991. The assessment and "weighing" of costs and benefits. In *Lives in the Balance,* edited by J. A. Smith and K. M. Boyd. New York: Oxford University Press. pp. 138–146.

Smith, Maggie. 1995. Rats: The road to her PhD was paved with dead rodents. *The Utne Reader* (May–June):85–87.

Spencer, Lea. 1994. In orbit: Fettman reaches new heights. *Journal of the American Veterinary Medical Association* 204(1):14–17.

Sperling, S. 1988. *Animal Liberators: Research and Morality.* Berkeley: University of California Press.

Sprigge, T. L. S. 1985. Philosophers and antivivisectionism. *Alternatives to Laboratory Animals (ATLA)* 13:99–106.

Stafleu, F. R., B. D. Baarda, F. R. Heeger, and A. C. Beynen. 1994. The influence of animal discomfort and human interest on the ethical acceptability of animal experiments. Paper read at Welfare and Science: Proceedings of the Fifth Symposium of the Federation of European Laboratory Animal Science Associations, June 8–11, 1993, Brighton, UK.

Stafleu, Frans Richard. 1994. The ethical acceptability of animal experiments as judged by researchers. PhD dissertation, Universiteit Utrecht, Utrecht, The Netherlands.

Stafleu, Frans R., F. Robert Heeger, and Anton C. Beynen. 1989. A case study on the impact of clinically-observed abnormalities in mice with gallstones on the ethical admissibility of a projected experiment with gallstone-bearing mice. *Alternatives to Laboratory Animals (ATLA)* 17:101–108.

Stephens, Martin L., Philip Mendoza, Adrianna Weaver, and Tamara Hamilton. 1998. Unrelieved pain and distress in animals: An analysis of USDA data on experimental procedures. *Journal of Applied Animal Welfare Science* 1(1):15–26.

Stephens, U. Kristina. 1987. Role of laboratory animal technicians as committee members. *Laboratory Animal Science* 37:103.

Stevens, Christine. 1968. Laboratory Animal Welfare. In *Animals and Their Legal Rights: A Survey of American Laws from 1641 to 1968,* edited by E. S. Leavitt. Washington, DC: The Animal Welfare Institute. pp. 46–66.

Stevens, Christine. 1990. Laboratory Animal Welfare. In *Animals and Their Legal Rights.* Washington, DC: Animal Welfare Institute. pp. 66–105.

Stricklin, W. R. 1995. Space as environmental enrichment. *Lab Animal* 24(4):24–29.

Subcommittee on Primate Standards, Institute of Laboratory Animal Resources, National Research Council. 1968. *Nonhuman Primates: Standards and Guidelines for the Breeding, Care, and Management of Laboratory Animals.* Washington, DC: National Academy of Sciences.

Subcommittee on Revision of Nonhuman Primate Standards, Institute of Laboratory Animal Resources, National Research Council, 1973. *Nonhuman Primates: Standards and Guidelines for the Breeding, Care, and Management of Laboratory Animals,* 2nd ed. Washington, DC: National Academy of Sciences.

Szymczyk, Jessica. 1995. Animals, vegetables and minerals. *Newsweek,* August 14, p. 10.

Takacs, David. 1996. *The Idea of Biodiversity: Philosophies of Paradise.* Baltimore, MD: Johns Hopkins University Press.

Tannenbaum, Jerrold. 1986. Animal rights: Some guideposts for the veterinarian. *Journal of the American Veterinary Medical Association* 188(11):1258–1263.

Tannenbaum, Jerrold. 1995. *Veterinary Ethics: Animal Welfare, Client Relations, Competition and Collegiality,* 2nd ed. St. Louis: Mosby.

Taub, E., J. E. Crago, L. D. Burgio, T. E. Groomes, E. W. Cook, IIIrd, S. C. DeLuca, and N. E. Miller. 1994. An operant approach to rehabilitation medicine: overcoming learned nonuse by shaping. *Journal of the Experimental Analysis of Behavior* 61(2):281–293.

Thomas, Elizabeth Marshall. 1993. *The Hidden Life of Dogs.* New York: Houghton Mifflin.

Toates, F. 2000. Multiple factors controlling behaviour: Implications for stress and welfare. In *The Biology of Animal Stress: Basic Principles and Implications for Animal Welfare,* edited by G. P. Moberg and J. A. Mench. Wallingford, UK: CABI Publishing. pp. 199–226.

Townsend, Paul, and David B. Morton. 1995. Laboratory animal care policies and regulations: United Kingdom. *ILAR Journal* 37(2):68–74.

U.S. Congress. 1966a. *Laboratory Animal Welfare Act of 1966,* Public Law 89-544.

U.S. Congress. 1966b. House. Conference Report to accompany H.R. 13881. 89th Cong., 2nd sess.

U.S. Congress. 1966c. Senate Committee on Commerce. Hearings on S. 2322, S. 3059, and S. 3138, 89th Cong., 2nd sess.

U.S. Congress. 1966d. House. Committee on Agriculture, Subcommittee on Livestock and Feed Grains. Hearings on H.R. 13406. 89th Cong., 2nd sess. pp. 103–110.

U.S. Congress. 1970a. *Animal Welfare Act of 1970*, Public Law 91–579, 91st Cong., 2nd sess.

U.S. Congress. 1970b. House. *Congressional Record.* 91st Cong., 1st sess., 1970. Vol. 116, pt. X. P. 40155.

U.S. Congress. 1981. House. *The Use of Animals in Medical Research and Testing. Hearings before the Subcommittee on Science, Research and Technology.* 97th Cong., 1st sess. Docket 68.

U.S. Congress. 1985a. *Food Security Act of 1985*, Public Law 99-198. Title XVII, Subtitle F–Animal Welfare.

U.S. Congress. 1985b. *Health Research Extension Act of 1985*, Public Law 99-158.

U.S. Congress. 1990. *Food, Agriculture, Conservation, and Trade Act of 1990*, Public Law 101-62. *Protection of Pets.* 101st Cong., 2nd sess.

U.S. Congress. 2002. Title X, Subtitle D Sec. 10301. *Definition of Animal under the Animal Welfare Act.*

U.S. Department of Agriculture. 1977. Animal Welfare: Definition of Terms. *Federal Register* 42(117):31022–31029.

U.S. Department of Agriculture. 1977. Code of Federal Regulations, 9.

U.S. Department of Health and Human Services. 1991. Protection of human subjects (45 CFR Subtitle A, Part 46). *Federal Register*:28012–28022.

U.S. Interagency Research Animal Committee. 1985. Principles for the utilization and care of vertebrate animals used in testing, research, and training. *Federal Register* 50(97):20864–20865.

Vanderwolf, C. H., G. Buzsaki, D. P. Cain, R. K. Cooley, and B. Robertson. 1988. Neocortical and hippocampal electrical activity following decapitation in the rat. *Brain Research* 451:340–344.

Veatch, Robert M. 1993. Benefit/risk assessment: What patients can know that scientists cannot. *Drug Information Journal* 27:1021–1029.

Veech, R. L., R. L. Harris, D. Veloso, and E. H. Veech. 1972. Freeze-blowing: A new technique for the study of brain in vivo. *Journal of Neurochemistry* 20:183–188.

Vierck, Charles J., Brian Y. Cooper, and Richard H. Cohen. 1983. Human and non-human primate reactions to painful electrocutaneous stimuli and to morphine. In *Animal Pain: Perception and Alleviation*, edited by R. L. Kitchell and H. E. Erickson. Baltimore, MD: American Physiological Society, Waverly Press.

Vyvyan, John. 1969. *In Pity and in Anger.* London: Michael Joseph.

Warbasse, James. 1910. *The Conquest of Disease through Animal Experimentation.* New York: Appleton.

Warren, A. L. 1979. Letter to the editor. *Journal of the American Veterinary Medical Association* 174(1):3.

Warren, Karen J. 2000. *Ecofeminist Philosophy: A Western Perspective of What It Is and Why It Matters.* London: Rowman and Littlefield.

White, William J. 1990. The effect of cage space and environmental factors. In *Guidelines for the Well-Being of Rodents in Research*, edited by H. N. Guttman. Bethesda, MD: Scientists Center for Animal Welfare. pp. 29–45.

White, William J., Melvin W. Balk, and C. Max Lang. 1989. Use of cage space by guinea-pigs. *Laboratory Animals* 23:208–214.

White, William J., Melvin W. Balk, and Lynnard J. Slaughter. 1974. Housing requirements–dogs and cats. In *CRC Handbook of Laboratory Animal Science,* edited by E. C. Melby and H. C. Altman. Boca Raton, FL: CRC Press. pp. 69–84.

Whitney, Leon F. 1950. The dog. In *The Care and Breeding of Laboratory Animals,* edited by E. J. Farris. New York: John Wiley & Sons. pp. 182–201.

Whitney, Robert A., Donald J. Johnson, and William C. Cole. 1973. *Laboratory Primate Handbook.* New York: Academic Press.

Wilder, R. L. 1996. Hormones and autoimmunity: animal models of arthritis. *Baillieres Clinical Rheumatology* 10(2):259–71.

Wilks, Samuel. 1881. Vivisection: Its pains and its uses. *Nineteenth Century* 10:936–948.

Williams, R. O. 1998. Rodent models of arthritis: Relevance for human disease. *Clinical and Experimental Immunology* 114(3):330–332.

Wolfle, T. L. 1987. Control of stress using non-drug approaches. *Journal of the American Veterinary Medical Association* 191(10):1219–1221.

Wolfle, T. L. 2002. Implications of human-animal interactions and bonds in the laboratory. *ILAR Journal* 43(1):1–3.

Woolverton, W. L., N. A. Ator, P. M. Beardsley, and M.E. Carroll. 1989. Effects of environmental conditions on the psychological well-being of primates: A review of the literature. *Life Sciences* 44:901–917.

Worden, Alastair N., ed. 1947. *The Care and Management of Laboratory Animals: Handbook of the Universities Federation for Animal Welfare.* Baltimore, MD: Williams and Wilkins.

World Medical Association. 1997. Declaration of Helsinki. *Journal of the American Medical Association* 277(11):925–926.

Yearley, Steven. 1991. *The Green Case: A Sociology of Environmental Issues, Arguments and Politics.* London: Routledge.

Yoder, J. T., B. W. Kingrey, and L. R. Dragstedt. 1964. Physical fitness in the confined dog: Criteria and monitoring of muscle performance. *American Journal of Veterinary Research* 26(106):727–738.

Zinn, Raymond D. 1968. The research dog. *Journal of the American Veterinary Medical Association* 153(12):1883–1886.

Zurlo, Joanne, Deborah Rudacille, and Alan M. Goldberg. 1994. *Animals and Alternatives in Testing: History, Science, and Ethics.* New York: Mary Ann Liebert.

Philosophy. *See also* ethics
    knowledge of animals in, 19–20, 49, 57
    as profession, 10
plants, moral status of, 53, 58–59, 63–64
Pollan, Michael, 192
pound animals in research. *See* random
    source animals in research
primates. *See* apes; baboons; head trauma
    research and; monkeys; Silver Spring
    monkeys
primatologists, 233–34, 263n.8
product testing. *See* toxicity testing
professions, sociology of. *See* sociology of
    professions
psychological well-being, 36–37, 92, 134,
    206–9, 213, 227–38, 263n.8
purpose-bred animals, 68, 85–86, 222, 224,
    262n.5

rabbits, 96, 100–1,103–7, 122, 235, 256n.3.
    See also Draize eye irritancy test
random source animals in research, 68,
    84–85, 210, 222, 262n.5
rats, exclusion from Animal Welfare Act,
    20, 26–27, 36, 53, 68–72, 239–42
Reader's Digest, 86
realism, 7, 10, 249n.3
reduction of animal numbers. *See* alter-
    natives
refinement of animal experiments. *See*
    alternatives
Regan, Tom, 44–45, 51, 53–56, 83, 89
Reinhardt, Viktor, 234, 237
religion and animal research, 89, 255n.9
replacement of laboratory animals. *See*
    alternatives
reporting requirements in Animal Welfare
    Act, 26–28
respect for persons, 178
reverence for life, 48, 50, 57, 152
Rich, Sigmund, 126
Richey, Judge Charles, 72, 83, 92, 227
rights of animals. *See* animal rights
rodents, public image of, 74, 77–79, 82, 88,
    92–93, 204. *See also* guinea pigs; ham-
    sters; mice; rats, exclusion from Ani-
    mal Welfare Act
Rollin, Bernard, 10, 45, 51–54, 59, 61–64,
    83, 150, 225

Rowan, Andrew, 26, 45, 72, 253n.11,
    261n.10
Russell, W. M. S., and R. L. Burch, 28, 65
Russow, Lilly-Marlene, 182
Ryder, Richard, 251n.2

Sapontzis, Steve, 181–82, 260n.5, 260n.2
Schweitzer, Albert, 48, 50
science, definitions of, 9
    versus common sense, 57–58, 62–65,
        95, 150, 154, 166, 169, 207, 210,
        216–19, 237–38, 244
science studies, 7, 16, 63, 65, 196
scientists, public perception of, 172–73
Scientists Center for Animal Welfare, 147,
    190–91, 259n.6
self-awareness, 64
self-regulation, 39, 104, 114, 147–48, 172
sentience, 48, 50–54, 58, 69, 83
Silver Spring monkeys, 75–77, 90–91, 141,
    255n.6, 257n.1
Singer, Peter, 44–45, 51, 53–55, 58–59,
    80–81, 83, 89, 252n.7
Smith, David, 49
Smith, Kenneth, and Jane Boyd, 57
Smith, Maggie, 204
social constructivism. *See* constructivism
social contract ethics. *See* contract ethics
    (contractarianism)
social housing of animals, 108, 110,
    113–15, 209–13, 228, 231–34,
    236–37, 243, 261n.1, 262n.6
social studies of animal issues, 6, 163
sociobiology and ethics, 48–49, 50, 57
sociology of professions, 8, 118–19, 138, 161
space flight, animal euthanasia during,
    186–87
space requirements in animal housing.
    See cages
species. *See also* individual kinds of animals
    biological differences, 121, 157, 161, 215,
        230, 253n.11
    differential treatment of, 67–68, 94,
        228–29, 242, 253n.1, 263n.7
    moral significance of, 20, 49–50, 52–53,
    role in rhetoric and philosophy, 67–68,
        73–95, 227
speciesism, 44–45, 49, 251n.2, 252n.7
spiders, 52, 54

Spinelli, Joe, 185
Spira, Henry, 23–24
Sports Illustrated magazine, 35, 75, 127–28
Sprigge, Timothy, 204
Stafleu, Frans, 94, 183
standards, engineering versus performance,
    20, 97–99, 103–7, 113–15, 164, 202,
    207, 212–13, 218, 226–28, 232
standing, legal, 176
stereotypies, 115, 136, 220, 253n.10
Stevens, Christine, 87, 128, 255n.8
stress, 136, 193, 204, 220, 222, 260n.7,
    261n.10
subject of a life criterion, 51, 53, 83
suffering, 56, 63, 240
surgery on animals, 32–33, 69, 93, 119–20,
    133, 251n.3, 257n.6

"3Rs": replacement, reduction, and refine-
    ment. *See* alternatives
Takacs, David, 7–8, 157
Tannenbaum, Jerrold, 45, 56, 59–61, 180,
    191, 260n.4
Taub, Edward, 90
technicians in laboratory animal care and
    use, 12, 33–34, 180–81, 192, 243
telos, 51–52, 83, 225–26
Thomas, Elizabeth Marshall, 9, 223–24
time, as a humane concern, 195–200, 202–4
toxicity testing, 23–24, 77–79, 169
transgenics, 25–26, 86–87, 117, 239–40,
    250n.2, 264n.1
Tuskegee syphilis studies, 177, 259n.2
twentieth century, first half, 74, 84, 88, 121,
    255n.7

United States Congress, 70–72, 90, 109,
    142–47, 166–67, 258n.5
United States Department of Agriculture
    (USDA)

correspondence, 13–14, 34, 72, 98, 131,
    135–36, 147–48, 150, 155, 165,
    199–201, 206–9, 212–14, 221–22,
    230
inspections, 33, 36, 90, 104, 122, 168,
    218, 227, 236–37, 242
science as basis of regulations, 9,
    110–11, 137, 213–16, 226
veterinary staff members, 41, 89, 109,
    165–67, 233
University of Chicago, 123–24
University of Pennsylvania, 90, 145
Unnecessary Fuss, 90
utilitarianism. *See* ethics

Vanderwolf, C. H., 197
Veatch, Robert, 178, 260n.4
vegetarianism. *See* meat-eating
vertebrate animals, moral status of, 68–69
Veterinarian's Oath, 165, 243, 264n.3
veterinarians. *See* American Veterinary
    Medical Association (AVMA); labora-
    tory animal veterinarians; United
    States Department of Agriculture
    (USDA)
vivisection, 22, 49, 75

warm-blooded animals, 69–70
Warren, A. L., 188–89
welfare, animal. *See* animal welfare, defi-
    nitions of
well-being, psychological. *See* psychological
    well-being
White, William J., 110, 112–13
Wilks, Samuel, 73

Yoder, J. T., 217

zoophilic psychosis, 88–89